卓越医学考博英语应试教材
ZHUOYUE ENGLISH TEST PREPARATION FOR FATMD

第 **10** 版

U0322837

2019 全国医学博士英语统考

综合应试教程

组　编　环球卓越医学考博命题研究中心

主　编　任　雁（首都医科大学）

副主编　李文斌（首都医科大学附属北京世纪坛医院）

参　编　王　京　张彦斌　蔺宏伟　吴兆红　周　全　李　珊　陈怡东

　　　　石　蕊　陈慧媛　梁莉娟　张秀峰　刘启升　初　萌　郑玉全

　　　　武瑞玲　(美)Xinyin Li

机械工业出版社
CHINA MACHINE PRESS

本书是卫生部组织的全国医学博士英语统一考试辅导丛书之一。

本书共分为五章，第一章为听力理解，第二章为词汇，第三章为完形填空，第四章为阅读理解，第五章为写作。本书具有讲解内容全面、针对性强、编写质量过硬三大特点。全书紧密围绕大纲要求和历年真题这一主线进行编写，包含最新医博考博真题，详细讲解各种题型的命题特点和应试方法，是一本很有针对性的应试辅导用书。

图书在版编目（CIP）数据

全国医学博士英语统考综合应试教程 / 任雁主编.
—10 版 . —北京：机械工业出版社，2018.7
卓越医学考博英语应试教材
ISBN 978-7-111-60590-4

Ⅰ . ①全… Ⅱ . ①任… Ⅲ . ①医学—英语—博士生入
学考试—教材 Ⅳ . ① R

中国版本图书馆 CIP 数据核字（2018）第 170976 号

机械工业出版社（北京市百万庄大街 22 号 邮政编码 100037）
策划编辑：孙铁军 责任编辑：王庆龙
版式设计：墨格文慧 责任印制：李 洋
天津嘉恒印务有限公司印刷

2018 年 8 月第 10 版第 1 次印刷
184mm×260mm · 31.25 印张 · 673 千字
0 001—5 000 册
标准书号：ISBN 978-7-111-60590-4
定价：69.80 元

丛 书 序

  这是一套由全国知名医学博士英语统考培训机构"环球卓越"策划，联手医学博士英语资深辅导专家，为众多志在考取医学博士的考生量身定做的应试辅导用书。

  全国医学博士外语统一考试共设置了听力对话、听力短文、词语用法、完形填空、阅读理解和书面表达6种题型。考试时间为3个小时。为了帮助广大考生在较短的时间内系统备考，在听、说、读、写4个方面得到强化训练，全面提高英语应用和交际能力，顺利通过考试，环球卓越为广大考生倾情奉献本套"卓越医学考博英语应试教材"。本丛书紧密结合卫生部组织的医学博士英语统一考试命题情况，针对最新考试大纲编写而成。丛书在《全国医学博士英语统考词汇巧战通关》《全国医学博士英语统考综合应试教程》和《全国医学博士英语统考实战演练》3个传统分册的基础上，特意增加了《医学考博阅读理解高分全解》和《医学考博听力、完形、写作高分全解》2个分册，专门解决不同基础读者的应试问题。传统分册从基础到综合再到真题实战演练，让考生在有限的时间里快速准确地把握进度，新增分册则根据医学博士英语试卷模块，专攻分项。对分值较大的阅读理解，则单立分册进行详解精练，使考生在考前做好全面细致的准备，顺利攻克考试难关，力求获得高分。

  本丛书的特点如下：

  一、名师执笔，实用性强

  策划编写本丛书的作者主要是设有医学院的综合性高校或者医科大学的教师，他们常年在环球卓越北京总校以及上海、杭州、南京、天津、郑州、广州等分校授课，是出色的医学博士英语辅导专家。丛书内容是他们多年辅导经验的提炼和结晶，实用性非常强，专为医学博士考生定制，是目前市面上较全面、系统的医学考博英语应试教材。

  二、紧扣新大纲，直击考试真题

  本丛书紧扣最新大纲，体例设置与大纲保持一致；各部分考点紧密结合最新历年真题，完全还原真题考场，命题思路分析透彻，重点突出，讲解精确；各部分内容严格控制在大纲规定的范围之内，让考生准确把握考试的重点、难点及命题趋势。本版修订特增加了全套2017年真题及其解析。另外，本书还为读者定制了2套2018年真题试卷，其中包含部分2018年真题。

  三、内容精练，讲练结合

  传统分册《全国医学博士英语统考词汇巧战通关》《全国医学博士英语统考综合应试教程》和《全国医学博士英语统考实战演练》简单精练，通过突破词汇基础关，学习各个题型应试方法以及在高质量实战中历练，考生可在有限的时间内进行全面复习，把握重点，比较系统地完成考前准备。新增的《医学考博阅读理解高分全解》和《医学考博听力、完形、写作高分全解》则是根据考生的具体情况，分模块予以详解，提升基础，总结技巧，各个击破，力争高分。

  四、超值服务，锦上添花

  本丛书附带超值赠送服务，由北京环球卓越在线（www.geedu.com）为每位购书读者提供专业的服务和强大的技术支持。具体为：

  1.《全国医学博士英语统考词汇巧战通关》附赠内容：环球卓越"2019医学博士统考英语辅导语词专项班（24学时，价值680元）"网络视频课程。使用方法：2018年8月20日后，刮开封面上的账号和密码，登录 www.geedu.com，按照"图书赠送课程学习流程"进行学习。

2．《全国医学博士英语统考综合应试教程》附赠内容：环球卓越"2019 医学博士统考英语辅导阅读专项班（12 学时，价值 680 元）"网络视频课程。使用方法：2018 年 8 月 20 日后，刮开封面上的账号和密码，登录 www.geedu.com，按照"图书赠送课程学习流程"进行学习。

3．《全国医学博士英语统考实战演练》附赠内容：环球卓越"2019 医学博士统考英语辅导模考串讲班（8 学时，价值 600 元）"网络视频课程。使用方法：2018 年 8 月 20 日后，刮开封面上的账号和密码，登录 www.geedu.com，按照"图书赠送课程学习流程"进行学习。

4．《医学考博阅读理解高分全解》附赠内容：环球卓越"2019 医学博士统考英语辅导阅读专项班（12 学时，价值 520 元）"网络视频课程。使用方法：2018 年 8 月 20 日后，刮开封面上的账号和密码，登录 www.geedu.com，按照"图书赠送课程学习流程"进行学习。

5．《医学考博听力、完形、写作高分全解》附赠内容：环球卓越"2019 医学博士统考英语辅导听力及写作专项班（12 学时，价值 520 元）"网络视频课程。使用方法：2018 年 8 月 20 日后，刮开封面上的账号和密码，登录 www.geedu.com，按照"图书赠送课程学习流程"进行学习。

环球卓越技术支持及服务热线：010-51658769；环球卓越医学博士英语统考试题与学习资料请登录 www.geedu.com。本丛书脉络清晰，内容丰富，针对性强，通俗易懂。相信广大考生在学习时会有在辅导班现场一般的感受；真诚希望本丛书能大大提高众考生的应试能力和实际水平，助每位考生在考场上轻松驰骋，快乐过关！

最后，感谢北京环球卓越为本丛书提供的专业服务和技术支持，愿他们精益求精，为社会提供更多、更好、更专的服务！

编　者
2018 年 4 月于北京

Preface 前　言

　　本书是卫生部组织的全国医学博士英语统一考试辅导丛书之一，在结合最新考试大纲和对最新真题进行分析的基础上，于2018年5月进行了修订。

　　为了帮助广大考生在较短的时间内系统备考，顺利通过考试，我们为广大考生量身定制了这本《全国医学博士英语统考综合应试教程》。修订版增加了2018年真题，以便考生掌握最新考试动向。

　　全书共分五章：

　　第一章为**听力理解**，通过真题讲解了听力理解部分的测试特点、应试技巧与方法以及听力常考用语，并配有专项练习和解析；修订版的听力部分将最新真题按照考试不同题型重新编排，解析部分更是精心制作，不仅含有听力原文和题目、选项对应的中文，还针对不同题型的解题技巧做出了详细讲解，真正做到讲练结合，旨在帮助考生有效地运用应试技巧，具有极强的指导性。

　　第二章为**词汇**，通过真题演练讲解了词汇部分测试内容和应试方法，并详细介绍了几种词汇记忆方法和重点的词根和词缀；结合例句对常考词组进行讲解，并配有专项练习和详细解析。此外，修订版将近三年真题作为词汇测试部分中的真题演练，并根据不同题型重新编排。这样，考生在掌握了必要的解题技巧后，能够最直接地将不同的解题技巧运用到相应的真题中，可大大增加考生的应试能力。

　　第三章为**完形填空**，结合最新真题讲解了完形填空的命题特点和应试方法，通过专项练习进行训练，并给出详细解析。

　　第四章为**阅读理解**，通过真题分析了阅读理解必备的语法知识、长难句结构、阅读理解各类题型应试方法，以及阅读理解整体答题方法。通过专项练习进行训练，练习部分附有详细解析，并重新修订配套练习的解析，附上题目、选项的中文详解，将答案出处清楚标明，并给予详细中文解释。考生认真练习后，能从答案、解题技巧等多方面得到有益帮助。

　　第五章为**写作**，依据真题对评卷人掌握的评分原则、写作常见问题和对策、写作常用词语和句子、写作常用医学词汇进行一一讲解，同时配有大量练习，并根据解题要领和步骤给出详细的解析和参考范文，有助于考生解决"不知如何写、写什么"的难题，让考生真正掌握正确完成英文摘要写作的要领。

　　本书具备以下特点：

　　1. **讲解内容全面**。本书根据考试题型，分专项编写，各章详细讲解了各个专项复习的要点和方法，内容全面，重点突出。

　　2. **配套最新真题及详解**。修订版将最新真题作为各项题目的配套练习，这样考生能直接接触真题，并在真题训练中，重点演练各项解题技巧。

　　3. **针对性较强**。本书各个部分都是在分析历年医学博士考试的基础上编写的，紧紧围绕考试要求进行讲解，完全为医博考生定制，是一本专业的医学博士应试教材。

4. 编写质量过硬。作者常年在医学院校任教，多年参与医学博士的阅卷工作，对医学博士英语考试的命题有比较深入的研究，对医学博士英语考试的材料来源有深入的追踪和分析。在这一背景下，作者进行了有效的选材，使本书非常适合医学博士英语考生的考前复习。

在编写过程中，本书始终围绕大纲要求和历年真题这一主线来讲解各个题型的命题特点和应试方法，提高了其作为应试教材的针对性。

由于编者水平有限，书中不妥之处在所难免，衷心希望广大读者批评指正！

编　者

2018 年 3 月于北京

Contents 目　录

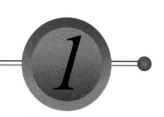

第一章 CHAPTER 1 听力理解

一、考试大纲要求、试卷结构与考试特点

（一）考试大纲要求及试卷结构

根据《全国医学博士外语统一考试英语考试大纲》（以下简称《考试大纲》）的有关规定，试卷中的听力部分包括两个模块：Section A 和 Section B。答题时间共约 30 分钟，听力部分共计 30 分。

Section A 为简短对话，旨在测试考生的英语听力能力。考试过程中，考生会听到每个简短对话和之后的提问，对话及问题只读一遍。然后，考生有 12 秒的作答时间，根据所听题目和对话，从四个选项中选出最佳答案。此部分共 15 个小题，每题 1 分，共计 15 分。

我们先来看看 2017 年真题的 Section A 部分：

1. A. To have a coffee.
   B. To hold her teddy bear.
   C. To take her medicine.
   D. To talk with the doctor.

2. A. They are ill-tempered.
   B. They rarely listen to him.
   C. They often give a wrong diagnosis.
   D. They always prescribe wrong medications.

3. A. His lovely voice.
   B. His Italian background.
   C. His attractive appearance.
   D. His patience with patients.

4. A. 2:30pm today.
   B. 2:00pm today.
   C. 2:30pm tomorrow.
   D. 2:00pm tomorrow.

5. A. He should take one pill 13 minutes before sleep for 30 days.
   B. He should take one pill 13 minutes before sleep for 13 days.
   C. He should take one pill 30 minutes before sleep for 13 days.

D. He should take one pill 30 minutes before sleep for 30 days.

6. A. Go to the cinema.   B. Eat out in a restaurant.

   C. Have a drink or bite in a bar.   D. Take a walk down the High Street.

7. A. Thursday, the 16th.   B. Friday, the 17th.

   C. Sunday, the 19th.   D. Monday, the 20th.

8. A. Mark De Weck.   B. Mark Te Weck.

   C. Marc De Weck.   D. Marc Te Weck.

9. A. It could be three days.   B. It could be three months.

   C. That's an easy question to answer.   D. That's an impossible question to answer.

10. A. The woman herself.   B. The woman's mother.

    C. The woman's husband.   D. The woman's sister-in-law.

11. A. It's a benign tumor.   B. It's a malignant tumor.

    C. It's an inherited disease.   D. It's on the man's right shoulder.

12. A. He is a hematologist.   B. He is a hepatologist.

    C. He is a psychologist.   D. He is a neurologist.

13. A. Because his wife, Sally, wants him to do so.

    B. Because his company has asked him to do so.

    C. Because he suspects that he might be infected.

    D. Because he is applying for emigration to Australia.

14. A. She used to handle her own luggage, but not anymore.

    B. She wants to take her luggage to the car by herself.

    C. She loves hauling her luggage around herself.

    D. She needs a hand from the man.

15. A. Shocked.   B. Nervous.   C. Annoyed.   D. Contented.

 录音原文

1. M: Good morning, Mrs. Evans, how are you today?

   W: Awful, doctor. They haven't brought me my morning coffee yet. I don't talk to anyone until I have had my morning coffee.

   M: Well, can you talk with me?

   W: Nope. I'm just a bear until I have my coffee.

   Q: What does the woman desperately want to do now?

2. W: So, you don't like doctors.

   M: Well, you may say so. You know, I have yet to meet a doctor who listens to me. And I think most of my troubles come from the medicines.

   Q: What is the man complaining about the doctors he has met?

3. W: I saw that nice doctor Matterrally again this morning.

   M: Oh, I do like him. He's lovely.

W: Very handsome. And what impressed me most is that he always takes his time with you not like some of the others. And lovely voice. Italian, you know.

Q: What does Dr. Matterrally impress the woman most with?

4. W: Hmm… Doctor Harris is off tomorrow. Do you think it can wait until Wednesday?

M: Oh, I was really hoping to get in today or tomorrow in case I need some antibiotics, maybe I'll have to go to the Wall King Clinic instead.

W: Actually we had a cancellation for two pm today if you can get away from the office.

M: Gee… it's almost one pm already! I think I can make it if I leave right now.

W: We're running a bit behind schedule, so you can probably count on seeing the doctor around two thirty.

M: That's great! Thanks for fixing me in.

Q: What time could the doctor probably see the man?

5. M: How often should I take the medicine?

W: Just take one pill about thirty minutes before you go to bed.

M: How long should I take them?

W: The prescription is for thirty days. If you're not sleeping well after thirty days, I'd like you to come back in.

Q: How should the man take the medicine?

6. M: Hi, Jenny! Are you doing anything tonight?

W: Err, I don't know. Why?

M: Well, we could have a bite to eat or we could take in a film. What do you fancy?

W: Well, that would be really nice. We could meet at the new bar on the high street and take it from there. What do you think?

M: Oh, that's nice. What time then?

Q: What are they going to do first?

7. M: Reservations, Robert speaking. I understand that you would like to book a room.

W: That's right. Four nights starting from Thursday, the 16th of this month.

Q: When is the woman supposed to check out at the hotel?

8. W: Could I have your first name please?

M: It's Marc. That's "Mar", and then "c" for "Charlie", not "k" for "kilo".

W: And your surname?

M: De Weck.

W: Could you spell that for me?

M: Yes, it's two words. First, De.

W: Is that "t" for "tango"?

M: No, "d" for "delta" and "e" for "echo". And then a separate word Weck.

W: Is that "V" for "Victor"?

M: No, it's "W" for "whiskey", and then "eck".

Q: What is the spelling of the man's name?

9. W: How long do we normally have to wait till they give us an answer?

M: How long is a piece of string. It could be three days or three months.

Q: What does the man mean?

10. M: Does your son now use a brown inhaler?

W: Yes, he uses it regularly.

M: Is there anyone else in the family with hay fever, eczema or asthma?

W: Oh yes, my mother had eczema all her life. I had eczema as a child. On my husband's side, several people including his sister have hay fever.

Q: Who else has got hay fever in the family?

11. W: I notice you've got this small lump on your shoulder.

M: I've had that for years. The GP says it's a fatty tumor.

W: Your left eyelid is lower than your right.

M: Yes, that seems to run in our family.

Q: What is true about the lump on the man's shoulder?

12. M: Good morning, Mrs. Beca Stump. I'm your doctor, Brown. Your GP asked me to see you at short notice because the blood test he did was abnormal. Did he explain this to you?

W: I didn't understand what he was saying. I'm very frightened because he told me to come here so quickly. It must be serious.

M: Yes, well, we're not yet certain about the diagnosis, but the blood test did show that you were very anemic and there seemed to be some abnormal white blood cells, We'll need to do some more tests and I'll explain about them later.

Q: What does the man do?

13. W: Well, is there any particular reason you feel you need to have an HIV test?

M: Yes, I am being sent by my company to Australia to head up a new subsidiary there. It's a great opportunity.

W: Sounds good. Congratulations!

M: Thanks. Yes, me and Sally, that's my wife. We've been wanting to emigrate there for a couple of years. So anyway, we filled in all the paperwork, just on the last hurdle now—might need proof of a negative HIV test. So I was wondering if you could arrange this for me.

Q: Why does the man ask for an HIV test?

14. M: Would you like me to help you get your bags into the car?

W: Don't bother. I need to be used to hauling these bags around myself.

Q: What does the woman mean?

15. W: Jack doesn't like his birthday present.

M: he's starting to get on my nerves. It's one thing to not like it, but it's another to complain about it. We tried our best to get him a good present.

Q: Which of the following can best describe the man's feeling towards Jack?

Section B 由一篇长对话和两篇短文组成，目的在于测试考生对英语篇章的听力理解能力。要求考生能理解所听材料的中心思想和主要内容，并能根据所听到的内容进行逻辑推理、分析概括和归纳总结。考试过程中，考生听完每个长对话或短文后会听到 5 个问题，且篇章及问题只读一遍。对每道题考生有 12 秒的作答时间，要根据所听题目和篇章从四个选项中选出一个最佳答案。此部分共 15 道题，每题 1 分，共计 15 分。

Section B

Conversation

16. A. A difficult case.   B. A trivial illness.
    C. A deadly disease.   D. A serious condition.

17. A. Cough.   B. Fever.
    C. Stuffed nose.   D. Sore throat.

18. A. A cold.   B. Allergy.   C. Sinusitis.   D. Pneumonia.

19. A. Whether the man should seek a second opinion.
    B. Whether the doctor's diagnosis is correct or not.
    C. Whether the doctor should prescribe an antibiotic.
    D. Whether Complicare should cover the man's expenses.

20. A. Nice and patient.   B. Rushed and impatient.
    C. Rational and eloquent.   D. Conservative and stubborn.

Passage One

21. A. Simply from the contents of their texts.
    B. Just from the number of texts they send.
    C. Merely from the books they read at leisure.
    D. Right from the way they spell certain words.

22. A. 2,030 sociology students.
    B. 2,300 sociology students.
    C. 2,030 psychologist students.
    D. 2,300 psychologist students.

23. A. Spiritual life.   B. Image and wealth.
    B. Academic success.   D. Morality and aesthetics.

24. A. 30% of the survey-takers texted more than 300 times a day.
    B. 30% of the survey-takers texted more than 400 times a day.
    C. 12% of the survey-takers texted at least 300 times a day.

D. 12% of the survey-takers texted at least 400 times a day.

25. A. Too much texting can make you shallow.

   B. Texting is nothing but a wonder of technology.

   C. Texting has more disadvantages than advantages.

   D. Too much texting results in poorly performing students.

Passage Two

26. A. Effective weight loss.　　　　B. Enhanced appetite.

   C. Improved health.　　　　　　D. Brain fitness.

27. A. A 12-week weight loss program.

   B. A 12-month weight loss program.

   C. A 12-week aerobic exercise program.

   D. A 12-month aerobic exercise program.

28. A. Exercise sometimes is just futile and not beneficial.

   B. Exercise should be encouraged, weight loss less emphasized.

   C. Aerobic exercise can do good to people both mentally and physically.

   D. Poor weight loss can inevitably result in disappointment and low self-esteem.

29. A. To control weight.

   B. To live well and long.

   C. To be together with friends.

   D. To enjoy the marvelous feeling of exercise.

30. A. Exercise: Value beyond Weight Loss.

   B. Exercise: the Way to Well-being.

   C. Exercise for a Better Life.

   D. Exercise for Weight Loss.

录音原文

Section B

M: Thanks for seeing me on short notice, doc. I wouldn't come in if I wasn't nearly dead.

W: Oh? How are you feeling bad?

M: I've been sick all week and I've scheduled to fly to Portland this weekend.

W: What sort of symptoms?

M: Mostly a sinus infection. I can't breathe and I've got this yellow stuff. I keep blowing out my nose.

W: How is it with your mouth open?

M: That's fine, but I can't go around like some kind of fish, you know.

W: OK, then, stuffy head, nasal drainage. What else?

M: That's it. That's enough. Usually I get these colds and they've gone in one or two days. This one I've had all week.

W: I see, and any other symptoms? Cough, fever, anything else?

M: Ah, maybe a tickle in my throat. I cough once or twice. No big deal, though.

W: OK, let's take a look at you. Hop up here on the examination table and slip off your shirt. Hmm. Well, Mr. George, the exam is entirely normal. All you've got is a cold. Take one of the over-the-counter decongestant, Dristan or Contac for example, maybe a couple of Aspirins. We'll see you for your physical in six months.

M: You mean you aren't going to give me something for this? I've got to go out of town in three days and I can't be sick then.

W: Yes, sometimes we use an antibiotic, but you aren't sick enough to make that worthwhile.

M: What? I am sick as I want to be. What is this? I'm not sick enough? What's going on? Is this because I'm capitation in Complicare? They tell you to save a few bucks by not prescribing penicillin.

W: That doesn't have anything to do with it. I treat you just like patients who pay right up front.

M: Hey, I pay plenty for this insurance, doc. And I don't see how I'm getting my money's worth.

16. How would you describe the man's illness?
17. What is the worst symptom of the man?
18. What is the doctor's diagnosis of the man?
19. What are the man and the doctor quarrelling about?
20. Which of the following can best describe the doctor's attitude and manner?

Passage One

Teenagers who text more than 100 times a day tend to be more shallow, image-obsessed and driven by wealth—not to mention pretty bad at spelling. The study from the University of Winnipeg suggests that a lot can be learned about a person's personality simply from the number of texts they send. The most incessant texters often turn out to be a slightly more racist than others.

The data was gathered over a period of three years from 2,300 psychology students at the University of Winnipeg. The theory the university study tried to test was that constant use of twitter and texting for communication results in a world where people have quick and shallow thoughts. The results indicate that students who text frequently place less importance on moral aesthetic and spiritual goals and greater importance on wealth and image. Strikingly the study states those who text more than 100 times a day were 30 per cent less likely to feel strongly that leading an ethical, principled life was important, in comparison to those who texted 50 times or less a day. In the most extreme cases, 30 per cent of the survey takers texted more than 200 times a day and 12 per cent texted at least 300 times a day.

21. According to the study, how can we learn about a person's personality?
22. Who are the participants of the study?
23. As indicated by the study, what do the students who text frequently value most?
24. About the most extreme cases mentioned in the study, which of the following is true?
25. What is the main idea of this talk?

Passage Two

Many, if not most, people start exercising because they want to lose weight. But very often they abandon exercise when the expected pounds fail to fall off. Study after study has found that, without major changes in eating habits, increasing physical activity is only somewhat effective for losing weight though. It helps people maintain weight loss. And shedding even a few pounds, especially around one's middle, can improve health.

For example, researchers in Brisbane, Australia, studied 58 sedentary overweight or obese men and women who participated in a closely monitored 12-week aerobic exercise program. Weight loss was minimal, but nonetheless the participants' waistline shrunk, their blood pressure and resting heart rate dropped, and their aerobic capacity and mood improved.

Exercise should be encouraged and the emphasis on weight loss reduced, the researchers concluded. "Disappointment and low self-esteem associated with poor weight loss could lead to low exercise adherence and a general perception that exercise is futile and not beneficial."

I walk three miles daily, or bike ten miles and swim three-quarters of a mile. If you ask me why, weight control may be my first answer, followed by a desire to live long and well. But that's not what gets me out of bed before dawn to join friends on a morning walk and then bike for my swim. It's how these activities make me feel: more energized, less stressed, more productive, more engaged and, yes, happier — better able to smell the roses and cope with the inevitable frustrations of daily life.

26. According to the research findings on exercise what can you achieve from increasing physical activity?
27. What kind of program did the participants of the study attend?
28. What is the conclusion that the researches of the Brisbane study reached?
29. What is the real reason that the speaker exercises every day?
30. What can be the best topic of this talk?

答案:	1. A	2. B	3. D	4. A	5. D	6. C	7. D	8. C	9. D	10. D
	11. A	12. A	13. D	14. B	15. C	16. B	17. C	18. A	19. C	20. A
	21. B	22. D	23. B	24. C	25. A	26. C	27. C	28. B	29. D	30. A

（二）听力理解考试特点

通过对历年考题的分析，可以看出听力理解考试有以下特点：

1. 听力材料内容兼顾日常交际与医学背景

在 Section A 里，多数题目围绕日常对话展开，大约 5～6 个题目涉及医学领域，如去医院看病；有时对话材料里也会提到医学常用词汇，如常见病或症状。因而，考生应该储备一定量的医学常用词汇，但医学词汇不作为听力测试第一部分的主要考点。在 Section B 中，医学为听力材料的主要背景，涉及常见病症、医学常识等。

2. 题型较为常见且为客观选择题

无论是第一部分还是第二部分，所有题目均为选择题，这样的题型是考生较为熟悉的形式。而且考试测试点与其他重大英语考试类似：Section A 的题目以测试习惯用语、特殊句式、词组含义、细节与推断题为主，详细的分析将在本章后面阐述；Section B 主要以测试细节为主。因而，从题型上看，考生不会有完全不适应的地方。

3. 口音较为固定、语速较快

对于考生来说，听力测试部分较为不适应的地方应该是听力材料的口音以及语速。每个考生可能对某一种英语口音较为熟悉，如英音或美音。医学博士英语统考听力测试中的发音常为标准的英音，因而，考生在平时应该多接触英音，这样才不至于在考试时觉得很陌生。另外，医学博士英语统考听力测试的语速也较快，连读处更是难点。因而，考生在平时听力训练时，应多加强发音规则和规律训练，以适应考试的语速和口音，这样在正式考试时，心理上就会占一定优势。

二、考查内容及相应的应试技巧

综观听力部分各类考题，考生要重视以下方面的问题：

1. 知识储备很必要

听力中经常会出现句式、词组、习语等，而这些表达往往是解题的关键，因而，考生应在考前注重积累与听力考试相关的语言知识点。

2. 语境信息是关键

无论是 Section A 还是 Section B，听力题目均在一定的语言环境下提出，无论听力材料的长或短，都会给考生足够的语言信息，因而抓住了关键信息或信号词（Cue Words）就等于找到了解题的密钥。

3. 预读选项有帮助

当听力录音中在播放 Directions 或者例子的时候，考生可利用这段时间预读选项。有些题目选项很有特点，考生通过预读选项可以提前知道考点，或者可以通过突出某个选项关键词对选项进行分类，或者还能够提前知道听力对话或短文的话语情景。所以，考生要养成提前看选项的习惯，做到料敌在先。

4．简单笔记是依靠

在听力考试过程中，由于极度紧张，人的记忆力在那时是有限的。考生经常会有这样的尴尬：在听对话或短文时，信息在脑海里清晰呈现，但是当问题提出后，即将解题时，却怎么也想不起来自己刚才所听到的信息了，结果无法正确解题，同时，紧张情绪增加，十分不利于考试。所以，考生在平时听力训练的时候，就应养成记笔记的习惯，边听边记是训练听力的好办法。

下面将针对听力理解考试的不同部分，结合部分真题，对考点和应试技巧进行有针对性的讲解。

（一）Section A 的主要考点及应试技巧

听力测试这一部分的考点大致有以下几个方面：细节题、特殊句式、固定词组、常用习语和推断题。下面就这些考点和应试技巧一一阐述。

1．细节题

细节题就是根据男女双方的对话细节提出问题，如时间、地点、事实等。细节题往往在选项上有特点，解题可以根据选项预先做出判断，如果选项都是表示时间或者数字的选项，就可以根据选项的指引，重点关注与数字或时间有关的信息，必要时要做简单的笔记。这种类型的考题重点较为单一，就是听力材料中的细节，解题切入点就是选项。

No. 1 Short Conversation

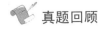 真题回顾

A. Tuesday.　　B. Wednesday.　　C. Thursday.　　D. Friday.

听力原文

M: Hi, Sherry. I wonder if it's possible to move the meeting to Wednesday. I can't make it on Tuesday. I'm tight up in the emergency room.

W: Eh... Wednesday is not good for me. How about Thursday?

Question: What is the original day for the meeting?

【解析】看到选项我们可以判断此题考点为时间，是细节题。题目的中文意思是："会议原定时间是在哪天？" original 是形容词，意思为"原先的，最初的"。对话中男士问："能否将会议改到周三，周二我不行，一天都在急诊室。"女士回答说："周三不行，周四如何？"此题就是要关注和时间相关的事件。

【答案】A

No.2 Short Conversation

真题回顾

A. To arrange an interview.
B. To get a part-time job on campus.
C. To take a course of pharmaceutics.
D. To apply for a job with the company.

 听力原文

M: I heard the Pharmaceutics Limited is going to hold an interview on campus next week.

W: Really? What day? I'd like to talk to them with my CV.

Question: What is the woman going to do?

【解析】题目问这位女士要做什么。录音对话中，男士提到他听说有个医药有限公司要在下周举办一场校园招聘会。Pharmaceutics 的含义为"制药学"。女士说到她要与这家公司谈谈她的 CV。CV 是这道题的关键信号词（Cue Word），全称为 curriculum vitae = resume，意思为"简历"。因而，这位女士是打算去应聘。

【答案】D

No.3 Short Conversation

真题回顾

A. Six.
B. Twenty-four.
C. Twelve.
D. Three.

 听力原文

W: How often should I take capsules and how many should I take?

M: Take 3 capsules every 6 hours.

Question: How many capsules should the woman take in 24 hours?

【解析】通过选项，我们可以清楚地知道该题的考点为细节，因而要关注听力材料中的数字。听力材料中 how often 为频率疑问词，capsules 的意思是"胶囊"。男士的回答是：每 6 小时吃 3 粒胶囊。问题是 24 小时内，这位女士应该吃多少粒胶囊。做一个简单的乘法运算就能得出答案。

【答案】C

No.4 Short Conversation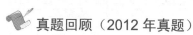

真题回顾（2012 年真题）

A. A broken finger.
B. A terrible cough.
C. Frontal headaches.
D. Eye problem.

听力原文

W: It's Mr. Cong, isn't it?

M: That's right. I saw you six months ago with a broken finger.

W: Yes, of course. And is that all healing well?

M: It's fine.

W: What can we do for you today?

M: Well, I've been having these headaches in the front, about my eyes. It started two months ago. They seem to come on quite suddenly, and I get dizzy spell as well.

Question: What is the trouble in the man now?

【解析】此题考点为细节信息再现。男士六个月前来看病是因为手指断了，今天来看病是因为头痛，故答案为 C。D 项为干扰项，男士在讲述病情时提到头疼，大概是眼周围的地方疼。

【答案】C

No. 5 Short Conversation

真题回顾（2012 年真题）

A. She needs a physical examination.　　B. She is in good health.

C. It's good to have a doctor friend.　　D. It's good to visit the doctor.

 听力原文

M: When you need a health checkup, just call me. It's totally free.

W: It's great having a doctor around.

Question: What does the woman mean?

【解析】此题为细节信息再现。男士说到需要体检打个电话给我，免费的。女士回答说有个医生在身边很好，所以答案为 C。

【答案】C

2. 固定词组

这类题型的解题关键就是某个多义词组在听力对话语境中的含义。这就需要考生对常用词组的含义有所准备，熟悉固定词组的常用含义是正确解题的保证。

No. 1 Short Conversation

 真题回顾

A. Her parents will let her stay in their house.

B.　Her parents' friends will accommodate her.

C.　She plans to visit some friends in San Diego.

D.　She is moving to San Diego with her parents.

 听力原文

M: So you'll spend the holiday weekends in San Diego?

W: Yeah, some friends of my parents live over there. And they will put me up.

Question: What does the woman mean?

【解析】根据听力材料，此题解题的关键在于女士回答中的 they will put me up 这句话。put up 这个词组的含义较多，但结合上下文可知其在本题中的意思是"解决住宿问题"。因而女士回答的含义就是"我父母的一些朋友住在那里，他们会为我解决住宿问题"。在四个选项中，选项 B 是听力原文的同义改写。accommodate = put sb. up，例如：The hotel can accommodate 500 tourists.（这家旅馆可住 500 名游客。）

【答案】B

No. 2 Short Conversation

 真题回顾（2012 年真题）

A.　He prefers to take pills to get anti-oxidants.

B.　He prefers to get anti-oxidants from food.

C.　He doesn't mind eating a lot every day.

D.　He is overcautious sometimes.

听力原文

W: We need anti-oxidants to prevent ourselves from developing cancer, but I don't like taking pills to get it.

M: But you need to eat a mountain of food every day to get all of the anti-oxidants you need.

W: I drink a lot of green tea; I eat onion, garlic and citrous food. I also get nine different colors of vegetables every day.

M: All those do have anti-oxidants, but I want to be on the safe side.

Question: What does the man mean?

【解析】对话中女士说抗氧化剂可以防癌，但她不想通过吃药来获取。男士告诉女士可以从每天的食物中获取所需的抗氧化剂。因而答案是 B。男士话语中的 on the safe side 的含义是"安全可靠，稳妥"。

【答案】B

No. 3 Short Conversation

 真题回顾（2011 年真题）

A. Four days.　　B. Ten days.　　C. One week.　　D. Two weeks.

听力原文

W: Well, Mr. Black, What brought you along today?

M: I've got a pain in my stomach.

W: How long have it been bothering you?

M: A fortnight.

Question: How long has the man's stomach ache?

【解析】此题考点为特殊表达式。对话中男士的回答是 "a fortnight"，这个词的意思是 "十四日，两周"。因而答案为 D。

【答案】D

No. 4 Short Conversation

真题回顾（2011 年真题）

A. To X-ray his chest.　　　　　B. To hospitalize him.

C. To perform a minor surgery.　D. To transfer him to a specialist.

 听力原文

W: What happened?

M: I was in a fight and got my head hurt.

W: Were you knocked out?

M: No.

W: I want you to go for an X-ray. And come back to me. You'll need some stitches for that wound.

Question: What is the doctor going to do for the man?

【解析】此题考点为细节再现。对话中医生最后告诉这位男士先去做个 X 光，然后回来，伤口需要缝几针。关键词为 stitch，这个词的意思为 "针脚，缝纫"，这里指的是缝合伤口，故答案为 C。

【答案】C

No. 5 Short Conversation

真题回顾（2012 年真题）

A. The woman's condition is critical.

B. The woman has been picking up quite well.

C. The woman's illness was caused by a mosquito bite.

D. The woman won't see the doctor any more.

 听力原文

M: Well, just keep your arm straight there. Fine, there will be a little prick like a mosquito bite. OK? There we go. OK, I will send that sample off and we'll check it. If the sample is OK, we won't need to go on seeing you anymore.

W: So you think I'm getting better?

M: Absolutely.

Question: What can be inferred from the conversation?

【解析】此题考点为细节信息再现。女士问医生自己是不是好转了，医生回答说当然，故答案为 B。选项 C 是干扰项，医生让女病人伸直手臂，并说会有像蚊子叮咬的刺痛，prick 的含义是"刺痛"。

【答案】B

3. 特殊句式

在听力考试中，特殊句式是一个重要考点，如反意疑问句、虚拟语气、双重否定等。这些句式的使用都是为了加强对话中说话人的语气，因而考生应从语气上把握这些特殊句式的含义。请看下面的真题：

No.1 Short Conversation

 真题回顾

A. She would go to the drug store.

B. She would go to see the doctor.

C. She would take medicine at home.

D. She would find the medicine cabinet.

听力原文

M: You don't look well. Are you sure you want to go out?

W: If there was some Aspirin in the medical cabinet, I would not need to go out to the drug store.

Question: What would the woman probably do?

【解析】听力对话中，男士说："你看上去不太好，你确定要出去吗？"女士回答说："如果药箱里有阿司匹林的话，我就不需要去药房了。"此题的重要句式就是虚拟语气中的 if 虚拟条件句。

【答案】A

No. 2　Short Conversation

真题回顾

A. The surgery was absolutely necessary for the patient.

B. The surgery could not have been more successful.

C. The necessity for the surgery was questionable.

D. The patient could not stand the surgery.

听力原文

W: Do you think the patient needs the surgery?

M: It couldn't be more necessary.

Question: What does the man mean?

【解析】此题的解题关键就在于男士话语中的句型，意思是"非常有必要"，也就是说，这个病人十分需要手术。如果考生对于这个句型的含义了解，解题就不难了。

【答案】A

4.　常用习语

此类型考题的考点主要是人们日常活动中常用到的一些短语和习语，这要求考生在备考期间，多积累这些习语，并且将这些表达式在语境中加深理解。

Short Conversation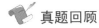

真题回顾

A. John is as clumsy as a pig.

B. John has never played a game like that.

C. John cannot win the game.

D. John has no confidence in himself.

听力原文

W: John says that he is confident that he can win the game.

M: He'll succeed when pigs fly.

Question: What does the man mean?

【解析】在女士的话中，be confident 的意思是"有信心"，女士告诉男士："约翰说他有信心赢得比赛。"男士的回答中有个习语：pigs fly 表示"不可能，除非出现奇迹"。所以男士的意思是说约翰根本不可能赢得比赛。

【答案】C

5. 推断题

推断题是听力考试中较为常见的题型，即根据听力对话中的细节内容、表达式或语气推测说话人的意图、引申含义或对话后可能发生的事情。这类题型较难，首先，考生要听懂对话中的细节内容，了解其含义，然后才能根据理解做出推断。请看以下真题实例：

No. 1 Short Conversation

 真题回顾

A. Larry will make other arrangements.

B. Larry will not go for the outing.

C. Larry will rearrange his plan.

D. Larry has changed his mind.

听力原文

W: I haven't heard whether Larry is going for the outing.

M: He made another arrangement before the outing was planned.

Question: What does the man mean?

【解析】此题要根据细节做出推断。问题是：What does the man mean?（这位男士的意思是什么？）在听力对话中，女士首先说："I haven't heard whether Larry is going for the outing.（我没听说 Larry 是否去郊游。）"男士回答："He made another arrangement before the outing was planned.（出游定下来之前他另有安排了。）"此题考点就是根据男士的这句话进行推断，Larry 在安排出游前就有别的安排了，可以推断出他将不去郊游。

【答案】B

No. 2 Short Conversation

 真题回顾

A. A question and answer section.   B. A self-introduction.

C. A presentation.   D. A seminar.

听力原文

M: Doctor Morris. That was a very interesting presentation. I enjoyed it very much.

W: It's very kind of you to say so. Thank you. Have we met before?

Question: What will most probably happen right then?

【解析】此题问对话后将发生什么事情。这类题型的关键在于对话中的最后一句：我们以前见过吗？根据这句话我们可以直接推断出说话人将要介绍自己了。

【答案】B

No. 3 Short Conversation

 真题回顾

A. It's overrated.　　　　　　　　B. It's rather boring.
C. It's hard to understand.　　　　D. It's extremely interesting.

 听力原文

W: Never have I read such interesting science fiction; you know, it's all about E.T.s.

M: That's understatement.

Question: What does the speaker imply about the fiction?

【解析】题目的意思是：说话人对小说想要表达什么态度？通过题目中的 imply 我们可知此题为推断题。对话中，女士说："从来没读过这么有意思的科幻小说，你知道的，它是关于外星人的。"随后男士说："That's understatement."考点关键词是 understatement，意思是"轻描淡写"。男士的回答暗示我们，他认为女士对于这部小说的评价仅用 interesting 这个词来形容是不够的，所以我们可以推断男士觉得这部小说很有意思。选项 A 意思是"评价过高了"。这类推断题是根据某个表达式或词语做出正确的推断，故应选 D。

【答案】D

No. 4 Short Conversation

 真题回顾

A. The man is working too hard.　　　B. The man needs to think it over.
C. The man is supposed to find a job.　D. The man has made a right decision.

 听力原文

M: Taking a long view, I'm leaving the company.

W: Why?

M: I often have to overwork which will do harm to my health.

W: But the job market is very tight, you know.

Question: What does the woman mean?

【解析】此题考点为推断。对话中男士打算离开公司。女士说道："但是就业市场紧张。"根据女士的回答可以推断出她的言外之意是劝男士考虑清楚再做决定，因而答案是 B。

【答案】B

No. 5 Short Conversation

 真题回顾（2011 年真题）

A. The woman's classmate.   B. The woman's boyfriend.

C. The woman's brother.   D. The woman's teacher.

 听力原文

M: I heard all the time that John is dating several girls.

W: But it's not true. He has explained everything to me.

M: Do you really believe what he said?

W: Yeah, I believe in our feelings for each other.

Question: Who is John?

【解析】此题考点为推断。对话中男士提到约翰正和几个女孩约会。女士答道："这不是真的，他已经向我解释了一切。"男士又问女士是否相信约翰所说的，女士说她相信两个人彼此的感情。从对话中我们可以推断出约翰是这位女士的男友，B 为答案。

【答案】B

No. 6 Short Conversation

 真题回顾（2011 年真题）

A. 250 yuan.   B. 450 yuan.   C. 650 yuan.   D. 850 yuan.

 听力原文

W: Good morning. Would you like the private hot spring room today? For 3 people, it would be 250 yuan per hour.

M: Are there any discounts?

W: Yes, it is 50 yuan cheaper for each additional hour.

M: Then we'll have 2 hours.

Question: How much will the man pay?

【解析】此题考点为推算。对话中提到私人温泉是三个人每小时 250 元。有打折，每增加一小时优惠 50 元。问题问两个小时多少钱。第一小时为 250 元，第二小时优惠 50 元，因而需要花费 450 元，B 为答案。

【答案】B

No. 7 Short Conversation

 真题回顾（2012 年真题）

A. The blouse is a bargain.   B. The blouse is too expensive.

C. The blouse is colorful.　　　　D. The blouse is so fashionable.

 听力原文

W: The blouse cost me like 8,000 yuan.

M: That's such a rip-off.

W: I really like it, the color, the design…

M: Fashion really kills women.

Question: What does the man mean?

【解析】此题考点为推断。女士说花了 8000 元买了这件上衣。男士提到 ripoff 这个词，含义是"骗人的东西"，他还提到时尚确实杀死女人。从上述信息可以推断出男士认为这件上衣太贵了，因此答案为 B。

【答案】B

（二）Section B 的主要考点及应试技巧

根据考试大纲的要求和规定，这一部分由一篇长对话和两篇短文组成，目的在于测试考生对英语篇章的听力理解能力。要求考生能理解所听材料的中心思想和主要内容，并能根据所听到的内容进行逻辑推理、分析概括和归纳总结。可以看出，这一部分的听力测试有别于 Section A，它主要测试听力材料中的细节。题型可以大致划分为：细节再现题、细节概括题和细节推理题。下面就按照具体题型进行讲述。

细节再现题：在 Section B 部分，由于听力材料比较长，因而考生可以获得的信息就会较丰富，在这种情况下，针对细节的考题就会比较多。这类题型就是对一些信息不做任何改变，或对其进行同义改写，再将其作为考试内容，以考查考生在听力过程中获得信息的能力。

细节概括题：这类题型是在细节再现题的基础上，更深一步地进行测试。考题一般测试听力材料中细节的汇总，比如提到说话人买的东西，然后分别说出了价格，再问这个人总共花了多少钱。或者类似于阅读理解中的主旨题。因此，考生应该将听力材料中的相关细节做一个简单的记录，让解题时有线索。

细节推理题：这类考题是在考听力细节的基础上再进一步要求考生根据所听内容进行符合逻辑的推理，主要测试点为推理。考生首先要理解听力细节，并且做一些简单的笔记，然后再进行推理。

在 Section B 中，虽然听力内容较多，对于考生来说不容易掌握，但是这部分考题都是根据某一篇材料进行考题设置，因而，题目之间的联系较大，从某种程度上来说这样也便于考生猜测和解题。另外，这部分的难点在于信息的收集，因而考生在平时复习备考的时候，应该着重注意细节的收集和记忆。从听力材料内容范围来说，一定会和医学场景或医学常识相关，所以这就要求考生必须具备一定量的医学常用词汇。下面，我们就通过一套真题来具体体会一下这三种题型的特点。

No.1 Long Conversation

真题回顾

16. A. For his dizziness.　　　　　　B. For his headaches.
    C. For his hurting eyes.　　　　　D. For his broken finger.
17. A. They have been going on for two weeks.
    B. They are hurting his eyes.
    C. They are hard to explain.
    D. They occur at any time.
18. A. In the morning.　　　　　　　B. In the afternoon.
    C. In the evening.　　　　　　　D. At night.
19. A. His night life.　　　　　　　　B. His broken finger.
    C. His work pressure.　　　　　　D. His irregular hours.
20. A. He feels cold.　　　　　　　　B. He feels faint.
    C. He feels nothing but sleepy.　　D. He feels himself falling down.

听力原文

M: Good morning, doctor.

W: It's Mr. Coleman, isn't it?

M: Right. I saw you about six months ago with a broken finger.

W: Yes, of course. And is that on heal now?

M: It's fine. No problem.

W: What can I do for you today?

M: Well, I've been having these headaches. They started about two months ago. They seem to come on quite suddenly and I got dizzy spells as well.

W: Right. Let's start with the headaches. Where is the pain exactly? Can you show me?

M: In the front. I thought it might be my eyes.

W: Do these headaches come on at any particular time?

M: Yeah. When I go to work in the morning, when I step outside my shop, I run the boutique. My shop is just nearby, so when I walk out, the headache comes on.

W: Do you ever have these headaches at night?

M: No. I am not sleepy at night. I wake up two or three times every night.

W: Why is that?

M: Well, I think I am a bit of worrier. I have staff problems at work, and the financial situation is tough at this moment.

W: I'm sorry to hear about that. Can I just come back for a moment to these dizzy spells? Can you describe them?

M: Well, they last a few seconds. I suddenly feel very dizzy.

W: This dizziness, to some people, is a sensation of the falling. To other people, it's a sensation of fainting. How would you describe your dizziness?

M: Well, I feel that I am going to fall down.

W: How about your health in general? How do you feel in general?

M: No problems. There are colds, but that's all about it.

W: OK, let me give you a check-over.

Questions 16 to 20 are based on the conversation you have just heard.

16. Why did the man visit the woman six months ago?

17. What can we learn about the man's headaches?

18. When does the man usually have his headaches?

19. What seems to have caused the man's headaches?

20. How does the man feel about his dizziness?

答案及解析

16. 【答案】D

【解析】细节再现题。题目是：为什么这位男士6个月前去看这位女医生？在听力材料中提到：I saw you about six months ago with a broken finger.（6个月前我来看骨折的手指。）所以答案为D。

17. 【答案】B

【解析】细节推理题。题目是：我们可以得知关于这位男士的头疼的什么情况？A项说他头疼已经两周了。但听力材料中提到：They started about two months ago.（开始于两个月前）因而不选A；C项意思是"很难解释头疼"。但是在听力材料中，我们可以知道这位男士对于头疼问题的表述，如时间、感受、疼痛处都很清楚，因而C错；D项是说疼痛在任何时候都发作。但是这位男士在描述病情的时候提到，早上的时候头疼，但晚上没有疼过，也就是说他头疼是在具体某个特殊时刻，所以D也不对。

18. 【答案】A

【解析】细节再现题。题目是：男士通常在什么时候头疼？文中提到：When I go to work in the morning, when I step outside my shop, I run the boutique. My shop is just nearby, so when I walk out, the headache comes on.（早上起来出门上班就开始头疼。）然后女士又问他晚上是否头疼，男士说道："No. I am not sleepy at night."所以答案为A。

19. 【答案】C

【解析】细节推理题。题目是：可能是什么引起这位男士的头疼？在听力中我们得知，这位男士是在早上出门上班的时候突然头疼，而且他也提到每天晚上都要起来两三次，因为他在工作上遇到了员工和资金的问题，故可知工作压力大使得他头疼。

20. 【答案】D

【解析】细节再现题。题目是：这位男士头晕时的感受如何？男士提到：I feel that I am going to fall down. 选项中只有 D 与原文信息一致，故为答案。

No.2 Passage

真题回顾

21. A. Easy to digest.　　　　　　　B. Rich in nutrition.
    C. High in blood cholesterol.　　D. Free of harmful substances.
22. A. A rise in egg price.　　　　　B. A high incidence of heart disease.
    C. A drop in egg sales.　　　　　D. The emergence of a new life style.
23. A. The reduced consumption of eggs.
    B. The development of substitute eggs.
    C. The improved ways of cooking eggs.
    D. The removal of nutritional substances in eggs.
24. A. The feeds.　　　　　　　　　B. The taste.
    C. The recipe.　　　　　　　　　D. The amount of cholesterol.
25. A. Eggs and their recipes.　　　　B. Eggs and their substitutes.
    C. Misconception about eggs.　　 D. The nutritional value of eggs.

 听力原文

Although there are extensive suppliers of vitamins, minerals and high-quality proteins, eggs also contain a high level of blood cholesterol, one of the major causes of the heart disease. One egg in fact contains a little more than 2/3 of the cholesterol the body needs daily. This knowledge has caused egg sales to drop in the recent years, which, in turn, has brought about the development of several alternatives to eating regular eggs. One alternative is to eat substitute eggs. These egg substitutes are not really eggs, but they look somehow like eggs when they are cooked. They have the advantage of having lower cholesterol weights, and they can be scrambled or used in baking. One disadvantage, however, is that they are not good for frying or boiling. A second alternative to regular eggs is a new type of eggs, sometimes called designer eggs. These eggs are produced by hens that are fed low-fat diets, including such ingredients as corn, flax and rice bran. In spite of their diets, however, these eggs contain the same amount of cholesterol as the regular eggs. Yet, the producers of these eggs claim that eating their eggs will not raise the blood cholesterol in humans.

Questions 21 to 25 are based on the passage you have just heard.

21. What is good about the eggs?
22. What happened when people came to know the high level of cholesterol in eggs?
23. What has been one of the approaches to the problems of cholesterol?
24. What makes the designer eggs different from the regular eggs?
25. What is the main idea of the talk?

答案及解析

21. 【答案】B

【解析】细节概括题。题目是：鸡蛋有什么好处？听力材料中提到：Although there are extensive suppliers of vitamins, minerals and high-quality proteins, eggs also contain a high level of blood cholesterol, one of the major causes of the heart disease.（尽管鸡蛋富含维生素、矿物质和高质量的蛋白质，但鸡蛋含有较多的胆固醇，而胆固醇是心脏病的主因之一。）A 项说易于消化；B 项指富含营养物质；C 项说胆固醇含量高；D 项说不含有害物质。故答案为 B。

22. 【答案】C

【解析】细节再现题。题目是：当人们认识到鸡蛋中含有较多的胆固醇时，发生了什么？A 项说鸡蛋价格上升；B 项说心脏病的发病率高；C 项说鸡蛋销量下降；D 项说新的生活方式出现。听力材料中"This knowledge has caused egg sales to drop in the recent years."表明，人们认识到这个问题后导致近年鸡蛋销售量下降。故答案为 C。

23. 【答案】B

【解析】细节再现题。题目是：解决胆固醇问题的方法之一是什么？A 项意为鸡蛋摄入下降；B 项意为鸡蛋替代物的发展；C 项意为鸡蛋烹调方式的改进；D 项意为鸡蛋中营养物质的去除。文中"This knowledge has caused egg sales to drop in the recent years, which, in turn, has brought about the development of several alternatives to eating regular eggs."告诉我们鸡蛋的替代品应运而生。所以答案为 B。

24. 【答案】A

【解析】细节概括题。题目是：designer eggs 与正常鸡蛋的不同之处在哪里？A 项意为喂养方式；B 项指口味；C 项指烹饪方法；D 项指胆固醇量。听力材料告诉我们：These eggs are produced by hens that are fed low-fat diets, including such ingredients as corn, flax and rice bran. 该句意为："鸡蛋是由用玉米、麻、糠麸等低脂肪食物喂养的母鸡下的。"根据这个信息，可知答案为 A。

25. 【答案】B

【解析】细节概括题。题目是：这篇短文的主旨是什么？A 项指鸡蛋和烹饪方法；B

项指鸡蛋和替代品；C 项指对鸡蛋的错误观念；D 项指鸡蛋的营养价值。听力全文都在说鸡蛋的替代品，故答案为 B。

No.3 Passage

 真题回顾

26. A. It is fun though not widely practiced.
    B. It is to benefit your dependents.
    C. It is getting popular.
    D. It is absurd.
27. A. The buying of life insurance is not the business of guessing.
    B. There must be a standard amount of life insurance for people.
    C. People are encouraged to buy more life insurance for more benefit.
    D. One has to rely on an agent to figure out the right amount of life insurance.
28. A. Following general estimates.
    B. Upgrading your quality of life.
    C. Making as much money as you can.
    D. Maintaining your current living standard.
29. A. The size of a family.   B. The source of income.
    C. The basic human needs.   D. The death of the bread-winner.
30. A. To present the advantages and disadvantages of life insurance.
    B. To encourage people to buy life insurance.
    C. To tell people how to buy life insurance.
    D. To help improve the quality of life.

 听力原文

Life insurance isn't fun to buy. It forces you to think about your death: a subject many prefer not to confront. But there's a single, overriding reason to buy life insurance: to provide an income for your dependents if you die. Don't depend solely on an agent to figure your life insurance needs. Rule-of-thumb estimates such as five or eight times your income are guessed: they may produce too little or too much insurance. Carry too little insurance and you may not provide a reasonable standard of living for your family after your death; carry too much and you may not enjoy a reasonable standard of living while you're alive.

According to statistics, most people who have life insurance don't have enough. Then how do you determine the amount of life insurance you will need to maintain your family's current lifestyle if the bread-winner died? First, think what your family's expenses will be if you die tomorrow? Then analyze your assets, the source of income that you can use to cover the expenses. Finally, subtract the assets from the needs. The result is the amount of the additional insurance you need to buy.

Questions 26 to 30 are based on the passage you have just heard.

26. What does the speaker think of buying life insurance?
27. Which of the following is true according to the speaker?
28. What is the most important thing to consider in buying life insurance?
29. What is the key element in determining the amount of life insurance?
30. What is the purpose of the talk?

答案及解析

26. 【答案】B
    【解析】细节再现题。题目是：说话人对于买人身保险的态度如何？A 项是说尽管没有广泛流行但很有意思；B 项是说对后代有好处；C 项指越来越流行；D 项是说荒谬可笑。听力材料的第一句话是：Life insurance isn't fun to buy.（买人身保险并不是一件快乐的事情。）因而排除 A。而听力材料的第三句 "… overriding reason to buy life insurance: to provide an income for your dependents if you die." 则告诉我们，买人身保险最重要的理由就是去世后给后代一些收入。最后又告诉人们该如何买保险。这些信息都说明说话人并没有觉得这件事情荒谬可笑，故排除 D。C 项在听力材料中没有提到，故答案为 B。

27. 【答案】A
    【解析】细节再现题。题目是：下面选项哪一个是正确的？A 项说买人身保险不是靠猜测就能决定的；B 项说人们必须有一定量的人身保险；C 项是鼓励人们多买保险多得利益；D 项是说人们不得不依靠代理算出人身保险的合适数额。此题用排除法会比较容易解题。听力材料中提到，购买的人身保险数额要合适，不能因此而影响现在正常的生活水平，并且告诉人们该如何自己算出该买多少，不要依靠代理。由这些信息可知答案为 A。

28. 【答案】D
    【解析】细节再现题。题目是：在买人身保险的时候，要考虑的最重要的问题是什么？A 项说依据大概的估计；B 项说提高生活质量；C 项说挣足够多的钱；D 项说保持目前的生活水平。听力材料中的 "carry too much and you may not enjoy a reasonable standard of living while you're alive." 表明了说话人的态度。答案为 D。

29. 【答案】B
    【解析】细节再现题。题目是：决定人身保险数额的主要因素是什么？A 项指家庭规模；B 项指收入来源；C 项是说人类的基本需要；D 项指养家糊口的人的去世。听力材料中提到该如何确定数额：First, think what your family's expenses will be if you die tomorrow? Then analyze your assets, the source of income

that you can use to cover the expenses. Finally, subtract the assets from the needs. The result is the amount of the additional insurance you need to buy.

（首先，考虑去世后家人的开销，分析财产和收入来源是否能支付这些费用。最后，从总需求金额中减去资产，剩下的就是你需要买的额外人身保险数额。）可知本题应选 B。

30. 【答案】C

【解析】细节推断题。题目是：这篇文章的写作目的是什么？A 项是呈现人身保险的优缺点；B 项是鼓励人们去买保险；C 项是告诉人们该如何买保险；D 项是帮助提高生活质量。通过前面几道细节再现题的解题，很容易得知本题答案为 C。

No.4 Passage

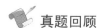 真题回顾

21. A. 35 million.   B. 34 million.   C. 25 million.   D. 20 million.
22. A. Author, professor and dreamer.
    B. Writer, professor and insomniac.
    C. Author, psychologist and insomniac.
    D. Dramatist, psychologist and scientist.
23. A. Sleeping in 8-hour consolidated blocks.
    B. Sleeping during day time.
    C. Going to bed soon after dark.
    D. Two blocks of 4-hour sleep with a waking break.
24. A. Because they have unnoticeable sleeping patterns.
    B. Because they sleep very little.
    C. Because they are insensitive.
    D. Because they can't complain.
25. A. Sleep is highly variable, and wears out with age.
    B. Falling asleep is a gradual process.
    C. Sleeping less will help you lose weight.
    D. People need to sleep eight hours a day.

 听力原文

Our culture is obsessed with sleep, and the lack of it, yet many of us don't know some basic facts. As many as 35 million Americans experience chronic insomnia, and yet in 2006 only $20 million was spent on research. In the 6 years that author, professor and lifelong insomniac Gayle Green spent researching and writing her book *Insomniac*, she learned almost all there is to know about sleep and the lack thereof. Here are 5 common myths about how we get our shut-eye and why:

1. Humans Need 8 Hours Sleep a Night

There are many ways of sleeping and few cultures sleep in 8 hours consolidated blocks like we do. Until the industrial era, many Western Europeans divided the night into "the first sleep" and "the second sleep". They'd go to bed soon after dark, sleep for 4 hours then wake for an hour or 2 during which they'd write, pray, smoke, have sex or even visit neighbors. In fact, there's some evidence to suggest that this sleep pattern maybe the one most in tune with our inherent circadian rhythms.

2. Sleep Isn't Just a Bodily Function

Sleep is a biological, physiological system, akin to the cardiovascular system, the nervous system and so on. Like any other system, it is highly variable, and it wears out and gets more fragile with age.

3. Animals Don't Have Sleep Problems

Insomnia occurs in animals and insects, too, sort of. Technically, insomnia is defined as a "complaint", and since animals can't complain, it's difficult to measure in them.

4. Falling Asleep Is a Gradual Process

Nope. Instead, for most people, it switches on and off like a light switch. But for insomniacs and narcoleptics, the switch doesn't work quite well. Instead they inhabit the space in between — never entirely awake, nor entirely asleep.

5. Sleeping Less Burns More Calories

In the short term, yes, but sleeping less probably won't help you lose weight. Lack of sleep suppresses our natural appetite-depressants, while fueling appetite-increasers, often leading to weight gain.

Questions:

21. According to the talk, approximately how many Americans suffer from chronic insomnia?
22. Which of the following can best describe Gayle Green?
23. Which of the following sleeping patterns might be the most in tune with our inherent biological system?
24. According to the talk, why is it difficult to measure insomnia in animals?
25. According to the talk, which of the following is true?

🕊 答案及解析

21. 【答案】A

【解析】此题为细节信息再现题。文章中提到：As many as 35 million Americans experience chronic insomnia，所以答案为 A。

22. 【答案】B

【解析】此题为细节信息再现题。文章中提到：In the 6 years that author, professor and lifelong insomniac Gayle Green spent researching and writing her book *Insomniac*... 答案为 B。

23. 【答案】C

　　【解析】此题为细节信息再现题。文章中提到：… there's some evidence to suggest that this sleep pattern may be the one most in tune with our inherent circadian rhythms. 而这里的 this sleep pattern 指的就是前一句话提到的睡眠模式：They'd go to bed soon after dark, sleep for 4 hours then wake for an hour or 2 during which they'd write, pray, smoke, have sex or even visit neighbors. 因而符合这一睡眠模式的是 C。

24. 【答案】D

　　【解析】此题为细节信息再现题。文章中提到：… insomnia is defined as a "complaint", and since animals can't complain, it's difficult to measure in them. 所以答案为 D。

25. 【答案】A

　　【解析】此题可以用排除法，文章中提出五个常见的对于睡眠的错误认识。B、C 和 D 正是其中的三个，因而 A 为答案。

三、听力考试常见用语

　　听力考试中，要求考生较好地了解常用的口语表达形式的含义，以下总结了常用口语表达，供考生复习参考。

1. **nothing but**

W: How dare you be so rude to me!

M: I'm so sorry. I didn't really mean to hurt you. It's nothing but a joke!

【解析】女士说："你怎么敢对我如此粗鲁！"句型"How dare you do sth."表达说话人的愤怒和不满，意思是"你怎么敢……"。男士道歉说没想伤害这位女士，这只是一个玩笑而已。nothing but 的含义是"仅仅"。

2. **anything but**

W: I heard you went to Paris for holidays last week. I believe it was bound to be a wonderful trip!

M: Not exactly. My visit to Paris was anything but a pleasure trip.

【解析】女士说她听说男士上周去巴黎度假了，她相信这绝对是一次不错的旅行。be bound to do sth. 表示"一定……"。在男士话语中，anything but 的含义为"绝不，绝非"，因而男士的意思是，他认为巴黎之行绝不是充满乐趣的旅行。

3. **How come?**

M: I have to tell you Sam failed the exam.

W: How come? Isn't he the best student in the class?

【解析】男士告诉女士 Sam 考试不及格。女士很诧异，how come 的含义相当于 why，意思是："怎么会这样？他难道不是班里最好的学生吗？"

4. **I'm up to my ears in…**

    M: Can you come over for dinner tonight?

    W: I'm up to my ears in works, so I'll have to take a rain check.

    【解析】男士问今晚能否顺便来吃个饭？女士说工作忙得不可开交，所以暂时来不了了。be up to one's ears in something 意思是"忙得不可开交"。rain check 表示"暂时拒绝，改日可以"的意思。

5. **be under the weather**

    W: Sam, what's wrong with you? I haven't seen you for several days.

    M: Oh, it's nothing. I was just a little under the weather. I feel better now.

    【解析】女士问男士，最近怎么啦，好几天没见到他了。男士回答说："没什么，有点不舒服，现在好多了。" be under the weather 表示"不舒服，生病了"。

6. **Don't bury your head in the sand.**

    W: I really don't want to do the work. It is so tough and I can't stand it anymore.

    M: Don't bury your head in the sand. You'll learn a lot more from the experience.

    【解析】女士抱怨道："我真的不想再做这项工作了，太难了，我再也忍受不了了。"男士安慰道："别逃避现实，你会从中学到很多东西。" don't bury your head in the sand 表示"不要逃避现实（即要勇于面对）"。

7. **be cut out for / to be**

    M: I heard Mary decided to study medicine.

    W: I don't think she is cut out for the medical profession.

    【解析】男士告诉女士，Mary 决定学医，女士说："我觉得她天生不是学医的料。" be cut out for sth. 表示"天生适合"。

8. **blow up**

    M: What's happened to Sam?

    W: When I told him the bad news that his son failed in the exam, he blew up.

    【解析】blow up 的含义为"很生气"。

9. 虚拟语气（**Subjunctive mood**）

    M: The dress you tried on was really nice, and reasonably priced.

    W: I'd bought it right away if they had had it in my size.

    【解析】男士说："你刚才试穿的衣服真漂亮，而且价格合理。"女士回答道："要是有我穿的号我会立马买走。"虚拟语气表示一种假设，实际情况是没有这位女士能穿的尺码。

10. **I will save my breath.**

    W: I know you need a lot of money for the project. But why don't you ask Sam for help?

M: Ask him? I'll save my breath.

【解析】女士问道："我知道这个项目你需要很多钱，但为什么不向 Sam 求助呢？"
男士回答道："向他借？我还是省省力气吧。"对话中，why don't you do
sth. 表示一种委婉的建议。I'll save my breath 的意思是"省省力气吧，没
用的"。

11. count on

W: I wonder to know whether Mary takes her camera.

M: You should never count on her. She is always forgetful.

【解析】女士说："我想知道 Mary 是否带相机了。"男士说："你永远不要指望她，
她总是丢三落四的。"count on 的意思是"依靠，指望"。

12. pigs fly

W: John says that he is bound to pass the exam.

M: He'll succeed when pigs fly.

【解析】女士说："约翰说他一定能通过考试。"男士幽默地说道："他能考试及格，
猪都能飞了。"pigs fly 表示"绝对不可能"。

13. count the days

M: Are you looking forward to going home for holidays?

W: Sure. I'm counting the days.

【解析】男士问女士："你盼着回家度假吗？"女士说："当然，我数着日子呢。"count
the days 暗示女士归心似箭，已经到了数着日子的地步了。

14. bite off more than one can chew

M: I've decided to take eight courses next semester.

W: Don't bite off more than you can chew.

【解析】男士告诉女士他决定下学期选八门课。女士的劝说意思是"别贪多，嚼不烂"。

15. cost sb. an arm and a leg

W: Did you see the pearl necklace Sam gave to Mary?

M: It must have cost him an arm and a leg.

【解析】女士问男士："你看到 Sam 给 Mary 买的珍珠项链了吗？"男士说："一定花
了他一大笔钱。"cost sb. an arm and leg 表示"让某人花了一大笔钱"。

16. not do anything / a lot / much for sb.

W: What do you think of my new hairstyle?

M: It doesn't do anything for you.

【解析】女士问男士，觉得她的新发型如何？男士认为这个发型并没有使她更漂亮。

17. hold water

W: I believe the wealthier you are, the happier you feel.

M: Your argument doesn't hold water.

【解析】女士认为，越富有，越快乐。男士反驳说："你的观点站不住脚。"hold water 意思是"说不通，站不住脚"。

18. cannot do…without…

W: Harry. You'd better forget Mary.

M: Impossible! I can't live without her!

【解析】女士劝男士忘了 Mary。男士答道；"不可能！没她我就没法活！"这个表达式的含义是"没有……就无法……"。

19. burn the midnight oil

W: What's wrong with you, John? You look very tired.

M: I have a big test today, so I burnt the midnight oil last night.

【解析】女士问男士："有什么不舒服吗？你看上去很疲惫。"男士说他今天有一个重要考试，昨天晚上熬夜了。burn the midnight oil 的含义就是 stay up，即"熬夜"。

20. put all one's eggs in one basket

M: I am now busy with job hunting.

W: You'd better apply for several jobs and don't put all your eggs in one basket.

【解析】男士告诉女士："我正忙着找工作。"job hunting 表示"找工作"。女士建议男士多申请几份工作，别孤注一掷。put all one's eggs in one basket 意思是"孤注一掷"。

21. if only

W: Have you found your wallet?

M: If only I could remember where I had left it.

【解析】女士问男士："找到钱包了吗？"男士说："要是我记得把它放在哪里了就好了。"if only 的意思是"要是……就好了"，表示一种假设，是虚拟语气的一种。

22. no wonder

W: I feel faint.

M: No wonder. You haven't had a bite all day.

【解析】女士说她感到头晕。男士说："不足为奇，你一整天都没有吃一口东西了。"no wonder 的含义是"不足为奇"。

23. in vain

W: As a friend, you should persuade him to accept the chance of going abroad for further study.

M: I had a talk with him about it, but in vain.

【解析】女士说道："作为朋友，你应该劝他接受这个出国进修的机会。"男士说："我和他就此事谈过，但没用。"in vain 的含义是"无用的，徒劳的"。

24. from scratch

M: It is reported that John Smith will have had 100 chain stores totally by the end of this year. He is the big cheese now.

W: But no one knows he started from scratch with 200 dollars he'd borrowed from his friend.

【解析】在男士话语中，it is reported that … 意为"据报道……"，chain stores 意为"连锁店"，the big cheese 指的是"大人物"。女士说道："但没人知道他是从一个朋友那里借来200美元白手起家的。"from scratch 的含义就是"白手起家"，相当于 from the beginning。

25. up to scratch

W: Mr. Smith, I'm wondering to know whether you are interested in our software.

M: Sorry, I have to say this software couldn't be up to scratch. It is not easy to use.

【解析】女士想要知道 Smith 对她们公司的软件是否感兴趣。在男士的话语中，be up to scratch 的含义是"达到标准"。

26. can't be too+ *a.*

M: Why are so many young girls obsessed with being thin?

W: As a man, you can't understand it. As for girls, they can't be too thin.

【解析】在男士的话语中，be obsessed with 的含义是"对……很痴迷"，男士意思是："为什么如此多的年轻女孩这么痴迷变瘦呢？"女士话语中，can't be too thin 的意思是："对于女孩子来说，再怎么瘦也不为过。"

27. It's written all over your face.

M: If you really like the purse, I will buy it for you.

W: How do you know I like it very much?

M: It's written all over your face.

【解析】 It's written all over your face 直译为"一切都写在你脸上了"，意思相当于 it's very obvious，即"太明显了"。

28. like peas and carrots

W: I admire Mary and Sam. They are always together whatever they do.

M: Exactly. They are like peas and carrots.

【解析】admire 意为"羡慕"，女士说很羡慕玛丽和山姆，无论做什么总是在一起。like peas and carrots 的含义是"形影不离"。

29. a third wheel

M: Mary and I would like to see a movie after work. Would you like to go with us?

W: Anyway, thanks. But I don't want to be a third wheel.

【解析】男士问女士，愿不愿意与他和玛丽下班后一起看电影？女士的回答中提到不想成为 a third wheel，意思是"多余的人"，即我们常说的"电灯泡"。

30. in one ear and out the other

W: As his father, you should persuade him to change his mind and choose medicine as his major.

M: Yes I did, but since he already made his decision, my advice went in one ear and out the other.

【解析】女士认为男士应该劝说儿子改变主意，选择医学专业。男士很无奈，说道："我劝过，但是因为他已经做了决定，我的建议也只能左耳朵进右耳朵出了。"意思是儿子不听劝。

31. be in sb.'s shoes

M: I really understand my son's decision that he persists in choosing maths as his major. Why doesn't he change his mind to learn accounting?

W: If you are in his shoes, you are likely to understand him.

【解析】在男士的话语中，persist in doing sth. 的意思是"执意要做什么"。accounting 指的是"会计专业"。女士回答中 be in sb.'s shoes 的含义是"设身处地，站在某人的立场上"。

32. pay lip service

M: Did you have a fine holiday? I remember you told me that your boyfriend had promised you to go abroad for holidays in the summer vacation.

W: He always pays lip service.

【解析】男士问女士假期过得是否愉快，因为女士曾说她男朋友答应假期带她去国外度假。在女士的回答中，lip 指的是"嘴唇"，pay lip service 的含义就是"光动嘴，不付诸行动"。

33. down-to-earth

M: I am determined to stop smoking since now.

W: Shouting slogans alone will never get things done. What you need is down-to-earth efforts.

【解析】男士信誓旦旦地说要戒烟。在女士的话语中，slogan 的意思是"标语"，down-to-earth 的含义是"脚踏实地的，实实在在的"，因而女士是在说，光喊口号没用，要实实在在地努力。

34. find fault with sb.

W: Recently, I'm not satisfied with my husband. He hasn't given me flowers for a week and I really hope he can be more romantic.

M: You shouldn't find fault with him all the time.

【解析】女士说她最近不满意她的丈夫，说丈夫已经有一周没有给她送花了，而且希望丈夫能更浪漫一些。find fault with 的含义是"挑剔，吹毛求疵"。

35. ups and downs

W: Mr. Smith was a successful investor before. But he is so unfortunate that he experienced a tough period recently. At first he was bankrupt, and then his wife died in a car accident.

M: Life is full of ups and downs.

【解析】unfortunate 意为"不幸的"，tough 意为"困难的"，bankrupt 意为"破产"。

女士认为史密斯先生最近很不幸，先是破产了，然后妻子死于一场车祸。男士也很感慨地说："生活有得意时也有失意时。"ups and downs 的含义就是"人生的起起伏伏"。

36. **odds and ends**

    M: I hear that you are moving in June. What can I do for you?

    W: Thanks. Everything is done except for a few odds and ends.

    【解析】男士听说女士要搬家，问是否需要帮忙。odds and ends 的含义就是"零零碎碎的东西"。女士的意思是，都准备好了，除了一些零碎东西。

37. **His (or her) bark is worse than his (or her) bite.**

    M: I really don't want to talk to my father any more. He is always shouting at me!

    W: Actually your father cares about you all the time. Don't worry, his bark is worse than his bite.

    【解析】男士说不愿意再和父亲说话了，因为他父亲总是对他大吼大叫。女士则告诉他其实他父亲一直都很在乎他。bark 原意指"大声的、愤怒的喊叫，狗的叫声"，his bark is worse than his bite 的含义就是"一个人外表看起来大吼大叫，但心地很善良"，接近汉语里的"刀子嘴，豆腐心"。

38. **at one's service**

    M: Madam, do you have anything I can do for you?

    W: No, thanks.

    M: If you need anything, I'm at your service.

    【解析】at one's service 的含义就是"随时可以提供帮助"，在上面这个情景中，意思是"如果您需要什么，尽管吩咐"。

39. **knock oneself out**

    W: You'd better go to bed now. Don't knock yourself out trying to finish the project today.

    M: I would like to, but there is not plenty of time!

    【解析】女士希望男士上床去睡觉，别让自己太累，别非得今天完成工作。knock oneself out 的意思是"使……筋疲力尽"。

40. **at one's finger's tips**

    W: Could you give me some advice on how to get along well with Jim?

    M: If it was at my finger's tips, I would give you all the information right now.

    【解析】get along well with sb. 意为"和某人愉快相处"。在男士的话语中，使用了虚拟语气，表示纯然假设，与现在事实相反；at one's finger's tips 的意思是"了如指掌"，这句话的意思是：如果这事我了如指掌的话，我会把全部情况立即告诉你（表明实际情况是"我不清楚"）。

41. **at stake**

    M: Mary, I'm afraid I can't go with you for dinner. I'm occupied with a big project now, and I have to finish it today, otherwise I'm likely to be fired.

W: Your health is at stake, not your job.

【解析】be occupied with 意为"忙于……"，fire 意为"开除"。女士的话中，at stake 的意思是"有风险，岌岌可危"，因而这句话的意思是：是你的健康受到损害，不是你的工作。

42. at one's wits' end

W: We have discussed the solution to the problem for a whole day. Who can put forward a feasible one now?

M: I'm afraid I can't. I'm at my wits' end now.

【解析】feasible 意为"切实可行的"。wit 原意是指"一个人的才智"，如果一个人的才智已经到头了，已经不知所措了，那么我们就可以用 at one's wits' end 来表示，意思相当于中文里的"江郎才尽"。

43. round the clock

W: I'm wondering whether you can go with me to see a movie today.

M: I'm afraid not. I have to finish a presentation and maybe I will work round the clock.

【解析】I'm wondering 是一种很委婉、客气地询问对方是否可以做某事的说法。round the clock 的含义是"昼夜不停"。

44. in good time

M: We hardly missed the train.

W: Yeah, thanks to the fast taxi driver, or we couldn't arrive at the station in good time.

【解析】thanks to 表示"多亏了……"，in good time 的意思是"及时"。

45. have one's hands full

W: Henry, here is a new order. Please deal with it right now.

M: Sorry, I can't accept the new order any more since I already have my hands full.

【解析】order 的意思是"订单"。have one's hands full 表示"让某人手里满满当当的"，意思就是"忙得不可开交"。

46. exclusive of

M: Hello, I would like to book a single room for Tuesday next week. What is the rate, please?

W: The current rate is $100 per night exclusive of breakfast.

【解析】book a single room 预订一个单人间。"What is the rate, please?"是在问房价是多少。exclusive of 的含义是"不包含"，所以女士的回答是说目前房价是一晚 100 元，不含早餐。

47. hang in there

M: Learning English is so tough that I don't want to learn it any more.

W: Hang in there!

【解析】男士认为英语学习太难了，不想再学下去了。hang in there 表示一种鼓励，意思是"别泄气，坚持下去"。

48. burn a hole in one's pocket

W: Jim, your shoes are cool. How much did it cost you?

M: 1,000 yuan.

W: It can really burn a hole in my pocket.

【解析】某物把一个人的口袋烧了个洞，意思是说"这样东西价格昂贵"。

四、听力专项练习及最新真题解析

2015 年真题

1. A. How to deal with his sleeping problem.
   B. The cause of his sleeping problem.
   C. What follows his insomnia.
   D. The severity of his medical problem.

2. A. To take the medicine for a longer time.
   B. To discontinue the medication.
   C. To come to see her again.
   D. To switch to other medications.

3. A. To take it easy and continue to work. B. To take a sick leave.
   C. To keep away from work. D. To have a follow-up.

4. A. Fullness in the stomach. B. Occasional stomachache.
   C. Stomach distention. D. Frequent belches.

5. A. Extremely severe. B. Not very severe.
   C. More severe than expected. D. It's hard to say.

6. A. He has lost some weight. B. He has gained a lot.
   C. He needs to exercise more. D. He is still overweight.

7. A. She is giving the man an injection. B. She is listening to the man's heart.
   C. She is feeling the man's pulse. D. She is helping the man stop shivering.

8. A. In the gym. B. In the office.
   C. In the clinic. D. In the boat.

9. A. Diarrhea. B. Vomiting.
   C. Nausea. D. A cold.

10. A. She has developed allergies. B. She doesn't know what allergies are.
    C. She doesn't have any allergies. D. She has allergies treated already.

11. A. Listen to music. B. Read magazines.
    C. Go to play tennis. D. Stay in the house.

12. A. She isn't feeling well.   B. She is under pressure.

     C. She doesn't like the weather.   D. She is feeling relieved.

13. A. Michael's wife was ill.

     B. Michael's daughter was ill.

     C. Michael's daughter gave birth to twins.

     D. Michael was hospitalized for a check-up.

14. A. She is absent-minded.   B. She is in high spirits.

     C. She is indifferent.   D. She is compassionate.

15. A. Ten years ago.   B. Five years ago.

     C. Fifteen years ago.   D. Several weeks ago.

Section B

*Directions: In this section you will hear one conversation and two passages, after each of which, you will hear five questions. After each question, read the four possible answers marked A, B, C and D. Choose the best answer and mark the letter of your choice on the **ANSWER SHEET**.*

Dialogue

16. A. A blood test.   B. A gastroscopy.

     C. A chest X-ray exam.   D. A barium X-ray test.

17. A. To lose some weight.   B. To take a few more tests.

     C. To sleep on three pillows.   D. To eat smaller, lighter meals.

18. A. Potato chips.   B. Chicken.   C. Cereal.   D. Fish.

19. A. Ulcer.   B. Cancer.   C. Depression.   D. Hernia.

20. A. He will try the diet the doctor recommended.

     B. He will ask for a sick leave and relax at home.

     C. He will take the medicine the doctor prescribed.

     D. He will take a few more tests to rule out cancer.

Passage One

21. A. A new concept of diabetes.

     B. The definition of Type 1 and Type 2 diabetes.

     C. The new management of diabetics in the hospital.

     D. The new development of non-perishable insulin pills.

22. A. Because it vaporizes easily.

     B. Because it becomes overactive easily.

     C. Because it is usually in injection form.

     D. Because it is not stable above 40 degrees Fahrenheit.

23. A. The diabetics can be cured without taking synthetic insulin any longer.

B. The findings provide insight into how insulin works.

C. Insulin can be more stable than it is now.

D. Insulin can be produced naturally.

24. A. It is stable at room temperature for several years.

B. It is administered directly into the bloodstream.

C. It delivers glucose from blood to the cells.

D. It is more chemically complex.

25. A. Why insulin is not stable at room temperature.

B. How important it is to understand the chemical bonds of insulin.

C. Why people with Type 1 and Type 2 diabetes don't produce enough insulin.

D. What shape insulin takes when it unlocks the cells to take sugar from blood.

Passage Two

26. A. Vegetative patients are more aware.

B. Vegetative patients retain some control of their eye movements.

C. EEG scans may help us communicate with the vegetative patients.

D. We usually communicate with the brain-dead people by brain-wave.

27. A. The left-hand side of the brain.   B. The right-hand side of the brain.

C. The central part of the brain.   D. The front part of the brain.

28. A. 31.   B. 6.   C. 4.   D. 1.

29. A. The patient was brain-dead.

B. The patient wasn't brain-dead.

C. The patient had some control over his eye movements.

D. The patient knew the movement he or she was making.

30. A. The patient is no technically vegetative.

B. The patient can communicate in some way.

C. We can train the patient to speak.

D. The family members and doctors can provide better care.

答案与解析

1. 【问题】男士想知道什么？

A. 如何解决睡眠问题。   B. 睡眠问题的起因。

C. 失眠后会如何。   D. 问题的严重程度。

【答案】A

【解析】细节信息题。通过对话我们得知这位男士睡眠不好，女士要给他开药，帮助他改善睡眠，因而 A 为答案。

2. 【问题】如果男士的问题持续的话，女士建议他做什么？

A. 加长服药时间。   B. 停止吃药。

C. 再次就诊。   D. 换药方。

【答案】C

【解析】细节信息题。通过对话我们知道药量是 30 天的，如果服药后患者还不好，建议他回来复诊。因而答案为 C。

3. 【问题】男士告诉女士怎么做？

    A. 放轻松，继续上班。   B. 请病假。

    C. 远离工作。   D. 跟进就医。

【答案】A

【解析】细节题。女士问她是否应该不工作（stay away from work），男士认为没有必要，只是要保持冷静即可。因此本题答案为 A（继续工作）。

4. 【问题】女士抱怨什么？

    A. 饱腹感。   B. 偶尔胃疼。   C. 胃胀。   D. 频繁打嗝。

【答案】B

【解析】推理题。女士说胃部在进食后会有疼痛的时候，但并非常态，所以她抱怨的是偶尔的胃疼。答案为 B。

5. 【问题】疼痛有多严重？

    A. 极端疼痛。   B. 不太严重。

    C. 比想象中疼。   D. 很难描述。

【答案】B

【解析】细节信息题。医生让女病人描述疼痛的级别。根据女士描述，大概级别为 2，且 not really bad，因而答案为 B。

6. 【问题】男士是什么意思？

    A. 他减重了。   B. 他增重了。

    C. 他需要更多的锻炼。   D. 他仍然超重。

【答案】C

【解析】细节信息题。女士认为男士没超重。男士提到如果跑上一段楼梯，他还是会过好一会儿，呼吸才能缓过来，需要加强锻炼（work out），因而答案为 C。

7. 【问题】女士正在做什么？

    A. 她正在为男士注射。   B. 她正在听诊心脏。

    C. 她正在把脉。   D. 她正在帮助男士止颤。

【答案】B

【解析】细节信息题，解题关键在于 stethoscope，意思是"听诊器"。因而答案为 B。

8. 【问题】这个对话可能发生在什么地方？

    A. 健身房。   B. 办公室。   C. 门诊。   D. 船上。

【答案】C

【解析】特殊短语理解题。男士提到 everything looks ship-shape，即"一切都很好，井井有条"。女士问何时再来复查，可知对话场景应为诊所。

9. 【问题】男士患了什么病？

    A. 腹泻。   B. 呕吐。   C. 恶心。   D. 感冒。

【答案】C

【解析】推理题。男士说既没有拉肚子也没有呕吐，只是觉得有点恶心，需要喝点热茶之类的东西。录音中出现了 sick 一词，因此本题最好的答案为 nausea（反胃）。

10. 【问题】女士是什么意思？

    A．她过敏了。   B．她不知道过敏源是什么。

    C．她没有过敏症状。   D．她的过敏已经得到治疗了。

【答案】C

【解析】此题为语义理解题。男士问女士过敏情况怎么样了，女士说不是认为的那样，意思是她没过敏，因而答案为 C。

11. 【问题】女士将要做什么？

    A．听音乐。   B．读杂志。

    C．打网球。   D．待在屋里。

【答案】C

【解析】细节信息题。女士在听音乐、看杂志。男士建议她出去打网球。因而答案为 C。

12. 【问题】女士是什么意思？

    A．她感觉不太舒服。   B．她压力很大。

    C．她不喜欢这个天气。   D．她觉得很放松。

【答案】A

【解析】语义理解题。解题关键在于女士说的词组：under the weather，意思是"身体不适"。因而答案为 A。

13. 【问题】从对话中可以得知什么？

    A．迈克的妻子病了。

    B．迈克的女儿病了。

    C．迈克的女儿生了一对双胞胎。

    D．迈克住院检查了。

【答案】C

【解析】细节信息题。解题信息是 Their daughter has just had twins，因而答案是 C。obstetrics and gynecology department 的含义是"妇产科"。

14. 【问题】关于女士的说法哪个是正确的？

    A．她健忘。   B．她很热情。

    C．她冷漠。   D．她有同情心。

【答案】D

【解析】细节信息题。女士要给男士再盖上一条毛毯，男士回应：You are so sweet. 由此可知这位女性很热心，答案为 D。

15. 【问题】女士什么时候骨折的？

    A．10 年前。   B．5 年前。

C. 15 年前。　　　　　　　　　　D. 几个星期前。

【答案】A

【解析】细节信息题。对话中有关这位女士的信息较多，根据问题：何时骨折的？原文信息是 I slipped on the ice and fractured my neck 10 years ago，因而答案是 A。

🎧 Section B

Dialogue

16.【问题】男士经历了什么样的医疗程序？

    A. 血液检查。　　　　　　　　　　B. 胃镜检查。

    C. 胸部 X 片检查。　　　　　　　　D. 钡餐透视检查。

【答案】D

【解析】题目问这位男士做了哪些检查。对话一开始就提到他做了钡餐检查，检查未显示他有溃疡。因而答案是 D。

17.【问题】下列哪一个不是医生的建议？

    A. 减重。　　　　　　　　　　　　B. 多做一些检查。

    C. 枕三个枕头睡觉。　　　　　　　D. 要少吃，要清淡。

【答案】B

【解析】题目问下列哪一项不是医生的建议。对话中，男士问是否还需要做其他检查以确诊（But are there other tests you can do to be absolutely sure?），医生说不用。因而答案是 B。

18.【问题】根据作者的建议，下列哪一种食物是男士要避免的？

    A. 薯条。　　　　B. 鸡肉。　　　　C. 麦片。　　　　D. 鱼类。

【答案】A

【解析】题目问医生建议病人应避免哪些食物。医生建议注意饮食，可以继续食用鸡肉和鱼肉，但不要吃薯条和煎蛋。因而答案是 A。

19.【问题】医生给出的诊断是什么？

    A. 溃疡。　　　　B. 癌症。　　　　C. 抑郁。　　　　D. 食管裂孔疝。

【答案】D

【解析】题目问医生的诊断是什么。对话一开始医生就说通过钡餐检查，未显示溃疡，但确实是食管裂孔疝（hiatus hernia）。因而答案为 D。

20.【问题】接下来 4 个星期，男士应该做什么？

    A. 他开始按照医生推荐的饮食方案进食。

    B. 他请病假并在家休息。

    C. 他服用医生开的药。

    D. 他另外做几个检查以排除癌症。

【答案】A

【解析】题目问接下来的四周这位男士要做什么。对话最后，男士说他愿意首先尝试改变饮食，然后服用上次医生给开的药。

Passage One

21.【问题】文章的主旨是什么？

    A. 糖尿病的新观点。

    B. 1 型和 2 型糖尿病的定义。

    C. 医院里糖尿病的新型管理。

    D. 不易坏的胰岛素丸的新发展

【答案】D

【解析】主旨题。文章一开始即点题：澳大利亚的化学生强化胰岛素化学键，以确保其在高温下稳定（不变质）。因而答案为 D。

22.【问题】根据文章，胰岛素为什么需要冷藏？

    A. 因为它很容易挥发。

    B. 因为它容易过度活跃。

    C. 因为它经常以注射形式保存。

    D. 因为它在 40 华氏度条件下不稳定。

【答案】D

【解析】细节信息题。题目问胰岛素要在低温下保存的原因。根据原文信息，胰岛素的化学结构较弱，在高温下会使得胰岛素失效，因而答案为 D。

23.【问题】什么使得这个研究前景不错？

    A. 不再依靠服用合成胰岛素便能治愈糖尿病。

    B. 研究成果告诉我们胰岛素是如何起效的。

    C. 胰岛素会更稳定。

    D. 胰岛素能得以天然生产。

【答案】B

【解析】此题为细节信息题。题目问什么使得该项研究前景更好。根据原文信息可以得知：研究结果可以有助于更好地了解胰岛素是如何起效的，因而答案为 B。

24.【问题】关于新型胰岛素的描述，哪一个是正确的？

    A. 它在室温条件下可以好几年保持稳定。

    B. 它可以直接进入血液。

    C. 它可以将葡萄糖从血液中输送到细胞中。

    D. 从化学成分上来讲，它更复杂。

【答案】A

【解析】细节信息题。题目问下列哪一个有关新型胰岛素的说法是正确的。根据原文信息可以得知：研究结果表明这种新型胰岛素可以在室温下放置几年（不变质），因而答案为 A。

25.【问题】根据文章所述，科学家们未知的是什么？

    A. 为什么胰岛素在室温下无法稳定。

B．理解胰岛素的化学联系是何等重要。

C．为什么1型和2型糖尿病人无法制造足够的胰岛素。

D．当胰岛素突破细胞从血液中获取糖分时是何种形态。

【答案】D

【解析】细节信息题。题目问哪一个是科学家还未知的。原文中提到当胰岛素"解锁"细胞，让血液中的葡萄糖进入细胞时，荷尔蒙的形态随之改变，但无人知晓呈何种形态。因而答案为D。

Passage Two

26．【问题】这篇文章主要讲了什么？

A．植物人更有意识。

B．植物人对眼部运动保留了一些控制。

C．脑波扫描帮助我们与植物人进行交流。

D．我们经常通过脑电波与脑死亡的人进行交流。

【答案】C

【解析】主旨题。文章开篇即点题：脑波扫描可能使得与脑死亡病人交流成为可能。因而答案为C。

27．【问题】在6个健康的志愿者中，挤压手部能激活大脑哪个部分？

A．大脑的左半部。　　　　　　　　　B．大脑的右半部。

C．大脑的中部。　　　　　　　　　　D．大脑的前部。

【答案】A

【解析】细节信息题。题目问六名健康的志愿者的攥手的想象激发大脑的哪个部位。根据文章可知实验结果大不相同：攥手激发大脑的左半部，而动脚趾激发大脑的中部。因而答案为A。

28．【问题】在23个植物人中，有多少能够持续回应"是-否"的问题？

A．31。　　　　　B．6。　　　　　C．4。　　　　　D．1。

【答案】C

【解析】细节信息题。题目问23名植物人病人中，有多少个被发现对问题持续有反应。原文信息是 4 patients were able to consistently respond to yes-or-no questions by changing their brain activity，因而答案为C。

29．【问题】从对两年前诊断为植物人的实验中我们可以得知什么？

A．病人已经脑死亡。

B．病人没有脑死亡。

C．病人对眼部运动有一些控制。

D．病人知道自己所做的活动。

【答案】B

【解析】细节信息题。根据文章描述，研究者通过EGG装置观察病人，最终得出结论：

从严格意义上讲，这些病人并不是真正的植物人。因而答案为 B。

30.【问题】当 EGG 信号表明植物人有反应时，下列哪一个表述不对？

      A．严格意义上来说，病人不是植物人。

      B．病人可以用某种方式沟通。

      C．我们可以训练病人讲话。

      D．家庭成员和医生能提供更好的照料。

【答案】C

【解析】细节信息题。通过主旨题与第 29 题的解答，我们可以排除选项 A 和 B。文章最后提到这一研究结果对于家属和医生护理有很好的借鉴意义，因而选项 D 也不是答案。最终答案为 C，文章中没提到。

 听力原文

Section A

1. M: What about the problem that I've been having in sleeping?

    W: I'm going to give you a prescription of some medicine to help you get a better night's sleep.

    Q: What does the man want to know?

2. M: How long should I take them?

    W: The prescription is for 30 days. If you're still feeling depressed after 30 days, I'd like you to come back in.

    Q: What does the woman advise the man to do if his problem continues?

3. W: Doc, should I stay away from work?

    M: No, I don't think that's necessary. Just remember to stay calm.

    Q: What does the man tell the woman to do?

4. M: How long have you been having this problem?

    W: It started in June, so for more than 5 months now. My stomach hurts after some meals but not always.

    Q: What does the woman complain of?

5. M: How strong is the pain exactly? On a scale of 1-10, how would you describe the intensity of the pain?

    W: Well, I'd say the pain is about a 2 on a scale of 1-10. Like I say, it's not really bad. It just keeps coming back.

    Q: How severe is the pain?

6. W: You don't seem to be overweight.

    M: No, not really. If I run up a flight of stairs, it takes me a while to get my breath back. I need to work out more.

Q: What does the man mean?

7.　M: Ooh, that's cold!

W: Don't worry; it's just my stethoscope.

Q: What is the woman doing?

8.　M: OK, everything looks ship-shape.

W: Great! When should I come again for a physical?

Q: Where did this conversation probably take place?

9.　M: I'm so sick in my stomach!

W: That's too bad. Have you been to the toilet? Any diarrhea or vomiting?

M: I've been to the toilet twice. But no diarrhea or vomiting. Perhaps I should drink something. Can I have a cup of hot tea?

Q: What is the man suffering from?

10.　M: How about allergies?

W: Not that I'm aware of.

Q: What does the woman mean?

11.　M: Louise, what are you doing now?

W: Oh, just listening to music, looking through magazines.

M: Staying in the house on a nice day like this? Come on, let's go to play tennis.

W: Oh great! You made my day.

Q: What is the woman going to do?

12.　M: Are you having any problems like weakness, fatigue, or headaches?

W: Well, I certainly felt under the weather.

Q: What does the woman mean?

13.　M: I saw Michael with his wife this morning, in the obstetrics and gynecology department. Is his wife ill?

W: No, she called me just now. Guess what? Their daughter has just had twins. And they were there for her.

Q: What can we learn from the conversation?

14.　W: Here's an extra blanket. Let me tuck you in.

M: You're so sweet. What is your name?

W: My name is Alice. I'll be on shift during the day for the next few days.

Q: What can be said of the woman?

15.　M: Now, I'd like to ask you about any illnesses you've had in the past. Could you tell me about this?

W: Let me think… I had my appendix out when I was 15. And I had a chest infection when I was on holiday in the USA 5 years ago. That's all.

M: Could you tell me if you've had any accidents or injured yourself at any time?

W: Well yes, I slipped on the ice and broke my neck 10 years ago. Actually I was in hospital then for several weeks. I'd forgotten that.

Q: When did the woman have a bone fracture?

Section B

Questions 16-20 are based on the following dialogue.

W: Well, your barium meal did not show an ulcer. But it did show that you have something we call a hiatus hernia. Do you know what that is?

M: I think my grandmother had one. But I haven't much of a clue, really.

W: Now I'm going to explain how we can try to get rid of your stomach and heartburn problems. I think it would help if you were able to lose a bit of weight. You'll be less likely to get the pain if you can eat smaller, lighter meals regularly. Standing upright after eating for a while helps so that your stomach is less likely to come up to your gullet than when you lie flat. Lastly, I'm going to give you some tablets that will stop your stomach from producing acid. Perhaps you could tell me what you feel about it.

M: Well, I worry that it might be difficult to eat the meals you suggest, because I'm a lorry driver and have to be on the road most of the day. And I'm not sure if I want to take those tablets.

W: Yes, I understand you might have some problems with the diet I'm suggesting, especially as roadside cafes usually sell meals with greasy food. However, perhaps you could keep to fish and chicken, and avoid chips and fried eggs. You say you're not keen on taking tablets. Why not?

M: A friend of mine had them, and then got worse. And 6 weeks later they found he had stomach cancer.

W: I see…so you were worried about having cancer?

M: Well, I was a bit. I suppose if my X-ray only showed a hernia, I must be clear. But are there other tests you can do to be absolutely sure?

W: Yes, there are. But I don't think it's necessary to do them at present. We'll want to see how you get on over the next few weeks with a change of diet. What about the tablets I suggested? I don't think it's possible that they caused your friend's cancer.

M: I think I'd rather try changing my diet first of all. Then, taking the medicine you prescribed for me last time.

W: Let's try that for the next 4 weeks. Then, I'll see you again.

16. What medical procedure has the man undergone?

17. Which of the following is NOT among the doctor's suggestions to the man?

18. According to the doctor's advice, which of the following foods should the man avoid?

19. What is the doctor's diagnosis of the man?

20. What will the man do for the next 4 weeks?

Questions 21-25 are based on the following passage.

Passage One

A team of Australian chemistry students have strengthened the chemical bonds of insulin to make it stable even at warm temperatures — a breakthrough that could simplify diabetes management. The finding could shed light on how insulin works and eventually lead to insulin pills, rather than injections or pumps.

Insulin needs to be kept cold because it is made of weak chemical bonds that degrade at temperatures above 40 degrees Fahrenheit, making it inactive. But using a series of chemical reactions, the research team, comprised of students from Monash University in Australia, replaced the unstable bonds with stronger, carbon-based ones.

The stronger bonds stabilize the insulin's two protein chains without interfering with its natural activity, according to a story about the findings at *SciGuru*. The so-called "dicarba" insulins were stable at room temperature for several years, *SciGuru* says.

Even more promising is that the findings provide insight into how insulin works.

People with Type 1 and Type 2 diabetes do not produce enough insulin, whether it's the result of an auto-immune disorder that stops producing it entirely (Type 1) or a condition brought on by other factors like obesity, in which the body can no longer use it properly (Type 2). Insulin is the mechanism that delivers glucose from the blood to the cells, so diabetics must take a synthetic form of the hormone.

When insulin unlocks cells to allow sugar to be taken up from the blood, the hormone's shape changes — but no one is sure what the shape looks like. If researchers knew that shape, they could design smaller, less-complex versions of insulin that don't use proteins.

Then it could be administered in pill form rather than directly into the bloodstream. Understanding the molecule's chemical bonds is a step toward unlocking that shape, the researchers say.

21. What is the main idea of the talk?
22. Why does insulin need to be kept cold, according to the talk?
23. What makes the research more promising?
24. What is true about the new type of insulin?
25. What is unknown to the scientists, according to the talk?

Questions 26-30 are based on the following passage.

Passage Two

Brain wave scanners might make it possible to communicate with people who are considered brain-dead, according to a new study reported in the *Economist*.

A couple of recent studies have shown that a small minority of vegetative patients might be more aware than they seem. Now, Damien Cruse, with the Medical Research Council's Cognition and Brain Sciences Unit in Cambridge, UK, thinks EEG machines will be able to help these patients communicate.

The team asked 6 healthy volunteers to wear EEG devices, which connect electrodes to a person's head. They were asked to respond to an audible tone by imagining that they were squeezing their right hands or wiggling the toes of both feet. The researchers found that the volunteers' brain responses were clearly different — the hand-squeezing activated the left-hand side of the brain, and the toe wiggling produced a response in the center of the brain.

Then they tested the procedure on a patient with locked-in syndrome, who was always completely paralyzed but retained some control of his fine movements. His brain responses were the same. Finally, they tested the procedure on a patient who had been declared vegetative 2 years earlier. They watched the EEG signals and were able to deduce which movement the patient was imagining.

The same team had studied 23 vegetative patients for 4 years and found 4 patients were able to consistently respond to yes-or-no questions by changing their brain activity. They were asked to imagine playing tennis when they wanted to give one response or walking around the house when they wanted to give the other.

Since the patients were responsive, they're not technically vegetative, the researchers say. Proof that they can communicate that they're not brain dead would have major implications for family members' and doctors' decisions about their care.

26. What does this talk mainly tell us?

27. For the 6 healthy volunteers, which part of the brain did the hand-squeezing imagination activate?

28. Of the 23 vegetative patients, how many were found to be able to consistently respond to yes-or-no questions?

29. What can we learn from the study on the patient declared vegetative 2 years earlier?

30. When EEG signals indicate that a vegetative patient is responsive, which of the following is NOT true?

2014 年真题

🎧 Section A

1.　A. About 12 pints.　　　　　B. About 3 pints.
　　C. About 4 pints.　　　　　D. About 7 pints.

2.　A. Take a holiday from work.
　　B. Worry less about work.

    C. Take some sleeping pills.

    D. Work harder to forget all her troubles.

3. A. He has no complaints about the doctor.

    B. He won't complain anything.

    C. He is in good condition.

    D. He couldn't be worse.

4. A. She is kidding.

    B. She will get a raise.

    C. The man will get a raise.

    D. The man will get a promotion.

5. A. Her daughter likes ball games.

    B. Her daughter is an exciting child.

    C. She and her daughter are good friends.

    D. She and her daughter don't always understand each other.

6. A. She hurt her uncle.   B. She hurt her ankle.

    C. She has a swollen toe.   D. She needs a minor surgery.

7. A. John likes gambling.

    B. John is very fond of his new boss.

    C. John has ups and downs in the new company.

    D. John has a promising future in the new company.

8. A. She will get some advice from the front desk.

    B. She will undergo some lab test.

    C. She will arrange an appointment.

    D. She will get the test results.

9. A. She's an odd character.   B. She is very picky.

    C. She is easy-going.   D. She likes fashions.

10. A. At a street corner.   B. In a local shop.

    C. In a ward.   D. In a clinic.

11. A. Sea food.   B. Dairy products.

    C. Vegetables and fruits.   D. Heavy food.

12. A. He is having a good time.

    B. He very much likes his old bicycle.

    C. He will buy a new bicycle right away.

    D. He would rather buy a new bicycle later.

13. A. It is only a cough.   B. It's a minor illness.

    C. It started two weeks ago. D. It's extremely serious.

14. A. The woman is too optimistic about the stock market.

    B. The woman will even lose more money at the stock market.

C. The stock market bubble will continue to grow.

D. The stock market bubble will soon meet its demise.

15. A. The small pills should be taken once a day before sleep.

B. The yellow pills should be taken once a day before supper.

C. The white pills should be taken once a day before breakfast.

D. The large round pill should be taken three times a day after meals.

Section B

Long Talk

16. A. Because he had difficulty swallowing it.

B. Because it was upsetting his stomach.

C. Because he was allergic to it.

D. Because it was too expensive.

17. A. He can't play soccer any more.　　B. He has a serious foot problem.

C. He needs an operation.　　D. He has cancer.

18. A. A blood transfusion.　　B. An allergy test.

C. A urine test.　　D. A biopsy.

19. A. To see if he has cancer.　　B. To see if he has depression.

C. To see if he requires surgery.　　D. To see if he has a food allergy problem.

20. A. Relieved.　　B. Anxious.

C. Angry.　　D. Depressed.

Passage One

21. A. The cause of COPD.

B. Harmful effects of smoking.

C. Men more susceptible to harmful effects of smoking.

D. Women more susceptible to harmful effects of smoking.

22. A. 954.　　B. 955.

C. 1909.　　D. 1955.

23. A. On May 18 in San Diego.　　B. On May 25 in San Diego.

C. On May 18 in San Francisco.　　D. On May 25 in San Francisco.

24. A. When smoking exposure is high.

B. When smoking exposure is low.

C. When the subjects received medication.

D. When the tobacco stopped smoking.

25. A. Hormone differences in men and women.

B. Genetic differences between men and women.

C. Women's active metabolic rate.

D. Women's smaller airways.

Passage Two

26. A. About 90,000.   B. About 100,000.

     C. Several hundred.   D. About 5,000.

27. A. Warning from Goddes Flight Centre.

     B. Warning from Health Ministry.

     C. Experience gained from the 1997 outbreak.

     D. Proper and prompt aid from NASA.

28. A. Distributing mosquito nets.

     B. Persuading people not to slaughter animals.

     C. Urging people not to eat animals.

     D. Dispatching doctors to the epidemic-stricken areas.

29. A. The higher surface temperatures in the equatorial part of the India.

     B. The short-lived mosquitoes that were the hosts of the viruses.

     C. The warm and dry weather in the Horn of Africa.

     D. The heavy but intermittent rains.

30. A. Warning from NASA.

     B. How to treat Rift Valley Fever.

     C. The disastrous effects of Rift Valley Fever.

     D. Satellites and global health—remote diagnosis.

答案与解析

Section A

1. 【A】男士说："I went up to the pub 4 times last week, and drank about 3 pints each evening."简单计算后可知，男士上周总共喝了 12 品脱的啤酒。故答案为 A。

2. 【B】男士说："Don't worry so much about things of work."即建议病人少想工作。故本题答案为 B。

3. 【C】男士说："Nothing to complain, really."意思是情况还不错，故本题的正确答案为 C。

4. 【C】女士说："Absolutely! He thinks you would!"肯定男士将涨薪水。因此本题答案为 C。

5. 【D】女士说："We are not always on the same wavelength."意思是母女俩经常无法沟通。因此本题的答案为 D。

6. 【B】本题考查的是 ankle 和 uncle 的发音区别。通过对话的上下文可知，女士扭伤的（twist）是 ankle（脚踝）。因此本题正确答案为 B。

7. 【D】男士说 John 在新公司十分胜任工作，老板十分器重他，并且肯定（bet）John

会在公司达成目标。因此本题答案为 D（在新公司前途光明）。

8. 【C】男士让女士拿着小条（slip）到前台去做检查的预约。因此本题答案为 C。

9. 【A】男士说：“Because she doesn't wear what everybody else wears.”即这个女孩儿的穿着从来都是与众不同的。由此可推理她的个性与常人迥异。因此 A 选项最贴切。

10. 【D】女士说：“I've been having some pains in my joints, especially the knees!”可知这个对话应该是就诊的场景，故本题选 D（门诊）。ward 意为“病房，监护室”，不合适。

11. 【D】男士说 heavy foods 通常会造成这种疼痛，故本题答案为 D。

12. 【D】男士说：“I think I need to buy a new one, but all in good time.”即考虑买新自行车，但得在适当的时候，故本题答案为 D。

13. 【C】女士说：“I have the cough for two weeks…”即该症状（symptom）是两周前开始的。故本题答案为 C。

14. 【A】女士说股市会反弹，男士说：“I'm sorry to burst your bubble…”即认为女士过于乐观。故本题答案为 A。

15. 【D】男士说：“The yellow one once a day before breakfast, the large round one three times a day after meals, the small ones when you need one for sleeping.”由此可判断本题答案为 D。

🎧 Section B

Long Talk

16. 【B】病人说自从换了药就不觉得恶心（sick）了。因此换药的原因是病人觉得恶心。故本题答案为 B。

17. 【C】医生说：“That means no soccer.”即不能踢球，但并非永远不能踢球，而是 3 个星期没法踢球。导致这个结果的原因是该病人腿部需要做一个手术。因此本题正确答案为 C。

18. 【D】通过对话内容可知，病人之前已经做了活组织切片检查（biopsy）。因此答案为 D。

19. 【D】医生告诉病人还需要做几个血液化验，来排除过敏（allergy）的问题。因此本题答案为 D。

20. 【A】医生说：“The biopsy shows the tumor is benign which means it is not cancerous. We're going to take it out anyway, just to be on the safe side.”病人排除了恶性肿瘤等问题，应该是比较放松的。因此本题答案为 A。

Passage One

21. 【D】从短文录音的第一句便可知道答案：Woman may be more susceptible to the lung-damaging effects of smoking than men。因此本题答案为 D。

22. 【C】根据录音中的 …including 954 subjects with chronic obstructive pulmonary disease

（COPD）and 955 controls 可知，总共招录的被试者（subjects）为 954+955=1909，故本题答案为 C。

23.【A】根据录音中的 …May 18, at the 105th International Conference of the American Thoracic Society in San Diego，可知本题的答案为 A。

24.【B】从录音中的 "but this gender effect was most pronounced when the level of smoking exposure was low" 可知，当 smoking exposure 较低时，性别差异最明显。

25.【C】从录音最后的 "Women have smaller airways, therefore each cigarette may do more harm. Also, there are gender differences in the metabolism of cigarette smoke. Genes and hormones could also be important." 可知，抽烟对男女不同性别的新陈代谢的影响是有差异的，女性狭窄的气道也是让女性更容易受到吸烟后果影响的因素，但其中并未说女性比男性的新陈代谢更活跃，因此 C 为正确答案。

Passage Two

26.【B】根据录音中的 "Some 100,000 stock animals succumbed and about 90,000 people were infected, hundreds fatally in five countries." 可知，本题答案为 B。

27.【D】从录音中的 "The difference was that the second time around there was warning… part of America's space agency, NASA, told the authorities in Kenya that they had a problem. They told them again in October. And again in November." 可知，第二次的区别在于有来自 NASA 及时而准确的警告。故本题答案为 D。

28.【D】从录音中的 "…the Kenyan health ministry had dispatched teams to the area to distribute mosquito nets and urge village leaders and religious authorities to stop people slaughtering and eating animals." 可知，只有 D 选项不是制止瘟疫肆虐的举措。

29.【D】从录音中的 "These higher temperatures brought heavy and sustained rains, cloud cover and warmer air to much of the Horn of Africa" 可知，D 是正确答案，B 选项应该改成 long-lived mosquitoes。

30.【D】该录音主要内容是 NASA 给予肯尼亚及时迅捷的警示，使其在 2007 年瘟疫爆发的时候避免了 10 年前的厄运。因此 D 选项是正确答案（卫星和全球健康——远程诊断）。

 听力原文

🎧 **Section A**

1. W: It would help me if you could go over last week and give me an idea how much beer you drank each evening.

    M: Well, let me see, I went up to the pub 4 times last week, and drank about 3 pints each evening.

    Q: How much beer did the man drink last week?

2. W: Is there anything else I can do to help me sleep tonight?

M: Don't worry so much about things of work. I know, I know, easier said than done.

W: Should I stay home from work?

M: No, I don't think that's necessary, just remember to stay calm.

Q: What did the doctor suggest the woman do?

3. W: How have you been feeling in general?

M: Nothing to complain, really.

Q: What does the man mean?

4. W: Our managing director is going to give you a raise.

M: Really? Are you kidding me?

W: Absolutely! He thinks you would!

Q: What does the woman say?

5. W: I've been so worried about my daughter. She's so different in temperament from me. We are not always on the same wavelength.

M: That's quite common with mothers and daughters.

W: She's a further personality and very much on the ball, but she is an excitable child.

Q: What does the woman mean?

6. M: Where is your injury?

W: Here, my ankle.

M: How did it happen?

W: I tripped over on the pavement and twisted it. It's swollen and very painful.

Q: What is true about the woman?

7. W: John wants to move upwards and onwards within his new company.

M: He is well qualified and the boss is into him.

W: So you think he will achieve his goal?

M: Yeah! I bet he will.

Q: What did the man mean?

8. M: Take the slip to the front desk and then arrange an appointment for the tests.

W: Thank you, doc! Have a nice day!

Q: What will the woman do?

9. M: There is one girl at my school whom everybody picks on.

W: Why?

M: Because she doesn't wear what everybody else wears.

Q: What can be inferred about the girl in question?

10. M: What are you coming for today, Ms. Anders?

W: I've been having some pains in my joints, especially the knees!

Q: Where did the conversation most probably take place?

11. W: How long does the pain last when you get it?

M: It comes and goes! Sometimes I hardly feel anything, and other times it can last up to half an hour or more.

W: Is there a type of food that seems to cause stronger pain than other types?

M: Um, heavy foods like steak or lasagna usually bring it on. I've been trying to avoid those.

Q: What type of food seems to cause stronger pain to the man?

12. W: Carl, your bicycle is too old. It's not safe to ride.

M: Yeah! I think I need to buy a new one, but all in good time.

Q: What does the man mean?

13. M: How long could you have these symptoms?

W: Oh, I have the cough for two weeks, but feeling ill just seemed the past a few days.

Q: What do we know about the woman's illness?

14. W: I think I could recover the cough at the end of the year.

M: I'm sorry to burst your bubble, but the stock index still ranges between 1,900 and 2,900 after a year.

Q: What does the man mean?

15. M: I just want to check if you understand which pills to take and when.

W: The yellow one in the morning and the others, oh, I think no, maybe, ah, best if I write it down! Then I won't forget!

M: Here is some paper. The yellow one once a day before breakfast, the large round one three times a day after meals, the small ones when you need one for sleeping.

Q: Which of the following statements is true?

🎧 Section B

Long Talk

W: Hi, Patrick, how are you feeling today?

M: A bit better.

W: That's good to hear. Are you still feeling nauseas?

M: No. I haven't felt sick to my stomach since you switched my medication.

W: Great, say, your test result came this morning.

M: It's about time. Is it good news or bad?

W: I guess it's a bit of both. Which do you want first?

M: Let's get the bad news over with.

W: OK. It looks like you are going to need surgery to remove your tumor from your leg. After the operation you're going to have to stay off your feet for at least 3 weeks. That means no soccer.

M: Well, I was afraid you were going to say that.

W: Now, for the good news. The biopsy shows the tumor is benign which means it is not cancerous. We're going to take it out anyway, just to be on the safe side.

M: Wow, that's a load off my mind. Thanks, doctor.

W: Don't get too excited. We still need to get to the bottom of all this way of loathing…

M: I probably have just been so worried about stupid lump.

W: These things often are stress-related, but we're still going to do a few blood test just to rule a few things out.

M: Things like what? Cancer?

W: Actually, I am thinking more along the line of food allergy.

Questions 16-20 are based on the conversation you have just heard.

16. Why did the man have to switch medication?
17. What is the bad news for the man?
18. What medical procedures has the man already undergone?
19. Why does the doctor ask the man to take a few blood tests?
20. Which of the following can best describe the man's feeling in the end?

Passage One

Women may be more susceptible to the lung-damaging effects of smoking than men, according to new research by Inga-Cecilie Soerheim, M.D., and her colleagues from Channing Laboratory, Brigham and Women's Hospital and University of Bergen, Norway. They analyzed data from a Norwegian case-control study including 954 subjects with chronic obstructive pulmonary disease (COPD) and 955 controls. All were current- or ex-smokers, and the COPD subjects had moderate or severe COPD.

"Overall our analysis indicated that women may be more vulnerable to the effects of smoking, which is something previously suspected but not proven," said Dr. Soerheim.

The study results will be presented on May 18 at the 105th International Conference of the American Thoracic Society in San Diego.

Examining the total study sample, there were no gender differences with respect to lung function (FEV1) and COPD severity, but the women were on average younger and had smoked significantly less than men.

To explore these differences further, they also analyzed two subgroups of the study sample: COPD subjects under the age of 60 (early onset group) and COPD subjects with less than 20 pack-years of smoking (low exposure group). In both subgroups, women had more severe disease and greater impairment of lung function than men.

"This means that female smokers in our study experienced reduced lung function at a lower level of smoking exposure and at an earlier age than men," said Dr. Soerheim.

It has long been suspected that the effect of smoking on lung function may be modified by gender. Interaction analysis confirmed that being female represents a higher risk of reduced lung function and severe COPD, but this gender effect was most pronounced when the level of smoking exposure was low.

"The gender difference in COPD susceptibility seems to be most important when smoking exposure is low. Women may tolerate small amounts of tobacco worse than men," Dr. Soerheim explained.

According to Dr. Soerheim, the reason why women may be more susceptible to the effects of cigarette smoke is still unknown, but there are several possible explanations: "Women have smaller airways; therefore each cigarette may do more harm. Also, there are gender differences in the metabolism of cigarette smoke. Genes and hormones could also be important."

Questions 21–25 are based on the passage you have just heard.

21. What is the most likely topic of this talk?
22. How many subjects did Dr. Soerheim recruit in her study?
23. When and where will Dr. Soerheim present their study results?
24. According to the talk, when is the gender difference most likely to be obvious in COPD susceptibility?
25. Which of the following is not an explanation for women's great susceptibility to the effects of smoking?

Passage Two

In December 1997 large numbers of cattle, goats and sheep began dying in the Garissa district of north-eastern Kenya. A month later people started dying, too. It was, at the time, the biggest recorded outbreak of Rift Valley fever in east Africa. Some 100,000 stock animals succumbed and about 90,000 people were infected — hundreds fatally — in five countries.

In December 2007 the same thing happened. Or, rather, it started to happen but was stopped in its tracks. The difference was that the second time around there was warning. In September researchers at the Goddard Space Flight Centre in Greenbelt, Maryland, part of America's space agency, NASA, told the authorities in Kenya that they had a problem. They told them again in October, and again in November. By the time the epidemic emerged, the Kenyan health ministry had dispatched teams to the area to distribute mosquito nets and urge village leaders and religious authorities to stop people slaughtering and eating animals. Though the outbreak still killed 300 people in Kenya, Somalia and Tanzania, it could have been a lot worse. According to Kenneth Linthicum of America's Department of Agriculture, the number of deaths would probably have been more than twice as high without the warning.

The warning itself was possible because of a model of how disease spreads that Dr. Linthicum helped design. And the data that were plugged into that model came from satellites.

What the researchers at Goddard had noticed at the time of the first outbreak was that in the months preceding it, surface temperatures in the equatorial part of the Indian Ocean had risen by half a degree. These higher temperatures brought heavy and sustained rains, cloud cover and warmer air to much of the Horn of Africa. Mosquitoes multiplied wildly — and lived long enough for the virus that causes the fever to develop to the point where it is easily transmissible. In September 2007 the researchers saw the same thing happening in the ocean, and suspected the same consequences would follow.

Questions 26–30 are based on the passage you have just heard.

26. How many stock animals died as a result of the outbreak of the Rift Valley fever in 1997?
27. What helped stop the outbreak of the Rift Valley fever in 2007?
28. Which of the following is not mentioned as a measure to prevent the 2007 outbreak from spreading?
29. What triggered the two outbreaks of the Rift Valley fever in Africa?
30. What is the talk mainly about?

2013 年真题

Section A

1. A. A cough.   B. Diarrhea.
   C. A fever.   D. Vomiting.
2. A. Tuberculosis.   B. Rhinitis.
   C. Laryngitis.   D. Flu.
3. A. In his bag.   B. By the lamp.
   C. In his house.   D. No idea about where he left it.
4. A. He's nearly finished his work.   B. He has to work for some more time.
   C. He wants to leave now.   D. He has trouble finishing his work.
5. A. A patient.   B. A doctor.
   C. A teacher.   D. A student.
6. A. 2.6.   B. 3.5.
   C. 3.9.   D. 136.
7. A. He is the head of the hospital.   B. He is in charge of Pediatrics.
   C. He went out looking for Dan.   D. He went to Michigan on business.
8. A. He has got a fever.   B. He is a talented skier.
   C. He is very rich.   D. He is a real ski enthusiast.
9. A. To ask local people for help.

B. To do as Romans do only when in Rome.

C. Try to act like the people from that culture.

D. Stay with your country fellows.

10. A. She married because of loneliness.　　B. She married a millionaire.

　　C. She married for money.　　D. She married for love.

11. A. Aspirant.　　B. Courageous.

　　C. Cautious.　　D. Amiable.

12. A. He was unhappy.　　B. He was feeling a bit unwell.

　　C. He went to see the doctor.　　D. The weather was nasty.

13. A. You may find many of them on the bookseller shelves.

　　B. You can buy it from almost every bookstore.

　　C. It's a very popular magazine.

　　D. It doesn't sell very well.

14. A. A general practitioner.　　B. A gynecologist.

　　C. An orthopedist.　　D. A surgeon.

15. A. Chemotherapy.　　B. Radiation.

　　C. Injections.　　D. Surgery.

Section B

Long Conversation

16. A. It is a genetic disorder.　　B. It is respiratory condition in pigs.

　　C. It is an illness from birds to humans.　　D. It is a gastric ailment.

17. A. Eating pork.　　B. Raising pigs.

　　C. Eating chicken.　　D. Breeding birds.

18. A. Running nose.　　B. Inappetence.

　　C. Pains all over.　　D. Diarrhea.

19. A. To stay from crowds.　　B. To see the doctor immediately.

　　C. To avoid medications.　　D. To go to the nearby clinic.

20. A. It is a debate.　　B. It is a TV program.

　　C. It is a consultation.　　D. It is a workshop.

Passage One

21. A. About 10,000,000.　　B. About 1,000,000.

　　C. About 100,000.　　D. About 10,000.

22. A. A cocktail of vitamins.

　　B. A cocktail of vitamins plus magnesium.

　　C. The combination of vitamins A, C and E.

D. The combination of minerals.

23. A. The delicate structures of the inner ear.

    B. The inner ear cells.

    C. The eardrums.

    D. The inner ear ossicles.

24. A. General Motors.　　　　　　　　　B. The United Auto Workers.

    C. NIH.　　　　　　　　　　　　　　D. All of the above.

25. A. An industrial trial in Spain.

    B. Military trials in Spain and Sweden.

    C. Industrial trials in Spain and Sweden.

    D. A trial involving students at the University of Florida.

Passage Two

26. A. The link between obesity and birth defects.

    B. The link between obesity and diabetes.

    C. The risk of birth abnormalities.

    D. The harmful effects of obesity.

27. A. Neural tube defects.　　　　　　　　B. Heart problems.

    C. Cleft lip and palate.　　　　　　　　D. Diabetes.

28. A. 20 million.　　　　　　　　　　　　B. 200 million.

    C. 400 million.　　　　　　　　　　　D. 40 million.

29. A. A weight-loss surgery.　　　　　　　B. A balanced diet.

    C. A change of lifestyle.　　　　　　　D. More exercise.

30. A. Why obesity can cause birth defects.　B. How obesity may cause birth defects.

    C. Why obesity can cause diabetes.　　　D. How obesity may cause diabetes.

答案与解析

Section A

1. 【问题】下列哪一个不是这个男孩儿的症状？

   　　A. 咳嗽。　　　　B. 腹泻。　　　　C. 发热。　　　　D. 呕吐。

   【答案】B

   【解析】此题为细节信息题，根据对话信息，男孩咳嗽、发烧，并且恶心、呕吐。因而
   选项 B 为答案。

2. 【问题】这位女士得的是什么病？

   　　A. 肺结核。　　　　B. 鼻炎。　　　　C. 喉炎。　　　　D. 流感。

   【答案】D

   【解析】此题为细节信息题，医生认为这位女士有流感的所有症状，因而答案为 D。

3. 【问题】男士的笔记本电脑在哪里？

      A．书包里。   B．台灯旁。   C．家里。   D．不知道。

【答案】C

【解析】此题为细节信息题，根据对话信息可知，男士将笔记本电脑落在家里了，因而答案为 C。

4. 【问题】有关这位男士可以推测出什么？

      A．他几乎要完成工作了。   B．他还得工作一会儿。

      C．他现在想走了。   D．他完成工作有困难。

【答案】B

【解析】此题为细节推断题。根据对话信息，男士说不会很快结束，还要做一会儿，因而答案为 B。

5. 【问题】这位男士是谁？

      A．病人。   B．医生。   C．老师。   D．学生。

【答案】D

【解析】此题为细节推理题。根据女士回答说的 "I have pathology class（病理学课）" 可知，他们均为学生。此处的 office hour 也可说明这是两个学生在谈论老师的办公时间。

6. 【问题】这位男士的钠的结果是多少？

【答案】D

【解析】此题为细节信息题。根据对话信息，答案为 D。Urea 为尿素，数值为 2.6，钾 Potassium 的数值为 3.9。

7. 【问题】关于 Doctor Wilson 哪个是正确的？

      A．他是这个医院的领导。   B．他负责儿科。

      C．他出去找 Dan。   D．他去密歇根出差。

【答案】D

【解析】此题为细节信息题。根据对话信息，Doctor Wilson 今早离开前往密歇根参加会议，因而答案为 D。对话中的 pediatrics 意为 "儿科"。

8. 【问题】哪一个是说这位男士的？

      A．他发烧了。   B．他是一个有天赋的滑雪者。

      C．他很有钱。   D．他是一个真正的滑雪爱好者。

【答案】D

【解析】此题为细节信息题。根据对话信息可知，这位男士用一个月的薪水买了滑雪板，女士表示很惊讶，认为这位男士太疯狂，对滑雪太狂热了，因而答案为 D。

9. 【问题】根据男士所言，出国旅游人们应该做什么？

      A．向当地人求助。

      B．只有在罗马时，才能像罗马人那样行事。

      C．像当地人那样行事。

      D．与本国人在一起。

【答案】C

【解析】此题为固定短语的理解。do as Romans do 的含义是"入乡随俗"，因而答案为 C。B 选项加上 only when in Roman 的状语后，则改变了这个习语的意思。

10. 【问题】关于 Cindy 这位女士暗示什么？

    A. 她因寂寞而结婚。   B. 她嫁给了百万富翁。

    C. 她因钱而结婚。   D. 她因爱而结婚。

【答案】C

【解析】此题为细节推断题。根据对话信息得知这位女士认为 Cindy 离婚的原因是她的丈夫没有她想象的那么有钱。因而答案为 C。

11. 【问题】哪个词能形容 Kate？

    A. 上进的。   B. 勇敢的。

    C. 谨慎小心的。   D. 和蔼可亲的。

【答案】B

【解析】此题为细节信息题。根据对话信息可知 Kate 敢于在会议上表达自己的想法，与会者有好多人也想如此，但因太害怕而沉默不语。故答案为 B。

12. 【问题】为什么这位男士昨天没去上班？

    A. 他不高兴。   B. 他身体不适。

    C. 他去看病。   D. 天气很不好。

【答案】B

【解析】此题为固定短语的理解。根据对话信息得知，男士没来上班是因为感觉 under the weather，含义为"身体不适"。因而答案是 B。

13. 【问题】关于《英语世界》这位女士暗示什么？

    A. 你可以在书店书架上看到很多。

    B. 你可以去任何书店买到。

    C. 它是一本很畅销的杂志。

    D. 这本书销量不好。

【答案】C

【解析】此题为固定短语的理解。flying off bookseller shelves 的含义是"热销"。因而答案为 C。

14. 【问题】这位女士是谁？

    A. 全科医生。   B. 妇科医生。

    C. 整形外科医生。   D. 外科医生。

【答案】B

【解析】此题为细节信息题。根据对话信息得知被送来的女患者患会阴囊肿，需要切除。因而答案是 B。

15. 【问题】这位男士首先要接受什么治疗？

    A. 化疗。   B. 放疗。

    C. 药物注射。   D. 手术。

【答案】C

【解析】此题为细节信息题。根据对话信息得知女士要先看看药物注射是否有效,患者的状况还不到进行化疗(chemotherapy)的程度。因而答案为 C。

🎧 Section B

Long Conversation

16. 【问题】有关猪流感我们知道什么?
   A. 遗传疾病。　　　　　　　　　　　B. 猪的呼吸疾病。
   C. 鸟类传染人的疾病。　　　　　　　D. 胃病。

【答案】B

【解析】此题为细节信息题。根据对话信息,专家说到猪流感就是一种常见的 respiratory ailment in pigs,因而答案为 B。

17. 【问题】什么情况下人会患猪流感?
   A. 吃猪肉。　　B. 养猪。　　C. 吃鸡。　　D. 养鸟。

【答案】B

【解析】此题为细节信息题。题目是人感染猪流感的原因。根据对话信息可知,病猪不允许进入市场,烹饪也可杀死病毒。只有养猪的人可能感染病毒。(Ill pigs are not allowed to enter the market. Cooking also kills the virus. Only people who work with pigs can catch the virus.)因而答案为 B。

18. 【问题】根据对话,下列哪一个是猪流感最常见的症状?
   A. 流鼻涕。　　B. 食欲不振。　　C. 全身疼痛。　　D. 腹泻。

【答案】B

【解析】此题为细节信息题。根据对话信息可得知最常见的症状有发热、疲劳、食欲不振和咳嗽。(The most common symptoms are fever, fatigue, lack of appetite and coughing.)因而答案为 B。

19. 【问题】说话人建议猪流感疑似患者做什么?
   A. 远离人群。　　　　　　　　　　　B. 立即就医。
   C. 不用吃药。　　　　　　　　　　　D. 去附近的诊所。

【答案】A

【解析】此题为细节信息题。根据对话信息可得知如果出现上述症状应该在家隔离,打电话给医生,但不要去医院就诊。(Stay home from work and school. To call your doctors to ask about the best treatment. Don't simply show up at the clinic or hospital that is unprepared for your arrival.)因而答案为 A。

20. 【问题】这个对话是什么?
   A. 一场辩论。　　　　　　　　　　　B. 一档电视节目。
   C. 一个咨询。　　　　　　　　　　　D. 一个研讨会。

【答案】B

【解析】此题为细节信息题。根据对话信息可得知这是一档健康生活的节目（Welcome to our program "Health Journey".），因而答案为 B。

Passage One

21. 【问题】根据文章，仅仅在美国有多少听力障碍患者？

【答案】A

【解析】此题为细节信息题。原文解题信息是：About 10 million people in the U.S. alone… are suffering from impairing noise-induced hearing loss.

22. 【问题】UM Cresgo 听力研究所开发什么以防听力丧失？

    A. 维生素鸡尾酒疗法。

    B. 维生素加镁鸡尾酒疗法。

    C. 维生素 A、C 和 E 的混合物。

    D. 矿物质混合物。

【答案】B

【解析】此题为细节信息题。原文解题信息是：… with the cocktail of vitamins and the mineral magnesium… to prevent hearing loss caused by loud noise.

23. 【问题】根据最新发现，大声噪音损伤什么？

    A. 微妙的内耳结构。   B. 内耳细胞。

    C. 耳鼓。   D. 内耳听骨。

【答案】B

【解析】此题为细节信息题。原文解题信息是：… noise … that damage the inner ear cells.

24. 【问题】根据文章，谁支持实验室研究？

    A. 通用汽车公司。   B. 美国汽车工人联合会。

    C. NIH。   D. 以上皆是。

【答案】C

【解析】此题为细节信息题。原文解题信息是：The laboratory research… was funded by NIH.

25. 【问题】下列哪一个没有包含在 Oral Quell 药物的多国人体临床试验中？

    A. 西班牙的工业试验。   B. 西班牙和瑞典的军事试验。

    C. 西班牙和瑞典的工业试验。   D. 佛州大学学生参与的试验。

【答案】C

【解析】此题为细节信息题。解题有效信息是：… military trials in Sweden and Spain, and industrial trials in Spain and the trial involving students at the University of Florida…

Passage Two

26. 【问题】这篇文章的主要内容是什么？

    A. 先天缺陷与肥胖的关系。   B. 肥胖与糖尿病的关系。

C. 先天异常的危险性。　　　　　D. 肥胖的危害。

【答案】A

【解析】此题为主旨题。题目是问这个独白的主要内容是什么。根据下列细节信息题可知独白主要讲述母亲肥胖对新生儿的影响。

27.【问题】母亲肥胖婴儿患病概率大的疾病，下列哪个除外？

A. 神经管畸形。　　　　　　　　B. 心脏问题。

C. 唇腭裂。　　　　　　　　　　D. 糖尿病。

【答案】D

【解析】此题为细节信息题。根据独白信息可得知，妈妈肥胖，婴儿患神经管畸形（neural tube defects）的概率高两倍，心脏畸形、唇腭裂（cleft lip and palate）、脑积水（water on the brain）、四肢发育问题的概率增大。因而选项D（糖尿病）是答案。

28.【问题】根据 WHO，世界上多少人被认定为肥胖？

【答案】C

【解析】此题为细节信息题。解题有效信息是 The World Health Organization classifies around 400 million people around the world as obese…

29.【问题】对于计划怀孕的肥胖妇女有何建议？

A. 减肥手术。　　　　　　　　　B. 饮食均衡。

C. 改变生活方式。　　　　　　　D. 多运动。

【答案】A

【解析】此题为细节信息题。解题有效信息是：… women who get pregnant after weight loss surgery tend to be healthier and less likely to deliver a baby born with complications compared to obese women.

30.【问题】根据文章，下一步研究的重点是什么？

A. 肥胖引起先天缺陷的原因。　　B. 肥胖如何引起先天缺陷。

C. 肥胖引起糖尿病的原因。　　　D. 肥胖如何引起糖尿病。

【答案】B

【解析】此题为细节信息题。解题有效信息是：Further study may show how obesity may cause these problems…

 听力原文

Section A

1.　M: What's the matter with this little boy?

　　W: He has a chesty cough all the time. His temperature is high. And he keeps telling me he wants to be sick.

M: Does he bring anything up?

W: No, because he has been off his food for the past two days. He just brings up bile.

Q: Which of the following is not the boy's symptom?

2. W: Good afternoon, doctor. I have a terrible headache. Yesterday I had a runny nose. Now my nose is stuffed up.

M: Let me give you an examination. First, let me have a look at your throat. OK, now let me examine your chest. Do you have a history of tuberculosis?

W: No, I don't think so.

M: Your throat is inflamed and your tongue is thickly coated. You have all the symptoms of influenza.

Q: What is the woman suffering from?

3. W: What are you looking for?

M: My laptop. I can't find it in my bag or anywhere.

W: I can't remember you carrying it here. Think about it one more time.

M: That's right. I left it at home.

Q: Where is the man's laptop?

4. M: How is your work going?

W: I think I will be finished soon.

M: Well, I won't be finished for a while.

Q: What can be inferred about the man?

5. W: When are Doctor Peterman's office hours?

M: Monday, Wednesday and Friday from 10 a.m. to noon.

W: That's not very convenient for me. I have pathology class then.

Q: What is the man?

6. W: Hello, Eric, what can I do for you?

M: I was wondering if you had the results.

W: Oh, yes, the results. We've got them.

M: Great.

W: Here we go. Urea 2.6, Sodium 136, and Potassium 3.9.

M: 3.5.

W: No, that's 3.9.

Q: What is the man's sodium level?

7. M: Hello, this is Don North from Pediatrics. I'd like a word with Doctor Wilson if it's possible.

W: I'm sorry, but he left for Michigan to attend a conference this morning. He was in fact looking for you just before he left.

Q: What is true about Doctor Wilson?

8. M: I spent my one-month salary buying a pair of skis.

   W: Are you crazy? You've got a ski fever.

   Q: What can we say about the man?

9. W: Most people feel culture shock when traveling to a foreign culture.

   M: That's for sure. But they should do as Romans do.

   Q: According to the man, what are people supposed to do when traveling to a foreign culture?

10. W: Cindy just got divorced.

    M: So soon! She got married only last summer.

    W: Well, she found out that her husband was not the millionaire she thought he was.

    Q: What does the woman imply about Cindy?

11. M: Kate was the only one brave enough to speak her mind at the meeting today.

    W: Yeah, a lot of people felt the same way, but were too scared to say anything. She just voiced the aspiration of them.

    Q: Which of the following words can best describe Kate?

12. W: Why didn't you come to work yesterday?

    M: I was feeling a little under the weather.

    W: Did you go to see the doc?

    M: No, nothing serious.

    Q: Why didn't the man go to work yesterday?

13. M: Have you heard of the magazine *The World of English*?

    W: Of course. It is one of many English magazines that are now flying off bookseller shelves.

    Q: What does the woman imply about the *The World of English*?

14. M: Hello Doctor Marks. It's Tim Tailor from ANNE at Edinburgh Centre.

    W: Hello.

    M: I've got a young woman, a 30-year-old woman referred up by her GP with a kind of perineal abscess for about 10-15 days.

    W: Right.

    M: She's been on antibiotics and basically it needs to be incised. Can you take her?

    W: Of course. What's the patient's name?

    Q: What is the woman?

15. W: What do you know about treatments of cancer?

    M: Chemotherapy. But that makes your hair fall out, doesn't it?

    W: Yes, there are some unpleasant side-effects. I'm not sure we need to consider that at this stage. We should see whether a series of injection will help.

    Q: What treatment will the man probably receive first?

Section B

Long Conversation

W: Hello Doctor Smith, welcome to our program "Health Journey". Could you tell us something about swine flu.

M: Well, it's a common respiratory ailment in pigs that doesn't usually spread to people.

W: But why are so many people infected?

M: Unlike most cases, this flu virus appears to be a sub-type not seen before in humans or pigs. It has genetic material from pigs, birds and humans, according to the WHO.

W: Then why is it called swine flu? Why pigs are the carriers of this virus?

M: Um. It's closer to say that pigs were the mixing balls for this virus.

W: What does it mean?

M: I mean birds cannot pass bird flu to people. But pigs are susceptible to getting flu viruses that infected birds. The virus inside the infected pig might mutate to a form that could also infect other mammals.

W: Wow, so complicated. By the way, can we catch swine flu from eating pork?

M: Actually, ill pigs are not allowed to enter the market. Cooking also kills the virus. Only people who work with pigs can catch the virus.

W: How do they feel if infected?

M: The most common symptoms are fever, fatigue, lack of appetite and coughing, although some people also develop runny nose, sore throat, vomiting or diarrhea.

W: What should we do if we have these symptoms?

M: Stay home from work or school. Don't get on a plane. Call your doctors to ask about the best treatment. Don't simply show up at the clinic or hospital that is unprepared for your arrival.

W: Say, the antiviral study. How is it going?

M: This strain of swine flu does appear sensitive to the antiviral drugs Relenza and Tami flu, but not to Amantadine and Remantadine.

W: We've learned a lot tonight. Thanks for your coming, Doctor Smith.

M: It's my pleasure.

Questions:

16. What do we know about swine flu?
17. What may cause people to have swine flu?
18. According to the dialogue, which is among the most common symptoms of swine flu?
19. What does the speaker advise the suspects of swine flu to do?
20. What can be said of the dialogue?

Passage One

Questions 21-25 are based on the following passage.

About 10 million people in the U.S. alone, from troops returning from war to students with music blasting through headphones are suffering from impairing noise-induced hearing loss. The rise in trend is something that researchers and physicians at the University of Michigan Cresgo Hearing Research Institute are hoping to reverse, with the cocktail of vitamins and the mineral magnesium（镁）that shall promise as a possible way to prevent hearing loss caused by loud noise. The nutrients were successful in laboratory tests. And now researchers are testing whether humans will benefit as well. The combination of vitamins A, C and E plus magnesium is given on pill form to patients who are participating in the research. Developed at the UM Cresgo Hearing Research Institute, the medication, called Oral Quell, is designed to be taken before a person is exposed to the loud noise. Until a decade ago, it was thought that noise damaged hearing by intense mechanical vibrations that destroyed delicate structures of the inner ear. There was no intervention to protect the inner ear other than reducing the intensity of sound reaching it, such as ear plugs which are not always effective. It was then discovered that noise caused intense metabolic activity in the inner ear and production of molecules that damage the inner ear cells. And that allows the discovery of intervention to prevent these effects. The laboratory research that led to a new understanding of mechanisms underlying noise-induced hearing loss was funded by NIH, the Preclinical Translation Research that led to the formulation of Oral Quell as effective preventative was funded by General Motors and the United Auto Workers. Now Oral Quell is being tested in a set of four multinational human clinical trials: military trials in Sweden and Spain, and industrial trials in Spain and the trial involving students at the University of Florida who listen to music at high volumes on their iPods and other PDAs.

Questions:

21. According to the talk, how many victims of hearing problem are there in the United States alone?
22. Which did UM Cresgo Hearing Research Institute develop to prevent hearing loss?
23. According to the latest findings, what does loud noise damage?
24. According to the talk, who supported the lab research?
25. Which of the following is not included as the multinational human clinical trials for Oral Quell?

Passage Two

Questions 26-30 are based on the following passage.

Catherine and other colleagues from Britain's New Castle University combined data from 18 studies to look at the risk of abnormalities of babies whose mothers were obese or overweight. Obese women were nearly twice as likely to have a baby with neural tube defects which are caused by the incomplete development of the brain or spinal cord, the study found. For one such defect, spinal bifida（脊柱裂）, the risk more than doubled. The researchers also detected increased chances of heart defect, cleft lip and palate, water on the brain（脑积水）and problems in the growth of arms and legs. The World Health Organization classifies around 400 million people around the world as obese, including 20 million under the age of 5, and the number is growing. Obesity raises the risks of diseases such as type II diabetes, heart problems and is a health concern piling pressure on an already overburdened national health system. Recent research has tight weight to other problems during pregnancy. A team from the Round Corporation Think Tank in California reported in 2008 that women who get pregnant after weight loss surgery tend to be healthier and less likely to deliver a baby born with complications compared to obese women. Further study may show how obesity may cause these problems, Juliet at New Castle University researcher who worked on the study said in a telephone interview. Women who are thinking about trying for a baby need to check their own weight first, and then think about seeking help if they are overweight.

Questions:

26. What is the talk mainly about?

27. Babies whose mothers are obese may have increased chances of the following diseases except which?

28. According to the WHO, how many people are classified as obese around the world?

29. Which of the following can be a suggestion for obese women who plan to have a baby?

30. According to the talk, what may be the focus of further studies?

以下为 2008 ～ 2012 年部分真题：

Part I Listening Comprehension (30%)

Section A

1.   A. The woman's condition is critical.
     B. The woman has been picking up quite well.
     C. The woman's illness was caused by a mosquito bite.
     D. The woman won't see the doctor any more.

2.   A. A broken finger.   B. A terrible cough.
     C. Frontal headaches.   D. An eye problem.

3. A. She needs a physical examination. B. She is in good health.
    C. It's good to have a doctor friend. D. It's good to visit the doctor.
4. A. He prefers to take pills to get anti-oxidants.
    B. He prefers to get anti-oxidants from food.
    C. He doesn't mind eating a lot every day.
    D. He is overcautious sometimes.
5. A. The blouse is a bargain. B. The blouse is too expensive.
    C. The blouse is colorful. D. The blouse is so fashionable.
6. A. To resign right away.
    B. To work one more day as chairman.
    C. To think twice before he makes the decision.
    D. To receive further training upon his resignation.
7. A. She didn't do anything in particular. B. She sent a wounded person to the ER.
    C. She had to work in the ER. D. She went skiing.
8. A. A customs officer. B. The man's mother.
    C. A school headmaster. D. An immigration officer.
9. A. It feels as if the room is going around.
    B. It feels like a kind of unsteadiness.
    C. It feels as if she is falling down.
    D. It feels as if she is going around.
10. A. John has hidden something in the tree.
    B. John himself should be blamed.
    C. John has a dog that barks a lot.
    D. John is unlucky.
11. A. The chemistry homework is difficult. B. The chemistry homework is fun.
    C. The math homework is difficult. D. The math homework is fun.
12. A. Whooping cough, smallpox and measles.
    B. Whooping cough, chickenpox and measles.
    C. Whooping cough, smallpox and German measles.
    D. Whooping cough, chickenpox and German measles.
13. A. Saturday morning. B. Saturday night.
    C. Saturday afternoon. D. Next weekend.
14. A. He's lost his notebook. B. His handwriting is messy.
    C. He'll miss class latter this week. D. He cannot make it for his appointment.
15. A. John failed the exam. B. John didn't take the exam.
    C. John passed the exam, but scored low.
    D. It took John a long time to pass the exam.
16. A. To travel by train. B. To go by taxi.

C. To go hiking.   D. To rent a car.

17. A. 1-231-555-1212.   B. 1-213-555-2112.
C. 1-213-555-1212.   D. 1-231-555-2112.

18. A. Morning sickness.   B. A frequent headache.
C. A pain in her right leg.   D. A boring hospitalization.

19. A. Doctor and patient.   B. Boss and secretary.
C. Agent and customer.   D. Driver and passenger.

20. A. To buy another pair of shoes.   B. To help his brother right away.
C. To turn to his brother for help.   D. To seek advice from the woman.

21. A. He is offering a piece of advice.   B. He is examining a patient.
C. He is attending his daughter.   D. He is taking a patient's history.

22. A. To ask the man to call her back.   B. To go to the botanic garden.
C. To do some gardening.   D. To play tennis.

23. A. Louise is not a new comer.   B. Louise loves being a nurse.
C. Louise did a lot of work for the man.   D. Louise has been waiting for a long time.

24. A. Two.   B. Three.   C. Four.   D. Seven.

25. A. She has thrown out of the car.
B. She was knocked down by the car.
C. She hit her head on the steering wheel.
D. She got the steering wheel in her chest.

26. A. She overacted to the man.   B. She cried over her failure.
C. She made a success of her diet.   D. She was jealous of the man.

27. A. He hates those who fool around.   B. He will never try the stuff.
C. He will shoot any drug dealer.   D. He regrets having tried the stuff.

28. A. The opposite to the man's expectation.   B. A quicker recovery than expected.
C. A pair of mismatching boots.   D. Her healthy pregnancy.

29. A. It was called off unexpectedly.
B. It raised more money than expected.
C. It received fewer people than expected.
D. It disappointed the woman for the man's absence.

30. A. In the housing office on campus.   B. In the downtown hotel.
C. At the rental agency.   D. In the nursing home.

31. A. Thrilled.   B. Refreshed.   C. Exhausted.   D. Depressed.

32. A. To travel with parents.   B. To organize a picnic in the country.
C. To cruise, even without his friends.   D. To take a flight to Maldives instead.

33. A. He's got a fever.   B. He's got nausea.
C. He's got diarrhea.   D. He's got a runny nose.

34. A. To suture the man's wound.   B. To remove the bits of glass.
C. To disinfect the man's wound.   D. To take closer look at the man's wound.

35. A. Mr. Lindley had got injured.　B. Mr. Lindley had fallen asleep.
    C. Mr. Lindley had fallen off his chair.　D. Mr. Lindley had lost consciousness.
36. A. She will apply to Duke University.
    B. She will probably attend the University of Texas.
    C. She made up her mind to give up school for work.
    D. She chose Duke University over the University of Texas.
37. A. Her boyfriend broke up with her.
    B. She was almost run over by a truck.
    C. One of her friends was emotionally hurt.
    D. She dumped her boyfriend's truck in the river.
38. A. It was more expensive than the original price.
    B. It was given to the woman as a gift.
    C. It was the last article on sale.
    D. It was a good bargain.
39. A. Excited.　B. Impatient.　C. Indifferent.　D. Concerned.
40. A. She regrets buying the car.　B. The car just arrived yesterday.
    C. She will certainly not buy the car.　D. This is the car she has been wanting.
41. A. He is seriously ill.　B. His work is a mess.
    C. The weather is lousy this week.　D. He has been working under pressure.

答案与解析

1. 【问题】从对话我们可以推测出什么？
    A. 女士的状况很严重。　B. 女士一直恢复得很好。
    C. 女士的病因蚊虫叮咬而起。　D. 女士不会再看医生了。
   【答案】B
   【解析】此题为细节信息再现。女士问医生是不是好转了，医生回答说当然，故答案为 B。选项 C 是干扰项，医生让女病人伸直手臂，并说会有像蚊子叮咬的刺痛，prick 的含义是"刺痛"。

2. 【问题】男士的问题是什么？
    A. 一根断了的手指。　B. 很严重的咳嗽。
    C. 前额疼痛。　D. 眼疾。
   【答案】C
   【解析】此题为细节信息再现。男士六个月前来看病是因为手指断了，今天来看病是因为头痛，故答案为 C。D 项为干扰项，男士在讲述病情时提到头疼，大概是眼周围的地方疼。

3. 【问题】女士是什么意思？
    A. 她需要体检。　B. 她健康状况良好。
    C. 有个当医生的朋友真好。　D. 看医生是有好处的。
   【答案】C

【解析】此题为细节信息再现。男士说到需要体检时就打个电话给他，是免费的。女士回答说有个医生在身边很好，所以答案为 C。

4. 【问题】男士是什么意思？

  A. 他想通过吃药来获取抗氧化剂。 B. 他想通过饮食来获得抗氧化剂。

  C. 他不介意每天多吃些。 D. 有时他过于谨慎。

【答案】B

【解析】对话中女士说抗氧化剂可以防癌，但她不想通过吃药获取这种物质。男士告诉女士说可以从每天的食物中获取所需的抗氧化剂。因而答案是 B。男士话语中的 on the safe side 的含义是"安全可靠，稳妥"。

5. 【问题】男士是什么意思？

  A. 裙子很便宜。 B. 裙子太贵了。

  C. 裙子很鲜艳。 D. 裙子很时尚。

【答案】B

【解析】此题为推断题。女士说花了 8000 元买了这件上衣。男士认为 "rip off"，这个词的意思是"骗人的东西"，他还说时尚确实杀死女人。从上述信息可以推断出男士认为这件上衣太贵了，因此答案为 B。

6. 【问题】这位男士要做什么？

  A. 马上辞职。 B. 再做一天主席。

  C. 决定前三思。 D. 接受辞职后的再培训。

【答案】C

【解析】此题为细节再现。解题有效信息是：I will give the second thought. 表示他会再考虑考虑，故选项 C 正确。"I've had it." 的含义是"我受够了"。

7. 【问题】周末这位女士做什么了？

  A. 没做什么特别的事儿。 B. 她送一名伤者去急诊。

  C. 她在急诊室工作。 D. 她去滑雪。

【答案】C

【解析】此题为细节再现。根据女士所说，她本打算去滑雪，但还是一直在急诊室工作。故选项 C 正确。

8. 【问题】这位女士是做什么的？

  A. 海关官员。 B. 男士的妈妈。

  C. 学校校长。 D. 移民官。

【答案】D

【解析】此题为细节判断题。对话中有效解题信息是：We are going to have to take away your visa.（我们将不得不收回你的签证。）可知这位女士是一名移民官。

9. 【问题】这位女士如何描述头晕？

  A. 好像房子在转。 B. 好像不稳。

  C. 好像她要摔倒了。 D. 好像她在转。

【答案】D

【解析】此题为细节再现。对话中有效解题信息是：I feel the latter.（我感觉是后者。）后者指的是她在转，故选项 D 正确。

10.【问题】这位男士暗示什么？

    A. 约翰在树里藏了东西。   B. 约翰自己应该受责备。

    C. 约翰有一条总是叫的狗。   D. 约翰倒霉。

【答案】B

【解析】此题为习语。男士说道约翰自己解释说是运气差，但他却认为（约翰）是"barking up the wrong tree"，这个习语的含义是"错怪人了"或"认错人了"。男士暗指约翰考试不及格不是运气差，而是他自己的问题，故选项 B 正确。

11.【问题】这位女士什么意思？

    A. 化学作业太难了。   B. 化学作业很有意思。

    C. 数学作业太难了。   D. 数学作业有趣。

【答案】A

【解析】此题为细节再现。对话中女士提到数学作业是 a piece of cake，即"小菜一碟"，但化学作业相当难，不是开玩笑的，故选项 A 正确。

12.【问题】女士小时候得过什么病？

    A. 百日咳、天花、麻疹。   B. 百日咳、水痘、麻疹。

    C. 百日咳、天花、德国麻疹。   D. 百日咳、水痘、德国麻疹。

【答案】B

【解析】此题考点为细节再现。女士提到她小时候得过麻疹、水痘和百日咳，但不是德国麻疹，故选项 B 正确。

13.【问题】男士打算何时学习？

    A. 周六早上。   B. 周六晚上。

    C. 周日下午。   D. 下周。

【答案】D

【解析】此题考点为细节再现。对话中有效解题信息是：on the weekend after this one（下周）。故选项 D 正确。

14.【问题】男士的麻烦是什么？

    A. 他丢了笔记本。   B. 他的字迹太潦草。

    C. 他将缺席这周后面的课。   D. 他因为有约，不能做到。

【答案】C

【解析】此题考点为细节再现。男士提到 be absent from class on Friday morning，说明他周五不来上课，故选项 C 正确。

15.【问题】这位女士暗示什么？

    A. 约翰考试没及格。   B. 约翰没参加考试。

    C. 约翰考试及格了，但分数低。 D. 约翰花费很长时间才考试及格。

【答案】D

【解析】此题考点为语气推测。对话中解题有效信息是 has passed … exam 以及 finally。

男性说道 John 考试过关了，女士的回答 finally 的含义是"终于（过了）"。因而可知选项 D 为正确答案。

16. 【问题】这位男士更喜欢做什么？
    A. 搭乘火车旅行。　　　　　　　　B. 乘出租车去。
    C. 远足。　　　　　　　　　　　　D. 租车。

【答案】B

【解析】此题考点为固定搭配。对话中解题有效信息是固定搭配词组 be up for。在对话中，男女就去哪里的交通工具进行讨论，说乘火车去大概 4 小时，打出租车去大约 2 小时。男士说："I'm up for that."这个词组表示他同意乘出租车去那里，所以答案是 B。

17. 【问题】电话号码是多少？
    A. 1-231-555-1212。　　　　　　B. 1-213-555-2112。
    C. 1-213-555-1212。　　　　　　D. 1-231-555-2112。

【答案】C

【解析】此题考点为细节信息再现。对话中电话号码一共被提到了 2 次。这种题型的解题要领就是跟着所说的号码直接进行判断。

18. 【问题】病人陈述病情时说了什么？
    A. （妊娠初期的）孕妇晨吐。　　　B. 经常头痛。
    C. 右腿痛。　　　　　　　　　　　D. 无聊的入院治疗。

【答案】C

【解析】此题考点为细节信息再现。根据四个选项的预读可知问题应该围绕病症或者症状等，故可以有针对性地听对话中相应的内容。对话中很清楚地提到病人说她自己右腿痛，故答案为 C。

19. 【问题】说话人可能是什么关系？
    A. 医生和病人。　　　　　　　　　B. 老板和秘书。
    C. 代理和顾客。　　　　　　　　　D. 司机和乘客。

【答案】B

【解析】此题考点是推断题。根据两个人之间对话的用词和语气可以推断关系。女士提到她要离开一周，希望男士 keep things straight around here，意思是"把这里的事情搞清楚"。男士回答道："你不用担心。"通过这个对话，我们可以推断两个人的关系是 B，女老板在交代并吩咐事情。

20. 【问题】这位男士可能做什么？
    A. 买另外一双鞋。　　　　　　　　B. 立即帮他哥哥。
    C. 向他哥哥寻求帮助。　　　　　　D. 向这位女士寻求建议。

【答案】C

【解析】此题考点为细节信息再现。对话中的有效信息是：I'll call him tonight. 对话中女士劝说男士应该靠他哥哥，哥哥会帮他，但男士不好意思向哥哥求助，女士就劝男士别这么想，男士最后答应，晚上打电话给哥哥。所以答案是 C。That's another pair of shoes. 的含义是"那就是另外一回事了"，例如：Making a promise and keeping it are quite a different pair of shoes.（做出承诺和实现承诺是完全不同的两回事）。

21.【问题】这位男士正在做什么？

    A. 他正给出建议。   B. 他正给病人做检查。

    C. 他正照顾他的女儿。   D. 他正记录病人病史。

【答案】B

【解析】此题考点是细节信息再现。此题通过男士让女士做的一系列动作可以做出判断。"请仰面躺在床上，我要抬抬你的左腿，看能抬多高，保持膝盖平直，这里疼吗？"故答案是 B。

22.【问题】这位女士要做什么？

    A. 让这位男士给她回电话。   B. 要去植物园。

    C. 要做一些园艺事情。   D. 去打网球。

【答案】D

【解析】此题考点为推断题。对话中男士邀请女士今天去植物园，女士说道："我真希望你早点儿给我打电话。已经安排去打网球了。"根据男士的回应"too bad, some other time（太糟了，改天吧）"可知女士要去打网球而不是去植物园。

23.【问题】男士暗示什么？

    A. 路易斯不是新来的。

    B. 路易斯愿意成为护士。

    C. 路易斯为这位男士做了很多事情。

    D. 路易斯已经等了很久了。

【答案】A

【解析】此题是推断题，对话中解题有效信息是：He's been here as long as I have.（我在这里多久，路易斯就在这里多久）。所以答案是 A。

24.【问题】这位女士现在有几个孩子？

    A. 2。   B. 3。   C. 4。   D. 7。

【答案】B

【解析】此题考点为细节信息再现。当被问是不是第一次怀孕时，女士回答说已经有三个，所以答案是 B。miscarriage 的含义是"流产"。

25.【问题】女士在车祸中怎么了？

    A. 她被抛出窗外。   B. 她被车撞倒了。

    C. 她头撞到了方向盘。   D. 方向盘撞到了她的胸部。

【答案】D

【解析】此题为细节再现题。根据男士所问，女士回答说："没被甩出去，但方向盘撞到了胸部，头撞到挡风板上。"可以判断选项 D 正确。

26.【问题】我们可以说这位女士怎么了？

    A. 她对男士反应过激。   B. 她为失败而哭。

  C．她节食成功。   D．她妒忌这位男性。

【答案】A

【解析】此题考点为推断题。男士说很抱歉听说女士节食 2 个月后体重增加 20 磅。女士的话语中 don't cry crocodile tears 的含义是"猫哭耗子假慈悲"；"You'd be jealous of my figure if I succeeded." 是虚拟语气句型，意思是"我要是成功了你肯定妒忌我的身材。"通过以上解释可知正确答案是 A。

27．【问题】这位男士什么意思？

  A．他讨厌那些鬼混、闲逛的人。

  B．他永远不会试那些东西。

  C．他会射杀任何一个毒品交易者。

  D．他后悔曾经试过那些东西。

【答案】B

【解析】此题为细节信息再现。对话中解题有效信息是男士说的"keep saying no … try the stuff"，意思是"我会对让我试这种东西的人永远说不"，所以答案是 B。fool around 的含义是"闲逛，鬼混"，所以 fool around with drugs 就是指"吸毒鬼混"。stick to my guns 的含义是"坚持自己的主张"。

28．【问题】这位女士是什么意思？

  A．与男士期望相反。   B．比预期恢复得快。

  C．一双不配套的靴子。   D．健康怀孕。

【答案】A

【解析】此题考点为习语。男士问女士术后感觉如何，是否有重生的感觉。女士答语中 the shoe is on the other foot 的含义是"恰恰相反"。例如：He says it was his brother who broke the window, but the boot is no the other foot.（他说打破窗的是他弟弟，但恰恰相反）。所以答案是 A。

29．【问题】关于筹款男士说了什么？

  A．活动意外取消了。   B．比想象中筹到更多的钱。

  C．比预期来的人少。   D．女士很失望男士缺席。

【答案】C

【解析】此题考点为细节再现。对话中解题的有效信息是男士话语中的"Fewer people came than we had expected."，意思是"比我们预期的来的人少"，故选项 C 正确。短对话听力测试中，一定要留意混淆项，通常对话中发音很清楚明显的词作为混淆项，但其相关信息却是错误的，如此题中的选项 A 和选项 D。

30．【问题】这个对话最可能发生在什么地方？

  A．校内住宿办公室。   B．市区饭店。

  C．租房中介。   D．养老院。

【答案】A

【解析】考点为细节推断。对话中解题有效信息是"… this office helps students with housing…"（这里是帮助学生住宿的办公室），以及"Are you a student in nursing program?"（你是护理专业的学生？）这些对话内容说明对话场景应该在校园里，且这个办公室针对护理专业的学生，所以 A 为正确选项。

31. 【问题】说话者的感受如何？

    A．兴奋，激动。   B．有精神的，清爽的。

    C．累极了。   D．郁闷的。

【答案】C

【解析】考点为常用习语。此题解题关键在于口语中的习语，但如果不是很清楚习语的确切含义，对话中的细节信息也可以帮助我们猜答案，如 "Let's get something to eat." "We'd be able to feel better with a little nutrition." 的含义是"找点儿东西吃""有一些营养，我们可以感觉好些"。这些有效信息可以确定他们现在的感受是 C。这个对话中的习语是最直接的解题信息："Let's call it a day."（我们今天到此为止吧）"I'm beat too."（我也累死了）。除此以外表示很累的说法还有："I'm exhausted." "I'm bused."

32. 【问题】这位男士打算做什么？

    A．和父母去旅行。

    B．安排一次乡村野餐。

    C．去乘船旅游，即使没有朋友（相伴）。

    D．改搭飞机去马尔代夫。

【答案】C

【解析】此题考点为细节再现。对话中解题有效信息是 "I'm still inclined to go. Alone if I have to."，意思是"我仍旧想去，如果必要的话我一个人去也行。"所以 C 项为正确答案。对话中 got off the ground 是一个习语，意思是"开始或取得进展"，说明男士和朋友乘船去马尔代夫的旅行没成。

33. 【问题】这位男士哪里不适？

    A．他发烧了。   B．他恶心。   C．他腹泻。   D．他流鼻涕。

【答案】C

【解析】此题考点为细节再现。对话中解题有效信息是：have the runs 和 going to the toilet。have the runs 的含义是"得痢疾"。所以选项 C 是答案。cereal 的含义是"麦片"。

34. 【问题】这位女士紧接着会做什么？

    A．缝合男士的伤口。   B．去除玻璃碎片。

    C．给男士伤口消毒。   D．靠近看男士的伤口。

【答案】A

【解析】此题考点为细节再现。对话中女士说到很多要做的事情：已经去除玻璃碎片，消毒了伤口，下一个要做的事情是缝合伤口。根据题目，可知考点是下一个要做的事情，关键词组是 stitch you up，意思是"缝合伤口"。尽管这个词组可能会给考生造成障碍，但根据 the next thing 可知，B 项、C 项以及 D 项都已经做完了。

35.【问题】从对话中我们可以得知什么？

A. Lindley 先生受伤了。

B. Lindley 先生睡着了。

C. Lindley 先生从椅子上摔下来了。

D. Lindley 先生失去知觉。

【答案】D

【解析】此题考点为固定词组含义。对话中解题有效信息是 pass out，其含义是"昏倒"。故选项D为答案。C项和对话中 found him in his chair（发现时他在椅子上）不符。

36.【问题】这位女士讲了 Jacky 的什么事？

A. 她将申请杜克大学。

B. 她很可能去得克萨斯大学上学。

C. 她下定决心辍学工作。

D. 她选择了杜克大学而不是得克萨斯大学。

【答案】B

【解析】此题为细节再现题。对话中的有效信息是：Jacky is considering attending the University of Texas in Houston.（Jacky 正考虑去休斯敦的得克萨斯大学上学。）故答案是 B。register 的含义是"报到，注册"。

37.【问题】这位女士是什么意思？

A. 她男朋友和她分手了。　　　B. 她差点儿被卡车碾过。

C. 她的一个朋友感情受伤。　　D. 她把男朋友的卡车丢到了河里。

【答案】A

【解析】此题的考点是固定搭配的含义和 dump 的含义。dump 的含义是"倾倒，倾销"。对话中最后女士所说的话 "My boyfriend just dumped me for another girl." 的含义是"我男朋友为了另外一个女孩抛弃了我"。故选项 A 为答案。选项 B 是原文信息 "You look like you've been run over by a truck" 的混淆项，原文含义是"你看上去就像被卡车碾过一样"，是一种比喻说法，不是事实，故选项 B 错误。

38.【问题】关于香奈尔的皮包，对话中说了什么？

A. 这个比原价贵很多。　　　　B. 这个是给女士的礼物。

C. 这是减价的最后一件。　　　D. 这是个很值的便宜货。

【答案】D

【解析】此题是细节再现题。解题有效信息是：the bag is so expensive（这个包很贵），以及 it was only one tenth of the original price（价格仅是原价的十分之一）。可以知选项 D 为正确答案。

39.【问题】下面哪个词可以很好地描述男士的感受？

A. 兴奋。　　　B. 没耐性。　　　C. 漠不关心。　　　D. 关注。

【答案】B

【解析】考点是细节再现。对话中的有效信息是：you have said that several times（你已经讲了很多遍了）。故选项 B 为正确答案。

40.【问题】这位女士什么意思？

        A．她后悔买了这车。   B．这车昨天刚到。

        C．她肯定不买这车。   D．这是她一直想要的车。

【答案】C

【解析】考点为意义推断题。女士所说的含义是"这车有很多毛病，如果你希望我买了，你一定认为我是昨天刚出生的"，这说明这位女士肯定不买这车。

41.【问题】这位男士什么意思？

        A．他病得很重。   B．他的工作一团糟。

        C．这周天气很糟糕。   D．他一直在压力下工作。

【答案】D

【解析】此题的考点是细节再现。当被问到最近工作如何时，这位男士说 lousy（很糟糕）以及 It's been a tense week（紧张的一周），故答案是 D。

听力原文

1. M: Well, just keep your arm straight there. Fine, there will be a little prick like a mosquito bite. OK? There we go. OK, I will send that sample off and we'll check it. If the sample is OK, we won't need to go on seeing you anymore.

     W: So you think I'm getting better?

     M: Absolutely.

     Q: What can be inferred from the conversation?

2. W: It's Mr. Cong, isn't it?

     M: That's right. I saw you six months ago with a broken finger.

     W: Yes, of course. And is that all healing well?

     M: It's fine.

     W: What can we do for you today?

     M: Well, I've been having these headaches in the front, about my eyes. It started two months ago. They seem to come on quite suddenly, and I get dizzy spell as well.

     Q: What is the trouble in the man now?

3. M: When you need a health checkup, just call me. It's totally free.

     W: It's great having a doctor around.

     Q: What does the woman mean?

4. W: We need anti-oxidants to prevent ourselves from developing cancer, but I don't like taking pills to get it.

     M: But you need to eat a mountain of food everyday to get all of the anti-oxidants you need.

     W: I drink a lot of green tea; I eat onion, garlic and citrous food. I also get nine different colors of vegetables every day.

M: All those do have anti-oxidants, but I want to be on the safe side.

Q: What does the man mean?

5.　W: The blouse cost me like 8,000 yuan.

M: That's such a rip-off.

W: I really like it, the color, the design…

M: Fashion really kills women.

Q: What does the man mean?

6.　M: I have had it! I am resigning from the job of chairman right now. I can't stand it another day.

W: Do you really mean you want to quit?

M: Well, maybe I will give it a second thought.

Q: What is the man going to do?

7.　W: Did you do anything over the weekend?

M: Not much, what did you do?

W: I had planed to going skiing, but I wound up working in the ER.

Q: What did the woman do over the weekend?

8.　W: We understand that you are not attending school.

M: I have been attending, but I have been sick recently.

W: You have attending only 3 days since last July.

M: 3 days? No, it's been more than that.

W: We are going to have to take away your visa.

Q: What is the woman?

9.　M: Does the dizziness feel like spinning or is it just a kind of unsteadiness?

W: It feels like spinning.

M: How would you describe it, is it as if, the room is going around or do you feel as if it's you that is going around.

W: I feel the latter.

Q: How does the woman describe her dizziness?

10.　W: Did you know that John failed in the math exam?

M: Yes, and he blamed it on bad luck, but I really think he's barking on the wrong tree.

Q: What does the man imply?

11.　M: Cathleen, how's the math homework coming?

W: That's a piece of cake, but the chemistry homework is really a hard nut to crack.

Q: What does the woman mean?

12.　M: I like to ask you about your past medical history. Can you tell me if you've had any childhood diseases?

W: When I was small, I had measles, chickenpox and whooping coughs. But I do not think I've ever had German measles.

Q: What diseases did the woman have when she was small?

13.　W: If you go to the football game on Saturday night and concerts or play on Sunday, you won't have much time to study.

M: Oh well, I can do that on the weekend after this one.

Q: When does the man plan to study?

14. M: I need to be absent from class on Friday morning, because I have a doctor's appointment. And I need to borrow someone's notes.

W: Well, you can certainly borrow mine if you do not mind my messy handwriting.

Q: What is the man's problem?

15. M: Did you hear that John has passed the Step One United States Medical Licensing Examination?

W: Finally.

Q: What does the woman imply?

16. M: It's a one-day trip. It must be pretty close.

W: It's about four hours by train.

M: Ha, OK. How else can we get there?

W: Well, I think, by taxi, it's only about two hours.

M: I'm up for that.

Q: What does the man prefer to do?

17. W: Information. What number do you need?

M: I need the number of German Embassy in Los Angeles.

W: You'll have to dial Information in Los Angeles. Dial 1-213-555-1212.

M: Sorry, could you say the number again?

W: Sure. 1-213-555-1212.

Q: What is the phone number?

18. W: Hello, Jim. I wonder if you could see a patient for me.

M: Certainly Anne. What's the story?

W: Well, it's a Miss Linda Holmes, a 35-year-old waitress. She is an infrequent visitor. She came to see me this morning complaining a pain in her right leg.

Q: What is the patient's complaint?

19. W: I will be gone for a week. So I hope you can keep things straight around here.

M: You have nothing to worry about.

Q: What is the probable relationship between the two speakers?

20. W: If you see he is your brother, that's another pair of shoes. I suppose you can rely on him to help you.

M: I know. But I feel ashamed to ask him for help.

W: Don't think that way. He is your dear brother!

M: OK, I will call him tonight.

Q: What will the man probably do?

21. M: Would you like to get into the couch and lie on your back, please? Now I am going to take your left leg and see how far you can raise it. Keep the knee straight. Does that hurt at all?

W: Yes, just a little. Just slightly.

Q: What is the man doing?

22. M: Hi, Jane, this is Peter. Such a nice day today. I thought we might go to the botanic garden.

    W: I wish you have called me earlier. I have just made plans to play tennis.

    M: Oh, that's too bad. Maybe some other time.

    Q: What is the woman going to do?

23. W: How do you like the nurse at the reception desk?

    M: You mean Louise? He's been here as long as I have.

    Q: What does the man imply?

24. M: Hello, Mrs. White. Is it your first visit to the clinic?

    W: Yes. But I've been to my doctor and he has checked me over.

    M: I see from his letter that he is satisfied with the way things are going. Is this your first pregnancy?

    W: Oh, no, I've had three. I lost two and had two miscarriages.

    Q: How many children does the woman have now?

25. W: I've just been in a road accident.

    M: Were you thrown out of the car, or did you get the steering wheel in your chest?

    W: I wasn't thrown out, but I got the steering wheel in my chest. And I hit my head on the wind screen.

    M: Were you knocked out?

    W: I don't remember anything after the accident.

    Q: What could be said about the woman in the car accident?

26. M: I'm sorry to hear that you've gained 20 pounds after going on a diet for 2 months.

    W: Don't cry crocodile tears. You'd be jealous of my figure if I succeeded.

    Q: What can we say about the woman?

27. W: Guess what! I hear some students of the school are fooling around with drugs.

    M: But you know I'll stick to my guns and keep saying no to those who want me to try the stuff.

    Q: What does the man mean?

28. M: How do you feel after the surgery? It seems that you've got a rebirth, right?

    W: I'm sorry, doctor, honestly, I think the shoe is on the other foot.

    Q: What does the woman mean?

29. W: How many people turned out at the fund raising event?

    M: Fewer people came than we had expected. It was disappointing, but we made a little money for our organization.

    W: Sorry, I wasn't able to attend. I intended to.

    Q: What did the man say about the fund raising event?

30. W: Excuse me, I understand that this office helps students with housing, is that right?

    M: Are you a student in nursing program? May I see your ID card? Um, yes, we can certainly help you. Where are you staying now?

    W: I just arrived yesterday. I'm staying at the hotel across the street.

    M: Will you be living alone or do you have a family, or would you be interested in sharing housing?

Q: Where does this conversation most probably take place?

31. M: Let's call it a day; we've acted for hours.

W: I'm beat too. Let's get something to eat.

M: We'd be able to feel better with a little nutrition.

Q: How are the speakers feeling?

32. W: I heard that you and some friends are organizing a cruise to Maldives.

M: It's never really got off the ground.

W: That's too bad. It sounded like fun.

M: Yeah, I'm still inclined to go. Alone if I have to.

Q: What is the man planning to do?

33. M: Doc, I'm afraid to have the runs.

W: Are you going to the toilet often?

M: Haven't stopped since every early this morning.

W: What did you have for breakfast?

M: Just cereal and a few cups of tea.

Q: What is the man's problem?

34. W: Take off your shirt and I will take a closer look.

M: Can you see any bits of glass?

W: Yes, I have removed them all, and disinfected the wound. The next thing I should do is to stitch you up.

Q: What is the woman going to do next?

35. M: Hello, Dr. Carbon here, what seems to be the problem?

W: It's Mr. Lindley. I found him in his chair, white as a sheet. I thought he passed out.

Q: What can we learn from the conversation?

36. W: Jacky is considering attending the University of Texas in Houston.

M: Really? I thought she was registered at Duke University.

W: That's true. But she decided that she didn't want to be so far away from home.

Q: What does the woman say about Jacky?

37. M: My gosh, you look like you've been run over by a truck. What's wrong?

W: My boyfriend just dumped me for another girl.

Q: What does the woman mean?

38. W: Did you like the Channel bag that I got?

M: You must have a rich boyfriend because that bag is so expensive.

W: I bought it on e-bay. It was only one tenth of the original price. And the purchase online is so easy.

Q: What is said about the Channel bag?

39. W: Bring some medicine when you go to picnic. Insects can transmit disease.

M: I see. You have said that several times.

Q: Which of the following can best describe the man's feeling?

40. M: Please look at this car, it's nice.

W: This car has a lot of faults. You must think that I was born yesterday if you expect me to buy it.

Q: What does the woman mean?

41. W: How are you doing these days with your new job?

M: Not very well, I'm afraid. I'm feeling lousy.

W: Really? Why?

M: It's been a tense week.

Q: What does the man mean?

Section B

Conversation One（2012 年真题）

1. A. White blood cell count.　　　　　B. Red blood cell count.
   C. X-ray.　　　　　　　　　　　　D. ECG.
2. A. Too much work to do.　　　　　　B. A heavy load of studying.
   C. Her daughter's sickness.　　　　　D. Her insufficient income.
3. A. Leukemia.　　　　　　　　　　B. Gastric ulcer.
   C. Immune disease.　　　　　　　　D. Gastric influenza.
4. A. Take the white tablets three times a day.
   B. Take the charcoal tablets three times a day.
   C. Take one or two white tablets at a time.
   D. Take two charcoal tablets a day.
5. A. Stay off work.　　　　　　　　　B. Drink plenty of liquids.
   C. Eat a lot of vegetables and fruit.　D. Postpone your exercise when sick.

【文章概要】医生和就诊的病人之间就检查结果发生的对话。

答案与解析

1. 【问题】根据女士的检查结果，下面哪一项是不正常的？

　　　　A. 白细胞数量。　　　　　　B. 红细胞数量。

　　　　C. X 光。　　　　　　　　　D. 心电图。

【答案】A

【解析】根据医生的判断，病人的 ECG 十分正常（perfectly normal），X 光片也没有问题，但是白细胞数量很高（white blood cell count is rather high）。因此本题答案为 A。

2. 【问题】下面哪一项不属于这位女士焦虑的原因？

　　　　A. 有太多工作要做。　　　　B. 沉重的学习任务。

　　　　C. 女儿生病。　　　　　　　D. 收入不高。

【答案】D

【解析】病人很焦虑，因为她本人工作很忙，女儿也生病了，学习压力也很大。只有
　　　　D（收入不高）不是她焦虑的原因，因此本题答案为D。

3. 【问题】医生对这位女士的诊断结果是什么？

    A．白血病。   B．胃溃疡。

    C．免疫系统疾病。   D．胃型流行性感冒。

【答案】C

【解析】医生说病人的白细胞数量高，证明身体正在跟病毒斗争，由此推理可知，病人
　　　　可能是免疫系统出了点问题。故本题选C。

4. 【问题】关于女士服用的药物，医生是如何嘱咐的？

    A．白色药片一日三次。   B．炭黑色药片一日三次。

    C．每次服用白色药片1片或2片。   D．每日服用2片炭黑色药片。

【答案】A

【解析】医生说，按照说明一天口服三次白色药片，而charcoal药片则需要根据肠胃
　　　　（bowels）的适应度来决定是服用一片还是两片了，因此本题正确答案为A。

5. 【问题】下列哪一项不属于医生的建议？

    A．请假在家休息。   B．多喝水。

    C．多吃蔬菜水果。   D．生病时暂缓健身。

【答案】D

【解析】医生对病人的建议是：不能上班，大量饮水，多食用蔬菜和水果。只有"生
　　　　病时暂缓健身"未被提及，故本题答案为D。

 听力原文

P:　Here is my result, doctor.

D:　Have a seat, and let's have a look. Well, your ECG is perfectly normal, and there is no problem with your X-ray, either. But your white blood cell count is rather high, which is what I expected, and it shows your body is fighting the virus.

P:　Is there anything here I can do so that I can feel better, doctor? I am really busy at work this week. And I have a lot of stuff to do, but I don't feel opt to it. Also my daughter is studying bad and…

D:　Don't worry. It's just against the feel. But I will give you some medicine for it to make you feel better. Three times a day take the white tablets as directed on the label after meals. And for the charcoal tablets, take one or two depending on how suitable your bowels are.

P:　Is there anything else I can do, Doctor Hunt?

D:　I know you are busy, but you really shouldn't go to work. However, that's up to you. Rest as much as possible, drink plenty of liquid, and eat plenty of vegetables and fruits. Remember, an apple a day keeps the doctor away. If there is no improvement after three days, come back and see me again.

P: Thank you, doctor.

Questions:

1. According to the women's test results, which of the following items is abnormal?

2. Which of the following is not the reason for the woman's anxiety?

3. What is the doctor's diagnosis of the woman?

4. How does the doctor say the medications are administered for the woman?

5. Which of the following is not one of the suggestions by the doctor?

Conversation Two（2010 年真题）

6. A. He is having a physical checkup.

   B. He has just undergone an operation.

   C. He has just recovered from an illness.

   D. He will be discharged from the hospital this afternoon.

7. A. He got an infection in the lungs.

   B. He had his gallbladder inflamed.

   C. He was suffering from influenza.

   D. He had developed a big kidney tone.

8. A. A bit better.   B. Terribly awful.

   C. Couldn't be better.   D. Okay, but a bit weak.

9. A. To be confined to a wheelchair.

   B. To stay indoors for a complete recovery.

   C. To stay in bed and drink a lot of water.

   D. To move about and enjoy the sunshine.

10. A. From 4 pm to 6 pm.   B. From 5 pm to 7 pm.

    C. From 6 pm to 8 pm.   D. From 7 pm to 9 pm.

【文章概要】医生在病人胆结石术后与病人之间的对话。

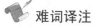 难词译注

gallstone ['gɔːlstəun] *n.*   胆结石

gallbladder ['gɔːlblædə] *n.*   胆囊

inflame [in'fleim] *v.*   发炎

答案与解析

6. 【问题】对话中有关这位男士的情况哪个选项是正确的？

            A. 他正接受体检。   B. 他刚经历了一场手术。

            C. 他已经从病症中恢复过来。   D. 他今天下午将出院。

   【答案】B

【解析】对话中提到男士有一块很大的胆结石，而且胆囊发炎，胆囊周围和里面都感染了。但现在都出来了，故可以推断他刚经历了一场手术。

7. 【问题】这位男士怎么了？

A. 肺部感染。　　　　B. 胆囊发炎。　　　　C. 流感。　　　　D. 肾结石。

【答案】B

【解析】对话中，女士提到：You have a pretty big gall stone and the gallbladder was quite inflamed. 即："你长了一大块胆结石，并且胆囊也发炎了。"由此可以判断 B 是正确选项。D 选项中 kidney stone 是"肾结石"的意思。

8. 【问题】现在这位男士感觉如何？

A. 好一些了。　　　　　　　　　　　　B. 很糟。

C. 很好。　　　　　　　　　　　　　　D. 还好，但还有点虚弱。

【答案】D

【解析】此题为细节再现。对话中解题有效信息是：I think I am OK. I'm feeling a bit of weak at the moment. 这说明病人仍旧感到虚弱，故选项 D 正确。

9. 【问题】根据医生指示，这个病人应该做什么？

A. 坐轮椅。　　　　　　　　　　　　　B. 为了痊愈，待在室内。

C. 卧床，多喝水。　　　　　　　　　　D. 来回走，晒太阳。

【答案】D

【解析】对话中，女士对男士说："But the sooner we have you on the move, the quicker you start to heal. So we'll help you sit in this chair this afternoon. Enjoy the sunshine." 即："你越早活动，就会越快痊愈。因此，我们今天下午会帮你坐在椅子上，享受一下阳光吧。"由此可以判断男士会四处活动一下。所以选 D。

10. 【问题】医院探视时间是何时？

A. 下午 4 点到 6 点。　　　　　　　　B. 下午 5 点到 7 点。

C. 晚上 6 点到 8 点。　　　　　　　　D. 晚上 7 点到 9 点。

【答案】C

【解析】此题为细节信息再现，根据最后医生所说探视时间是晚上 6 至 8 点。

📝 听力原文

W: Hello.

M: Hello.

W: So, did you have a comfortable night?

M: No, not really.

W: Sorry to hear that. And how are you feeling at the moment?

M: A bit better.

W: You don't feel sick at all?

M: No, I am OK.

W: That's good! Are you having sips of water?

M: No.

W: Would you like some?

M: Well, I do not really feel like.

W: Oh, you can't drink anything at the moment.

M: The nurses have been giving me mouth washes.

W: Yes I think you begin to pick up as the day goes on and we'll carry on giving you something to ease the discomfort. Does it hurt much?

M: Well, it does when I move about.

W: Right, but the sooner we help you on the move, the quicker you start to heal. So we'll help you sit in the chair this afternoon. Enjoy the sunshine.

M: OK, I can't say I am really looking forward to that.

W: You had a pretty big gallstone, and your gallbladder was quite inflamed, with a lot of infection around it and inside it. Well it is out now. So, no need to worry about it. It won't cause you any more trouble.

M: Uh.

W: Any more questions or anything we can do for you?

M: No, I think I am OK. I'm feeling a bit of weak at the moment. When will my wife be able to come and see me? The nurses told me before, but I can't remember.

W: The visiting hours are from 6 to 8 in the evening.

M: OK, thank you. She will be here tonight in that case.

W: Fine, well I will stop in to see you tomorrow.

M: Thank you.

Questions:

6. What is true about the man in the conversation?

7. What was wrong with the man?

8. How is the man feeling now?

9. What is the man supposed to do according to the doctor's orders?

10. What is the hospital's visiting hour?

🎧 Conversation Three（2009 年真题）

11. A. For the purpose of diagnosis confirmation.
    B. For the possibility of legal trouble.
    C. For the doctor's investigation.
    D. For the patient's future use.

12. A. He has got cancer in his pancreas.   B. He falls with a stomach problem.
    C. He suffers from fatigue.   D. He has a loss of weight.

13. A. See a dietician.　　　　　　　　B. Have an operation.
　　 C. Start chemotherapy.　　　　　　D. Take medication for pain relief.
14. A. A couple of years.　　　　　　　B. More than 5 years.
　　 C. A couple of months.　　　　　　D. Approximately 5 years.
15. A. Suspicious.　　　　　　　　　　B. Anxious.
　　 C. Hesitant.　　　　　　　　　　　D. Factual.

【文章概要】医生和病人就胰腺癌复发进行讨论，谈话涉及治疗方案以及还能活多长时间。

难词译注

scan [skæn] v.　　　　　　　　　　　　扫描
recurrence [ri'kʌrəns] n.　　　　　　　复发
pancreas ['pænkriəs] n.　　　　　　　　胰腺
chemotherapy [ˌkəməu'θerəpi] n.　　　化疗
dietician [ˌdaiə'tiʃən] n.　　　　　　　营养师
life expectancy　　　　　　　　　　　　寿命预期

答案与解析

11.【问题】为什么要对问诊进行录音？
　　　　　A. 为了确认诊断。　　　　　　B. 为了可能出现的法律纠纷。
　　　　　C. 为了医生调查。　　　　　　D. 为了病人今后使用。
　　【答案】D
　　【解析】此题考点为细节再现。对话一开始就提到医生想要对问诊进行录音，这样病人及他太太可以在今后回放今天还不太清楚的事情。所以选项 D 为正确选项。

12.【问题】根据医生诊断，斯考特先生怎么了？
　　　　　A. 他得了胰腺癌。　　　　　　B. 他有胃病。
　　　　　C. 他感到疲劳。　　　　　　　D. 他体重下降。
　　【答案】A
　　【解析】此题考点为细节再现。对话中医生说："It's likely that you got a recurrence of cancer in your pancreas.（很可能你的胰腺癌复发了。）"所以答案是 A。

13.【问题】下面哪一个不是给斯考特先生的建议？
　　　　　A. 见营养师。　　 B. 手术。　　 C. 开始化疗。　　 D. 吃药缓解疼痛。
　　【答案】B
　　【解析】此题考点为细节再现。医生说："Surgery isn't an option at this stage.（这个阶段手术不是一个选择。）"因而 B 项不是医生给出的建议。

14.【问题】根据医生所说，斯考特先生能活多久？
　　　　　A. 几年。　　 B. 5 年以上。　　 C. 几个月。　　 D. 大约 5 年。
　　【答案】C

【解析】此题考点为细节再现。医生说："I'd say it's a matter of months rather than years.（这是几个月的问题但不是几年的事情。）"所以可知病人还能活几个月，故答案 C 正确。

15.【问题】下面哪个词最能描述医生话语的语气？

      A．怀疑。   B．担心。   C．犹豫。   D．讲事实的。

【答案】D

【解析】此题考点为推断。整个对话我们可以得出医生一直在很坦白地告诉病人真实情况，他自己也说："…it's always good to be honest with people…（坦白相告总是好的）"所以选项 D 正确。

 听力原文

W: Mr. Scot. I like to record this consultation, so you and Mrs. Scot can play back later for anything that may not be clear to you today. I'm afraid that the scan results aren't very good. It's likely that you got a recurrence of cancer in your pancreas. That would explain why you've been feeling so tired, and your loss of appetite and weight.

M: Doctor Smith, do I need surgery?

W: Surgery isn't an option at this stage. Although we cannot operate, there's still a lot we can do to help you. You've got tablets for pain relief, and we can give you something stronger if you need it. We can also start you on a course of chemotherapy to help you with your symptoms. This won't cure you, but will make you feel more comfortable. It's unusual to have any advice on what you eat and to help you get your appetite back.

M: What's my life expectancy? How long have I got?

W: One can never be certain about these issues. People with this condition vary a great deal. I would be wrong to give you a definite time scale. But I'd say it's a matter of months rather than years. I'm sorry to have to tell you all this, but my feeling is that it's always good to be honest with people, then you know what's what. If you are in agreement, I'd like to book you into Ward 2 to start your chemo. You'll need to come in every week for the next month.

Questions:

11. What is the recorded consultation for?

12. According to the doctor's diagnosis, what's happened to Mr. Scot?

13. Which of the following is not a suggestion for Mr. Scot?

14. According to the doctor, what might be Mr. Scot's life expectancy?

15. Which of the following can best describe the tone of doctor's words?

Conversation Four（2008 年真题）

16. A. He has got bowel cancer.　　　　B. He has got heart disease.
    C. He has got bone cancer.　　　　　D. He has got heartburn.
17. A. To have a colonoscopy.　　　　　B. To seek a second opinion.
    C. To be put on chemotherapy.　　　D. To have his bowel removed.
18. A. A pretty minor surgery.　　　　　B. A normal life ahead of him.
    C. A miracle in his coming years.　　D. A life without any inconveniences.
19. A. Thankful.　　　　　　　　　　　　B. Admitting.
    C. Resentful.　　　　　　　　　　　　D. Respectful.
20. A. It was based on the symptoms the man had described.
    B. It was prescribed considering possible complications.
    C. It was given according to the man's actual condition.
    D. It was effective because of a proper intervention.

【文章概要】医生和病人就病情进行讨论，医生认为病人要做截肠手术，病人还咨询了术后对生活的影响。

难词译注

bowel ['bauəl] *n.*	肠道
colostomy bag	结肠造瘘袋
seal [si:l] *n.*	密封
odor-free ['əudə-fri:] *a.*	无味的
colonoscopy [ˌkəulə'nɔskəpi] *n.*	结肠镜检查

16.【问题】这位男士哪里不适？
　　　　A. 他得了肠癌。　　　　　　　B. 他得了心脏病。
　　　　C. 他得了骨癌。　　　　　　　D. 他感到胃灼热。
　　【答案】A
　　【解析】对话一开始医生就告诉病人可能要做截肠手术。并且在对话中，病人也得知自己患的是 cancer of the bowel，即"肠癌"，故答案是 A。
17.【问题】医生建议这位男士做什么？
　　　　A. 做一个结肠镜检查。　　　　B. 再咨询别人。
　　　　C. 做化疗。　　　　　　　　　D. 截去肠子。
　　【答案】D
　　【解析】对话一开始医生就告诉病人可能要截掉肠子或者一段肠子。所以答案是 D。
18.【问题】医生说了什么来安慰这位男士？
　　　　A. 这是一个很小的手术。　　　B. 生活正常。
　　　　C. 未来几年的奇迹。　　　　　D. 生活不会有任何不便之处。
　　【答案】B

【解析】文章中最后医生对病人提到 you will be able to live a pretty normal life and go work, and everything，说明病人会过正常的生活，故选项 B 正确。

19.【问题】这位男士对医生是什么态度？

    A．感谢。   B．钦佩。   C．愤慨。   D．尊敬。

【答案】C

【解析】对话中男士得知自己患的是肠癌时，他提到医生一直给他开的药是针对胃灼热的，虽然他口头说的是千谢万谢，但这位男士的真正意图不是感谢医生，而是表达出自己的气愤。

20.【问题】医生就他以前给病人的治疗说了什么？

    A．这个治疗是依据这位男士所描述的症状的。

    B．考虑到可能的并发症开的药。

    C．根据病人的实际状况给开的药。

    D．因为适当的介入，这个治疗很有效。

【答案】A

【解析】当病人针对医生以前的治疗提出质疑时，医生解释说他所开具的药都是根据病人自己描述的症状开的，而且只有结肠镜检查才能真正看到他的情况。所以正确答案是 A。

听力原文

W: Well, you'll probably have an operation to remove the bowel, or some of it. It's too diseased to save, I'm afraid.

M: How will I go without a bowel? How can I live without a bowel?

W: During the operation, they will fit you externally with a colostomy bag.

M: You mean the bag of shit hanging inside of my clothes?

W: Well, that's perhaps an unnecessarily cruel way of putting it. But, broadly speaking, yes. It is sealed and odor-free. They'll show you how to empty it and change it for yourself. And nobody need ever know that you've got one unless you tell them.

M: Well, thanks a lot. Cancer of the bowel! All this time you have been prescribing tablets for heart burn, and it turns out that I got cancer of the bowel? Oh, thanks a million. What next? How long will I go on now? Will I be able to live any kind of normal life? Tell me!

W: I prescribed for you on the basis of the symptoms you yourself described to me. Only a colonoscopy can reveal your condition. No doctor could diagnose your condition without the hospital tests that I arranged for you. And yes, you will be able to live a pretty normal life and go work, and everything. Nobody need ever know a thing unless you choose to tell them. And you have full life ahead of you.

Questions:

16. What is wrong with the man?

17. What does the doctor recommend the man to do?

18. What does the doctor assure the man of?

19. What is the man's attitude towards the doctor?

20. What does the doctor say about the previous treatment for the patient?

🎧 Passage One（2011 年真题）

21. A. Liver failure.　　　　　　　　　B. Breast cancer.
　　C. Kidney failure.　　　　　　　　D. Diabetes out of control.

22. A. Shape.　　　　　　　　　　　　B. Color.
　　C. Price.　　　　　　　　　　　　D. Size.

23. A. It is much smaller than a microwave.　B. It leaves much room for reduction.
　　C. It is widely used in the clinic.　　D. It is perfect.

24. A. It is under a clinical trial.　　　　B. It is available in the market.
　　C. It is widely used in the clinic.　　D. It is in the experimental stage.

25. A. The commercial companies have invested a lot in the new machine.
　　B. The further development of the machine is in financial trouble.
　　C. The federal government finances the research.
　　D. The machine will come into being in no time.

【文章概要】短文讲述一种能够模仿人类嗅觉感知疾病的机器。

🚩 答案与解析

21.【问题】哪种疾病是闻不出来的?
　　　　A. 肝功能衰竭。　　　　　　　B. 乳腺癌。
　　　　C. 肾衰竭。　　　　　　　　　D. 糖尿病失控。
　　【答案】B
　　【解析】从短文开始可知，能通过嗅觉感知的有 diabetes（糖尿病）病人的存在，紧跟着又提到如果病人的 kidney（肾脏）或者 liver（肝脏）功能有问题他也能感知到。因此未被提及的病只有 B（乳腺癌）。

22.【问题】这种机器过去存在什么问题?
　　　　A. 形状。　　　　B. 颜色。　　　　C. 价格。　　　　D. 尺寸。
　　【答案】D
　　【解析】文中提到过去使用的机器是 enormous（巨大的），由此推理可知，过去机器的问题是尺寸太大，故 D 选项是正确答案。

23.【问题】下列哪项陈述是正确的?
　　　　A. 比微波炉都要小好多。　　　　B. 尚有很大浓缩的空间。
　　　　C. 在临床得到广泛应用。　　　　D. 完美。
　　【答案】B

【解析】根据最后一句可知，新款机器还 very much in the experimental stage（很大程度上处于试验阶段），由此可推理得知这款机器还有很大的改进空间。故选 B。

24.【问题】新款机器现在处在什么阶段？

    A．处在临床试验阶段。   B．已经开始在市场上销售。

    C．在临床上得到广泛应用。   D．尚处在试验阶段。

【答案】D

【解析】根据上文的解析可知，D 为正确答案。

25.【问题】和过去的机器相比，这台机器有何不同？

    A．商业公司在新机器上投入巨大。

    B．机器的进一步研究面临财务困难。

    C．联邦政府资助了该项研究。

    D．这台机器很快就会大功告成。

【答案】C

【解析】短文最后说："与商业公司生产的药品不同，这次是由联邦政府做的。"由此可知，该产品是由联邦政府支持研发并提供资金支持。故本题选 C。

 听力原文

A lot of doctors can tell what's wrong with you by sleeping, and I can do this by smelling. This actually goes back to the day of ancient Greece. For example, you can walk into a room or get close to a patient who had diabetes that is not well controlled. There is a kind of sweetish smell. That means I can walk into a room and tell if a patient has kidney failure or liver failure. And now there is a machine that can do that too. It is fascinating that there have been these machines in the past, but they were just enormous. These machines are impossible to use clinically, because, you know, in a whole room for the equipments. So in the past, they were not used in therapy. But the newly-invented ones are very small and concise. They use new laser technology and now available given the size of the machine. Unlike the previous, they are just of the size of microwave. However, they are very much in the experimental stage. Interestingly, unlike any of these things which are produced by commercial company, this work is being done by the federal government.

Questions:

21. What disease can't be smelt?

22. What was the problem of the machine in the past?

23. Which of the following statements is true?

24. What stage is the new machine in now?

25. What is the difference about the machines from the past ones?

Passage Two（2010 年真题）

26. A. The link between weight loss and sleep deprivation.
    B. The link between weight gain and sleep deprivation.
    C. The link between weight loss and physical exercise.
    D. The link between weight gain and physical exercise.

27. A. More than 68,000.   B. More than 60,800.
    C. More than 60,080.   D. More than 60,008.

28. A. 7-hour sleepers gained more weight over time than 5-hour ones.
    B. 5-hour sleepers gained more weight over time than 7-hour ones.
    C. Short-sleepers were 15% more likely to become obese.
    D. Short-sleepers consumed fewer calories than long sleepers.

29. A. Overeating among the sleep-deprived.
    B. Little exercise among the sleep-deprived.
    C. Lower metabolic rate resulting from less sleep.
    D. Higher metabolic rate resulting from less sleep.

30. A. Exercise every day.   B. Take diet pills.
    C. Go on a diet.   D. Sleep more.

【文章概要】睡眠多少和减肥的关系。

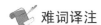 难词译注

obese [əu'bi:s] *a.*	肥胖的
overturn [ˌəuvə'tə:n] *v.*	推翻
the sleep-deprived	缺乏睡眠的人群

答案与解析

26. 【问题】Patel 的研究表明什么？
    A. 减肥和缺乏睡眠的关系。   B. 增肥和缺乏睡眠的关系。
    C. 减肥和锻炼的关系。   D. 增肥和锻炼的关系。
    【答案】B
    【解析】推断题。原稿第一段"His study of more than 68,000 women has found that those who sleep less than 5 hours a night gain more weight over time than those who sleep 7 hours a night."意思为：他对 6.8 万名女性的研究表明，晚上睡觉少于 5 小时的人与睡 7 小时的人相比体重会增加。所以应该讲的是睡眠不足与体重增加的问题，因此答案为 B"体重增加与睡眠少的关系"。

27. 【问题】Patel 的研究中有多少个受试者？
    A. 多于 68000。   B. 多于 60800。

C. 多于 60080。 D. 多于 60008。

【答案】A

【解析】此题为细节再现题。文章第一段提到他针对 68000 位女性进行研究。

28. 【问题】根据 Patel 的观点，下面哪一个不是正确的？

A. 睡 7 小时的睡眠者比睡 5 小时的人增重更多。

B. 睡 5 小时的人比睡 7 小时的人增重更多。

C. 睡眠少的人有 15% 的可能会肥胖。

D. 睡眠少的人比睡眠多的人消耗的热量少。

【答案】A

【解析】根据第一段研究结果做出判断：His study of more than 68,000 women has found that those who sleep less than 5 hours a night gain more weight over time than those who sleep 7 hours a night. 意思是睡眠不足 5 小时的人要比睡眠 7 小时的人增重更多，故本题选 A。

29. 【问题】根据 Patel 的观点，体重差异的原因是什么？

A. 睡眠不足者大都饮食过量。 B. 睡眠不足者大都很少锻炼。

C. 睡眠不足导致的低代谢率。 D. 睡眠不足导致的高代谢率。

【答案】C

【解析】根据文章中的这句话 "This finding overturns the common view that overeating among the sleep-deprived explains such weight differences." 可以得知研究结果推翻了普遍的观点——睡眠缺乏群体中的过激反应可以解释这样的体重差异，这可知选项 A 错误。"Lower metabolic rate or less fidgeting resulting from less sleep may be the reason behind the weight gain." 告诉我们代谢率低或者因为睡眠少造成的烦躁可能是原因，故选项 C 正确。

30. 【问题】如果想减肥，Patel 会给出什么样的建议？

A. 每天锻炼。 B. 服用饮食药片。

C. 控制饮食。 D. 睡得多一些。

【答案】D

【解析】此题可根据文章主旨进行解题，全文围绕睡眠和减肥的关系，指出睡眠不足会比睡眠较多的人增重更多，故选项 D 正确。

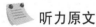 听力原文

Here's a dreamy weight-loss plan: take a nap. That's the message from work by Sanjay Patel at Case Western Reserve University in Cleveland, Ohio. His study of more than 68,000 women has found that those who sleep less than 5 hours a night gain more weight over time than those who sleep 7 hours a night.

Controlling for other differences between the groups, Patel found that women who slept 5 hours or less gained 0.7 kilograms more on average over 10 years than 7-hour sleepers. The short-sleeping group was also 32 percent more likely to have gained 15 kilograms or more, and 15 percent more likely to have become obese.

Significantly, the short-sleepers consumed fewer calories than those who slept 7 hours, says Patel, who presented his results this week at the American Thoracic Society International Conference in San Diego, California. This finding overturns the common view that overeating among the sleep-deprived explains such weight differences.

Lower metabolic rate resulting from less sleep may be the reason behind the weight gain, Patel suggests. "It obviously also suggests that getting people to sleep more might be a relatively easy way to help people lose weight," he says.

Questions:

26. What did the Patel's study indicate?

27. How many subjects did Patel have in his study?

28. According to the Patel's study, which of the following is not true?

29. According to Patel, what might be the reason behind the weight differences?

30. What is the suggestion Patel will give to those who want to lose weight?

🎧 Passage Three（2009 年真题）

31. A. Life evolution.　　　　　　　　　　B. Space exploration.
　　C. Extraterrestrial life.　　　　　　　　D. Unknown flying objects.

32. A. His 50th birthday.　　　　　　　　　B. NASA's 50th anniversary.
　　C. The university's 50th anniversary.
　　D. The US Cosmology Association's 50th Anniversary.

33. A. Even primitive life is impossible.　　　B. Intelligent life is fairly common.
　　C. Intelligent life is less likely.　　　　　D. Any form of life is possible.

34. A. Nuclear weapons.　　　　　　　　　B. Alien kidnapping.
　　C. Human extinction.　　　　　　　　　D. Dangerous infection.

35. A. Ironic.　　　B. Negative.　　　　　　C. Indifferent.　　D. Supportive.

【文章概要】文章通过 Stephen Hawking 在大学的报告讨论太空探索的重要性。

✏️ 难词译注

cosmic ['kɔzmik] a.　　　　　　　　　　宇宙的

stumble ['stʌmbl] v.　　　　　　　　　　困惑

extraterrestrial life　　　　　　　　　　外星生命

abduction [æb'dʌkʃən] n.　　　　　　　劫持

weirdo ['wiədəu] n.　　　　　　　　　　古怪的人

答案与解析

31. 【问题】文章主要讲什么？

   A. 生命进化。   B. 太空探索。

   C. 外星生命。   D. 未知飞行物。

   【答案】C

   【解析】此题为主旨题。通过完成细节题就可以得出主旨题的答案。

32. 【问题】霍金在乔治·华盛顿大学演讲时是什么重大事件？

   A. 他 50 岁生日。   B. NASA 50 周年。

   C. 大学 50 周年。   D. 美国宇宙协会 50 周年。

   【答案】B

   【解析】此题为细节再现。文中解题有效信息是：Hawking's comments were part of the lecture at George Washington University on Monday in honor of NASA's 50th anniversary（霍金的言论是为了庆祝 NASA 50 周年周一在乔治·华盛顿大学所做的演讲的一部分）。所以选项 B 正确。

33. 【问题】就外星生命而言，霍金支持的观点是什么？

   A. 甚至原始生命都不可能。   B. 智能生命相当普遍。

   C. 智能生命可能性较小。   D. 任何形式的生命都有可能。

   【答案】C

   【解析】此题为细节再现。文中解题有效信息是：Hawking said he prefers the third opinion, "Primitive life is very common, and intelligent life is fairly rare." 含义是他更倾向第三种观点：原始生命很普遍，但有智能的生命极其稀少。所以选项 C 正确。

34. 【问题】关于遇到外星人，霍金给出的警告是什么？

   A. 核武器。   B. 外星人绑架。

   C. 人类灭绝。   D. 危险的感染。

   【答案】D

   【解析】此题为细节再现。文中解题的有效信息是：Hawking warned, "Watch out if you would meet an alien. You could be infected with a disease to which you have no resistance." 即霍金警告说，如果遇到了外星人要小心，你可能被感染上你没有抗体的疾病。所以选项 D 正确。

35. 【问题】霍金对太空探索的态度是什么？

   A. 讽刺。   B. 反对。   C. 漠不关心。   D. 支持。

   【答案】D

   【解析】此题为推断题。文中解题的有效信息是：Hawking compared people who don't want to spend money on human space exploration to those who opposed to the journey of Christopher Columbus in 1492. "The discovery of the new world made a difference to the old. Just think we won't have had a Big Mac or KFC."这句话的意思是：霍金把不希望花钱进行人类太空探索的人比作那些 1492 年反对哥伦布航海的人。"新世界的发现影响到旧世界。想象我们还没有巨无霸或肯德基吧。"从这句话可知霍金对于太空探索的观点是支持的。注意，有关态度题，尤其是问说话人或作者态度时，类似选项 C 的不可能是正确答案，因而可以排除，因为漠不关心的态度与作者写作意图不相符。

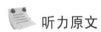 听力原文

Stephen Hawking

Life on other planet is likely, but intelligent life is less likely. Famed astrophysicist, Stephen Hawking has been thinking a lot about the cosmic question: Are we alone? "The answer is probably not," he says. "If there is life elsewhere in the universe," Hawking says, "why haven't we stumbled onto some alien broadcasts in space? Maybe something like 'alien quiz show'?" Hawking's comments were part of the lecture at George Washington University on Monday in honor of NASA's 50th anniversary. He theorized that there are possible answers to whether there is extraterrestrial life. One option is that there likely isn't any life elsewhere or maybe there is intelligent life elsewhere. But when it gets smart enough to send signals into space, it's also smart enough to make destructive nuclear weapons. Hawking said he prefers the third opinion, "Primitive life is very common, and intelligent life is fairly rare." He then quickly added: "Some would say it has yet to occur on earth." So should you worry about aliens? Alien abduction claims come from the "weirdos" and are unlikely. However, because alien life might not have DNA like us, Hawking warned, "Watch out if you would meet an alien. You could be infected with a disease to which you have no resistance." The 66-year-old British cosmologist who suffers from ALS and must speak through a mechanical device believes if the human race is to continue for another million years, we would have to boldly go where no one has gone before. Hawking compared people who don't want to spend money on human space exploration to those who opposed to the journey of Christopher Columbus in 1492. "The discovery of the new world made a difference to the old. Just think we won't have had a Big Mac or KFC."

Questions:

31. What is the passage mainly about?
32. What is the event when Hawking delivered his lecture at the George Washington University?
33. What is the idea Hawking favors in terms of extraterrestrial life?
34. What is Hawking's warning to the encounter of an alien?
35. What is Hawking's attitude towards human space exploration?

🎧 **Passage Four**（2009 年真题）

36. A. Obese people need more food.

    B. Obese people require more fuel.

    C. Obesity contributes to global warming.

    D. Obesity is growing as a global phenomenon.

37. A. Limited living space.

    B. Crowded shopping malls.

    C. Food shortage and higher energy prices.

    D. Incidence of diabetes and cardiovascular diseases.

38. A. Over 700 million.　　　　　　　　B. Over 400 million.

    C. Over 2.3 billion.　　　　　　　　D. Over 3 billion.

39. A. 1,800 calories.　　　　　　　　B. 1,280 calories.

    C. 1,680 calories.　　　　　　　　D. 2,960 calories.

40. A. Climate change.　　　　　　　　B. The fall of food prices.

    C. A rise in energy prices.　　　　　　D. An increasing demand for food.

【文章概要】肥胖也导致全球变暖。

✍ 难词译注

swell　[swel] v.　　　　　　　　　　　　　　增长

surpass　[səˈpɑːs] vt.　　　　　　　　　　　超越

🌱 答案与解析

36.【问题】下面哪一个能描述谈话主旨？

　　　　A. 肥胖者需要更多食物。　　　　B. 肥胖者要求更多的燃料。

　　　　C. 肥胖导致全球变暖。　　　　　D. 肥胖是一个日益严重的全球现象。

　　【答案】C

　　【解析】此题为主旨题。参见文章概要。

37.【问题】根据这个讲话，下面哪一个会因为肥胖人群增多变得更糟？

　　　　A. 有限的生存空间。

　　　　B. 拥挤的购物商场。

　　　　C. 食物短缺和更高的能源价格。

　　　　D. 糖尿病和心血管疾病的发病率。

　　【答案】C

　　【解析】此题为细节再现。短文提到：This adds to the food shortage and higher energy prices. 意思是"人口增长还加重了食物短缺和能源价格上涨。"因而选项 C 正确。

38.【问题】据世界卫生组织说，直到 2015 年，估计全球肥胖人数是多少？

A. 超过 7 亿。　　　　　　　　　B. 超过 4 亿。

C. 超过 23 亿。　　　　　　　　D. 超过 30 亿。

【答案】A

【解析】此题为细节再现。短文提到："At least 400 million adults worldwide are obese. The World Health Organization (WHO) projects by 2015, 2.3 billion adults will be overweight and more than 700 million will be obese. 含义是"现在全世界有至少 4 亿成年人肥胖。世界卫生组织认为到 2015 年将会有 23 亿人超重，并且有 7 亿多人肥胖。"故选项 A 正确。

39. 【问题】根据研究，一个肥胖人每天需要多少热量？

A. 1800 卡路里。　　　　　　　B. 1280 卡路里。

C. 1680 卡路里。　　　　　　　D. 2960 卡路里。

【答案】D

【解析】此题为细节再现。短文中提到：The researchers found that obese people require 1,680 daily calories to sustain normal energy and another 1,280 calories to maintain daily activities. 含义是"研究者发现肥胖人每天需要 1680 卡路里热量维持正常能量，还需要 1280 卡路里的热量维持日常活动。所以一个肥胖的人每天总共需要 2960 卡路里的热量。"故答案为 D。

40. 【问题】据爱德华和罗伯特的观点，如果我们改善了 BMI 的正常分布，会发生什么事？

A. 气候变化。　　　　　　　　　B. 食品价格下降。

C. 能源价格上涨。　　　　　　　D. 食品需求增加。

【答案】B

【解析】此题为细节再现。短文中提到：Promotion of a normal distribution of BMI would reduce the global demand for, and thus the price of, food. 含义是"改善 BMI 的正常分布可以降低全球需求，进而降低食品价格。"所以选项 B 正确。

 听力原文

Obesity Contributes to Global Warming Too

Obese and overweight people require more fuel to transport them, and the problem will worsen as the population grows, a team at the London School of Hygiene & Tropical Medicine says.

This adds to the food shortage and higher energy prices, the school's researchers wrote in the journal *Lancet* on Friday.

At least 400 million adults worldwide are obese. The World Health Organization (WHO) projects by 2015, 2.3 billion adults will be overweight and more than 700 million will be obese.

In their model, the researchers pegged 40 percent of the global population as obese with a body mass index of near 30. Many nations are fast approaching or have surpassed this level.

BMI is a calculation of height to weight, and the normal range is usually considered to be 18 to 25, with more than 25 considered overweight and above 30 obese.

The researchers found that obese people require 1,680 daily calories to sustain normal energy and another 1,280 calories to maintain daily activities, 18 percent more than someone with a stable BMI.

Because thinner people eat less and are more likely to walk than rely on cars, a slimmer population would lower demand for fuel for transportation and for agriculture.

This is also very important because 20 percent of greenhouse gas emission stems from agriculture.

The next step is quantifying how much a heavier population is contributing to climate change, higher fuel prices and food shortage.

"Promotion of a normal distribution of BMI would reduce the global demand for, and thus the price of, food," Edwards and Roberts wrote.

Questions:

36. Which of the following can best describe the main idea of the talk?
37. According to the talk, which of the following can be made worse by the growing obese population?
38. According to WHO, by 2015, what would be the estimated figure of the global obese population?
39. According to the researchers, how much energy would an obese person need for a day?
40. According to Edwards and Roberts, what would happen if we promote a normal distribution of BMI?

🎧 Passage Five（2008 年真题）

41. A. Smoking and lung cancer.   B. Lung cancer and the sexes.
    C. How to quit smoking.   D. How to prevent lung cancer.
42. A. Current smokers exclusively.   B. Second-hand smokers.
    C. With a lung problem.   D. At age 40 or over.
43. A. 156.   B. 269.
    C. 7,498.   D. 9,427.
44. A. Smoking is the culprit in causing lung cancer.
    B. Women are more vulnerable to lung cancer than men.
    C. Women are found to be more addicted to smoking than men.
    D. When struck by lung cancer, men seem to live longer than women.
45. A. Lung cancer can be early detected.
    B. Lung cancer is deadly but preventable.

    C. Lung cancer is fatal and unpredictable.

    D. Smoking affects the lungs of men and women differently.

【文章概要】讨论有关吸烟对男女肺部影响的差异，以及男女患肺癌的概率差异等。

 难词译注

compelling [kəm'peliŋ] *a.*	令人信服的
to date	到现在为止
be vulnerable to	易受……的伤害
twist [twist] *n.*	转变，转折
tumor ['tju:mə] *n.*	肿瘤
estrogen ['estrədʒən] *n.*	雌激素
ovary ['əuvəri] *n.*	卵巢

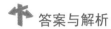 答案与解析

41.【问题】这个演讲主要是关于什么的？

    A. 吸烟和肺癌。   B. 肺癌和性别。

    C. 如何戒烟。   D. 如何预防肺癌。

【答案】B

【解析】这是很典型的长文章的题目，主旨题。考生可以最后解答这道题，因为把下面相关的细节题解决了，主旨就很容易概括归纳了。短文一开始就点题，讨论吸烟对女性和男性的影响，随后大篇幅介绍有关对男女吸烟者的研究，以及这个研究所得出的男女吸烟者患肺癌的情况。所以最贴切的主题是B。

42.【问题】这个研究的参与者的要求之一是什么？

    A. 不包含目前的吸烟者。   B. 吸二手烟者。

    C. 肺部有毛病的。   D. 年龄 40 岁以上的。

【答案】D

【解析】此题是细节题，短文中提到研究参与者的要求是健康，40 岁以上，现在或者以前是吸烟者。根据这些信息可知 D 为答案。

43.【问题】在整个历时八年多的过程中，有多少参与者得了肺癌？

    A. 156。   B. 269。   C. 7498。   D. 9427。

【答案】B

【解析】此题从选项上就可以知道题目和数字有关，因而在听短文时就应该特别留心和数字有关的信息，并加以记录。短文中提到研究过程中，研究者们发现有 113 名男性和 156 名女性出现肺肿瘤，相加可知答案是 B。

44.【问题】下面哪一个是研究的发现之一？

    A. 吸烟是肺癌的罪魁祸首。   B. 女性比男性更容易患肺癌。

C．发现女性比男性吸烟更上瘾。　　D．患上肺癌，男性似乎比女性活得久。

【答案】B

【解析】短文中提到 "… researchers determined that women are twice as vulnerable to lung cancer as men."，这句话表明女性比男性更易得肺癌，所以选项 B 为答案。

45．【问题】吸烟方面的调查者一致同意的是什么？

A．肺癌可以早期发现。　　　　　　B．肺癌致死但可以预防。

C．肺癌致死但不可预测。　　　　　D．吸烟对男女肺部的影响有差异。

【答案】B

【解析】短文最后提到所有调查者都愿意承认：肺癌尤其致命，但几乎完全可以预防。所以选项 B 为答案。

 听力原文

For years researchers have debated whether smoking effects the lungs in men and women differently. In a most compelling study on the topic to date, researchers determined that women are twice as vulnerable to lung cancer as men. But in a surprising twist, they die at half the rate of men.

The study, which was published last week in the Journal of the *American Medical Association*, included 9,427 men and 7,498 women from throughout North America who were healthy, at least 40 years old and either current or former smokers. Over the course of more than 8 years, a group of investigators led by Dr. Claudia Henschke of the Weill Medical College in New York City identified lung tumors in 113 of the men and 156 of the women. Then the researchers kept track of who lived and for how long, as well as the treatment participants were given. The study showed that both sexes tended to be in their late 60s when they received a lung-cancer diagnosis but that the women usually had smoked considerably less than the men. Still, at each stage of lung cancer, the women lived longer than the men.

If the reported results are confirmed, there are a few hints from other research that might explain the sex difference. Women's bodies appear to have greater difficulty repairing the damage to their genes caused by smoking, but there is also some evidence that estrogen, which is found in women's lungs as well as their ovaries, may interfere with some tumors' ability to grow.

There is one thing about which all investigators are ready to agree: lung cancer is particularly deadly and almost entirely preventable. So the take-home message is clear: Don't smoke! If you do smoke, quit!

Questions:

41. What is the talk mainly about?

42. What was one of the requirements for the participants of the study?

43. Over the course of more than eight years, how many of the participants developed lung cancer?

44. Which of the following is one finding of the study?

45. What is the consensus among all the investigators on smoking?

Passage Six（2008 年真题）

46. A. A hobby.
    C. A learning experience.
    B. The whole world.
    D. A career to earn a living.

47. A. Her legs were broken.
    B. Her arms were broken.
    C. Her shoulders were seriously injured.
    D. Her cervical vertebrae were seriously injured.

48. A. She learned a foreign language.
    C. She learned to be a teacher.
    B. She learned to make friends.
    D. She learned living skills.

49. A. She worked as a skiing coach.
    B. She was a college instructor.
    C. She was a social worker in the clinic.
    D. She worked as an elementary school teacher.

50. A. Optimistic and hard-bitten.
    B. Pessimistic and cynical.
    C. Humorous and funny.
    D. Kind and reliable.

【文章概要】介绍一个名叫 Jill Kinmont 的女孩，作为多项全国青年和成年滑雪赛事的获胜者，由于滑雪事故成为残疾人，并且如何不气馁地面对生活的故事。

难词译注

avid skier	滑雪爱好者
collapse [kə'læps] n.	崩塌
slope [sləup] n.	斜坡
cervical vertebrae	颈椎
hover ['hɔvə] v.	徘徊，翱翔
paralyze ['pærəlaiz] vt.	残疾
rehabilitation ['ri:(h)ə,bili'teiʃən] n.	康复

答案与解析

46. 【问题】发生事故前，滑雪对于 Jill 来说意味着什么？
    A. 爱好。　　　B. 全部。　　　C. 学习经历。　　D. 赚钱的事业。

【答案】B

【解析】短文中一开始提到 Jill 自述滑雪是一切，是全部，所以选项 B 为答案。

47. 【问题】当 Jill 从 Alta 山上滑下来的时候，发生了什么？

    A．腿断了。   B．手臂断了。

    C．肩部严重受伤。   D．颈椎严重受伤。

【答案】D

【解析】短文中提到她滑下来时落地不稳，导致第 4、5、6 节颈椎断裂，生死徘徊后，最终肩部以下残疾。故选项 D 为答案。如果对于颈椎这个词不了解，根据后文提到她残疾了也可以做出正确猜测。

48. 【问题】康复阶段 Jill 学习什么？

    A．她学外语。   B．她学习交朋友。

    C．她学做老师。   D．她学习生活技能。

【答案】D

【解析】短文提到，康复治疗期间她学习写字、打字以及如何吃饭。掌握了生活技能后，她又进入加利福尼亚大学学习艺术、德语和英语。根据以上提到的信息，选项 D 为正确答案。

49. 【问题】Jill 把什么当作新的事业？

    A．做滑雪教练。   B．大学老师。

    C．诊所的社工。   D．小学老师。

【答案】D

【解析】短文中提到她选择了新的工作目标，那就是教小学的孩子。所以选项 D 为正确答案。

50. 【问题】Jill 性格中最令人印象深刻的是什么？

    A．乐观且坚忍不拔。   B．悲观且吹毛求疵。

    C．幽默有趣。   D．热心肠且可靠。

【答案】A

【解析】此题是概括总结题。根据以上题目的解题答案很容易得出 Jill 是一个很乐观向上不服输的女孩，故选项 A 最符合。此外，短文中也提到康复治疗期间她一直乐观、坚定。

 听力原文

Jill Kinmont was an avid skier, competing and winning numerous titles in junior and senior national skiing events. As Jill says, "Skiing was it — everything — my world." Jill's world collapsed on Jan 30, 1955 when she skied off the Alta run and landed helplessly on the slope. Her fourth, fifth, and sixth cervical vertebrae were broken. For days, Jill hovered between life and death. By April, it became clear that she would be paralyzed from the shoulders down.

Jill underwent rehabilitation therapy with cheerful determination. She learned to write, to type, and to feed herself. Once she had mastered daily living skills, she enrolled in the University of California at Los Angeles, where she studied art, German, and English. After overcoming yet another personal tragedy, the death of her boyfriend in a plane crash, Jill graduated in 1961.

By this time, Jill had chosen a new career goal: teaching elementary school children. Officials at UCLA, however, rejected her application for admission to the graduate school of education because of her paralysis. But she persevered, working with children in the UCLA Clinic School. When her family moved to Seattle, Jill was able to fulfill her new dream. She attended the School of Education at the University of Washington and began her new life's work as a teacher.

She taught school first in Washington, then Beverly Hills in California. Finally moving back to Bishop in 1975 where she taught special education in Bishop Union Elementary School until her retirement in 1996.

Questions:

46. What did skiing mean to Jill before the accident?

47. What happened to Jill when she skied from the Alta run?

48. What did Jill learn during her rehabilitation?

49. What did Jill do as her new career?

50. What is the most impressive about Jill's personality?

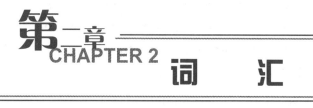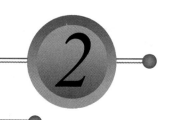

第一章 CHAPTER 2 词 汇

一、考试大纲的要求及试卷结构

　　根据考试大纲的要求，词汇用法部分旨在测试考生对英语词汇和短语的理解及使用能力。从试卷结构来看，这部分考试分为两个部分：Section A 和 Section B。考试时间约为10分钟。

Section A

　　这部分考题的题干中有一处空白，要求考生从四个备选项中选出一个最佳答案，使得题干语法正确、逻辑合理、意义完整。此部分一共10题，每题0.5分，共计5分。例如：

This environment can also affect a person's mental and _____ health.

A. conventional

B. personal

C. physical

D. impersonal

（答案：C）

Section B

　　这部分考题的题干有一个词或短语下面画有横线。要求考生从四个备选项中选出一个与画线部分的意义相同或近似的最佳答案。本部分测试的词或词组不超出考试大纲所要求掌握的单词、词组表。这部分一共有10题，每题0.5分，共计5分。例如：

The queer woman kept over one hundred cats in her house.

A. odd

B. energetic

C. generous

D. subtle

（答案：A）

二、真题演练与解析

Part II Vocabulary (10%)

Section A

Directions: *In this section all the sentences are incomplete. Four words or phrases, marked A, B, C and D, are given beneath each of them. You are to choose the word or phrase that best completes the sentence. Then, mark your answer on the **ANSWER SHEET**.*

1. There was no _____ but to close the road until February.
    A. dilemma
    B. denying
    C. alternative
    D. doubt

2. I _____ when I heard that my grandfather had died.
    A. fell apart
    B. fell away
    C. fell out
    D. fell back

3. I'm _____ passing a new law that helps poor children get better medicine.
    A. taking advantage of
    B. standing up for
    C. looking up to
    D. taking hold of

4. In front of the platform, the students were talking with the professor over the quizzes of their _____ subject.
    A. compulsory
    B. compulsive
    C. alternative
    D. predominant

5. The tutor tells the undergraduates that one can acquire _____ in a foreign language through more practice.
    A. proficiency
    B. efficiency
    C. efficacy
    D. frequency

6. The teacher explained the new lesson _____ to the students.
    A. at random
    B. at a loss
    C. at length
    D. at hand

7. I shall _____ the loss of my reading-glasses in newspaper with a reward for the finder.
    A. advertise   B. inform   C. announce   D. publish

8. The poor nutrition in the early stages of infancy can _____ adult growth.
    A. degenerate   B. deteriorate   C. boost   D. retard

9.   She had a terrible accident, but _____ she wasn't killed.
     A. at all events   B. in the long run
     C. at large   D. in vain

10. His weak chest _____ him to winter illness.
     A. predicts   B. preoccupies   C. prevails   D. predisposes

Section B

Directions: *Each of the following sentences has a word or phrase underlined. There are four other words or phrases beneath each sentence. Choose the word or phrase which would best keep the meaning of the original sentence if it were substituted for the underlined part. Mark your answer on the* **ANSWER SHEET**.

11. The company was losing money, so they had to lay off some of its employees for three months.
     A. owe   B. dismiss   C. recruit   D. summon

12. The North American states agreed to sign the agreement of economical and military union in Ottawa.
     A. convention   B. conviction
     C. contradiction   D. confrontation

13. The statue would be perfect but for a few small defects in its base.
     A. faults   B. weaknesses   C. flaws   D. errors

14. When he finally emerged from the cave after thirty days, John was startlingly pale.
     A. amazingly   B. astonishingly   C. uniquely   D. dramatically

15. If you want to set up a company, you must comply with the regulations laid down by the authorities.
     A. abide by   B. work out   C. check out   D. succumb to

16. The school master applauded the girl's bravery in his opening speech.
     A. praised   B. appraised   C. cheered   D. clapped

17. The local government leaders are making every effort to tackle the problem of poverty.
     A. abolish   B. address   C. extinguish   D. encounter

18. This report would be intelligible only to an expert in computing.
     A. intelligent   B. comprehensive   C. competent   D. comprehensible

19. Reading a book and listening to music simultaneously seems to be a problem for them.
     A. intermittently B. constantly   C. concurrently   D. continuously

20. He was given a laptop computer in <u>acknowledgement</u> of his work for the company.

A. accomplishment　　　　　　　B. recognition

C. apprehension　　　　　　　　D. commitment

✝ 答案及解析

1. 【答案】C

【解析】dilemma 困境，进退两难；denying 否认，拒绝；alternative 选择；doubt 怀疑。but 表示"除了……"。there was no denying or doubt 的含义为"毋庸置疑"，不符合句意。

题干译文：除了等到二月份封路，此外别无选择。

2. 【答案】A

【解析】fall apart 破碎，破裂，崩溃；例如：My bike is falling apart. 我的自行车要散架了。fall away 减少，消散；例如：All our doubts fell away gradually. 我们的一切疑虑逐渐消失了。fall out 掉落，脱落；例如：Due to extreme fatigue, his hair is falling out. 由于极度疲劳，他的头发在脱落。fall back 后退，撤退；例如：The army received the order that they would fall back tomorrow. 部队接到明天撤退的命令。

题干译文：当我听说我祖父去世的时候，我崩溃了。

3. 【答案】B

【解析】take advantage of 利用，例如：He took advantage of every opportunity to show himself in public. 他利用每一个机会在公众场合展示自己。stand up for 支持，维护；例如：You should learn to stand up for your rights. 你应该学会维护自己的权益。look up to sb. 钦佩，仰慕；例如：He is the only president looked up to by all people. 他是唯一受所有人钦佩的总统。take hold of "抓住，握住"，例如：Let's move the table. You take hold of that end. 我们来移开桌子，你抓住那一端。

题干译文：我支持通过一项新的法律，帮助穷苦的孩子获得更好的药品。

4. 【答案】A

【解析】compulsory 必修的；compulsive 强制的，强迫的；alternative 选择性的；predominant 卓越的，支配的，突出的。

题干译文：在讲台前，学生正在和教授讨论他们必修科目的测验。

5. 【答案】A

【解析】proficiency 熟练，精通；efficiency 效率；efficacy（药物，治疗）功效；frequency 频率。此题关键的突破点在于题干中的介词 in，以上这些词只有 proficiency 与介词 in 连用，表示"在……方面熟练"，例如：proficiency in English 精通英语。

题干译文：辅导教师告诉本科生，通过不断的练习，一个人就能精通一门外语。

6. 【答案】C

【解析】at random 随意地，任意地，胡乱地，例如：Names were chosen at random from the list. 名字是从名单中随意选择的。at a loss 不知所措，例如：His comments left me at a loss for words. 他的评论让我不知道该说什么好。at length 详尽地，例如：Please tell me what happened to you at length. 请详尽地告诉我在你身上发生了什么事情。at hand 接近，例如：Help is always at hand. 援助总是近在咫尺。

题干译文：老师给学生详细地讲授新课。

7. 【答案】A

【解析】advertise 作为动词的含义是"登广告"。inform 通知某人某事，常用表达式为：inform sb. of sth.；announce 宣布；publish 出版。

题干译文：我要在报纸上刊登眼镜的寻物启事，发现者将有奖金。

8. 【答案】D

【解析】degenerate 退化；deteriorate 使恶化；boost 促进；retard 阻碍，妨碍。infancy 幼年；nutrition 营养。

题干译文：幼年早期营养不良会阻碍成年成长。

9. 【答案】A

【解析】at all events 不管怎么样，无论如何，例如：At all events you should listen to your parents' opinions. 无论如何你应该听听你父母的意见。in the long run 最终，从长远观点来看，例如：In the long run, it is worthwhile to make an investment in education. 从长远来看，在教育上投资是值得的。at large 整个，全部，未被捕获的，例如：A few years ago there was unrest in the country at large. 几年前整个这个国家处于动荡中。The killer is still at large. 这个杀手仍然逍遥法外。in vain 徒劳，白费力气，例如：He tried to persuade her not to go out, but in vain. 他试图劝说她不要出去，但没用。

题干译文：她发生了可怕的意外，但不管怎么样，她没死。

10. 【答案】D

【解析】predict 预测；preoccupy 使全神贯注，迷住；prevail 流行，盛行；predispose 使预先有……倾向，易于感染，常与介词 to 连用，例如：Frustration predisposes him to look at things pessimistically. 挫折使他很悲观地看待事物。Fatigue predisposes one to cold. 疲劳使人容易感冒。此题的关键在于题干中的介词 to。

题干译文：他肺部很弱，冬天容易患病。

11. 【答案】B

【解析】题干中画线词组 lay off 的含义为"解雇"。owe 欠（债）；dismiss 解散，开除；recruit 招募；summon 召集。

题干译文：公司资金流失，他们不得不让一些员工停职 3 个月。

12. 【答案】A

【解析】题干中画线词 agreement 的含义是"协议，协定"。convention 惯例，习俗，协定；conviction 深信，定罪；contradiction 反驳，矛盾；confrontation 面对。

题干译文：北美国家同意在渥太华签署经济和军事联盟协议。

13. 【答案】C

【解析】题干中画线词 defect 的含义是"瑕疵"。fault 故障，毛病；weakness 弱点；flaw 瑕疵；error 过失，错误。题干中 statue 的含义是"雕像"，but for 意思是"要不是"，例如：But for your help, I couldn't have finished the work on time. 要不是你的帮忙，我们不可能按时完成工作。

题干译文：要不是底座上的一些小瑕疵，这个雕像会是完美的。

14. 【答案】B

【解析】题干中画线词 startlingly 意思是"令人吃惊地，大吃一惊地"。amazingly 令人惊讶地，令人惊奇地；astonishingly 惊讶的程度比 amazingly 强，与 startlingly 意思相近；uniquely 独特地，独一无二地；dramatically 极大地，相当地。故 B 为正确选项。

题干译文：约翰 30 天后终于从洞穴中出来，他脸色苍白，让人大吃一惊。

15. 【答案】A

【解析】题干画线词组 comply with 的意思是"顺从，遵从"。abide by 坚持，遵守；例如：It is very necessary to abide by your promises. 遵守你的承诺十分必要。work out 锻炼身体，计算出；例如：I used to work out regularly to keep fit. 过去我常常定期运动，保持身体健康。She was very disappointed because she couldn't work out the math problem. 因为没能解出这道数学题，她很失望。check out 调查，核实；例如：The police are checking out evidence they found. 警察们正在调查他们发现的证据。succumb to 屈服，屈从；例如：At last he succumbed to cancer and died. 他最终放弃抗争，死于癌症。

题干译文：如果要成立公司，就必须得遵守权力机构制定的条规。

16. 【答案】A

【解析】题干画线词 applaud 的意思是"鼓掌，赞许"。praise 表扬；appraise 估量，估价；cheer 兴高采烈；clap 鼓掌（表示赞许或欣赏），通常与 for 连用。

题干译文：学校校长在公开讲话中称赞这个女孩的英勇。

17. 【答案】B

【解析】题干画线词 tackle 的意思是"解决（问题）"。abolish 废除，废止（制度，法律等）。address 作为名词，意思是"地址，演说"；作为动词，意思为"写地址，发表演说，处理，对付"；extinguish 熄灭；encounter 遭遇。

题干译文：当地政府领导正千方百计解决贫穷问题。

18. 【答案】D

【解析】题干画线词 intelligible 的意思是"易懂的"。intelligent 聪明的；comprehensive 综合的；competent 有能力的，能胜任的；comprehensible 易于了解的。

题干译文：这篇报道只有计算方面的专家容易懂。

19. 【答案】C

【解析】题干画线词 simultaneously 的意思是"同时发生地"。intermittently 断断续续地，间歇地；constantly 经常地；concurrently 并存地，同时发生地；continuously 连续地。

题干译文：同时看书和听音乐对他们来说似乎是个问题。

20. 【答案】B

【解析】题干画线词 acknowledgement 的意思是"承认"，题干词组 in acknowledgement of 的意思是"感谢，谢礼"，例如：I was rewarded a medal in acknowledgement of my contribution to our company. 我被授予一枚奖章，以表彰我对公司的贡献。题干中的 laptop 指的是笔记本电脑。accomplishment 成就，完成；recognition 承认；apprehension 理解；commitment 承诺，允诺，奉献。

题干译文：为感谢他为公司所做的贡献，公司奖励他一台笔记本电脑。

三、考查内容及相应的应试技巧

（一）考查内容与解题步骤

医学考博英语词汇部分主要测试考生对单词和词组的识别和应用能力。Section A 与 Section B 两部分的考查内容分别具有以下特点：

1. Section A（填空题）

1) 考查考生对句意的理解和词汇含义的记忆能力。这类考题选项方面的特点是：备选词汇多为较高级词汇或较高级的高频词，要求考生选择与句意吻合的单词，例如上面试题中的第 1、4、8、10 题。

2) 考查考生对形近词的辨别能力，这类考题的选项特点鲜明：备选词汇在拼写上很相似或者都具有相同的前缀或后缀，例如上面试题中的第 5、10 题。

3) 考查考生对同义词、近义词的识别能力，这类考题的选项往往是意思相近的单词，例如上面试题中的第 7 题。

4) 考查考生对短语或词组的熟悉程度，例如上面试题中的第 3、9 题。

5) 考查考生对短语或词组搭配的掌握，这类考题的选项具有的特点是：四个备选项的动词都是同一个单词，如 go, come, fall, break 等，但它们各自的介、副词不同；或者四个选项的介、副词相同，但与之搭配的名词或动词不同，例如：上面试题中的第 2、6、9 题。

Section A 部分的解题步骤：

1) 仔细阅读题干，理解句子的大概含义，推测所填单词的含义；

2) 通过题干所提供的信息，看是否涉及搭配关系；

3) 根据对选项单词的掌握，先选择一个可能的答案，并放入题干中，通读全句，以验证所选词汇是否符合句意和题干中的搭配；

4) 如果题干存在某种逻辑关系，如因果、转折、对比等，还要注意自己的选择是否符合这些逻辑关系的表述；

5) 如果遇到选项中有自己不认识的单词，不要轻言放弃，要利用排除法解题。寻找题干中的解题信息，然后看看自己所熟悉的单词是否符合，如果不符合就可以排除，然后再在不熟悉的单词中判断最佳答案，例如：

Mary was so _____ with her money that she never spent a single extra penny.

A. rich   B. frugal   C. pretentious   D. stupid

【解析】根据对选项的分析，考生有可能不熟悉 B 选项，而可以通过构词法猜测 C 选项的大概含义，然后根据题干中的句型 so...that...（如此……以至……）来判断所熟悉的 A，C 和 D 是否符合句意。然后就可以排除这三个选项，因而答案为 B。

2. Section B（画线替换题）

1) 题干中画线词汇考生较为熟悉，但四个备选词汇中有的单词较生僻。或者题干画线词汇为常用单词，但在题中的含义是考生不熟悉的。

2) 题干中画线词汇考生不熟悉，但四个备选词汇多为考生认识的单词，例如上面试题中的第 15、18、19、20 题。

3) 选项中经常出现形近词，例如上面试题中的第 12、18 题。

4) 选项中可能出现近义词，例如上面试题中的第 13、14 题。

根据两部分词汇测试的不同特点，考生应该采用不同的解题步骤。

Section B 部分的解题步骤：

1) 先看画线单词或词组是否熟悉；

2) 然后再通读题干，确定画线部分的含义；

3) 最后根据自己对选项词义的理解，选择与画线部分含义最接近的一个，此部分注意解题要领为画线词的近义词而不是哪一个符合句意；

4) 同样，如果出现不认识画线单词的情况，一定要沉着冷静，在题干中寻找解题信息。例如：

Applicant will be asked to provide information on how they will <u>disseminate</u> information to other students at their university or college.

A. disclose   B. deliver   C. spread   D. analyze

【解析】考生可能不熟悉画线单词，但是题干中，我们可以判断这个单词为动词，它所在的句子部分为 they + V. information to other students... 这样，我们就可以判断大概含义就是他们给其他学生信息，因而画线部分有可能是"传递"的意思，可以判断选项应该在 B 和 C 中，最后再区分两个近义词的含义，B 的含义为"递送"，如递送包裹、报纸等，因而正确答案应该为 C。

（二）考生复习提示

无论掌握了什么样的解题技巧，在词汇测试中，考生的词汇知识毋庸置疑是解题的根本。因而各位考生应该加强自己对词汇知识的掌握。但是，考生们在进行词汇部分复习的时候，并非要机械简单地按照大纲词汇表记忆每个单词的拼写和含义，这样的复习收效也不会很好，而是要注意以下几个方面：

1. 根据自身水平，合理安排复习进度。在复习过程中，切忌按照大纲词汇表，从字母 A 开始，一个一个单词地进行。应该根据自己的词汇水平和词汇难易程度、考查范围有的放矢地进行复习。词汇难易程度和考查范围级别可以参看本丛书的词汇巧战通关。

2. 词汇的具体复习要做到广而精。根据上述考查内容的分析，考生在记忆单词含义和拼写的时候，要额外注意一词多义、派生词等。对于考试中的重点词汇，不能仅停留在认识的层次，要对这样的单词做到全面掌握。

3. 注意单词、词组之间的关系。复习过程中，要学会联想，也就是说要关注同义词、反义词以及形近词或词组。这样，复习的单词就不是单一、零散的，这对考试解题也大有帮助。

4. 记忆单词的方法要多样且有效。记忆单词的拼写绝对不意味着是死记硬背单词的字母组合，要寻求甚至自己创造记忆单词的方法，目的是能够准确且牢固地记住单词。本章下面的内容将会介绍几种单词记忆的方法。

5. 固定搭配要记牢。单词搭配，尤其是介、副词的搭配尤为重要，这在解题时有可能是关键点。

6. 培养自己对词汇语境含义的理解和认识。任何单词都不是孤立存在的，都会在一定的语境中充当一定成分，体现某个含义。这就需要考生在语境中理解单词的含义，这样不仅能更加准确地理解单词，而且对于阅读也有很大帮助。

7. 对于常用医学词汇要注意积累。虽然词汇测试部分不涉及医学词汇的考查内容，但是我们也要注意词汇在医学博士英语考试中的服务作用。考生有必要积累常用医学词汇，这对于其他考试部分尤其是阅读、写作都有很大帮助。

8. 勤复习、多运用。记忆单词绝对不是一遍就可以做到的，考生在记忆单词的时候要根据自身情况分阶段反复进行复习。此外，还要借助各种手段来巩固单词的拼写、发音和使用。

四、词汇记忆方法

这里介绍几种记忆单词的方法，供各位考生参考。

（一）词根词缀记忆法

在英语中，有很多词根是单词含义的根本，在词根的基础上增加前缀或者后缀，使得这个单词的含义发生转变。例如：cycl 相当于 circle，意思是"圆圈"，在这个词根的基础上增加前缀或后缀，就可以记忆很多词，如：

前缀 bi- 的含义是 two（两个），因而 bicycle 就是指两个圆圈，即为自行车。

cycle 作为名词含义为"周期"。

cyclic，后缀 -ic 为形容词的词缀，因而含义就是"周期的"。

recycle 是动词，前缀 re 的含义为 again（再次），因而这个单词的含义为"再生，回收"。

在复习中，考生要掌握一些常用词根、词缀，这样记忆单词就不再会毫无头绪，而是有规律可循，同时也可以减轻需要记忆的单词量。此外，这种记忆方法也有助于考生熟悉形近词。本节稍后会罗列一些常用词根、词缀。

（二）联想法

联想的形式和方法很多，比如派生词、形近词、同义词，这些都会帮助考生按照单词群去记忆。例如：

imagine, image, imaginable, imaginative, imaginary

（三）拆分法

拆分法就是将单词根据特定的特点拆分，利用它们之间的意义进行联想，从而达到记忆的效果。例如：

status — state + us   bonus — bone + us   campus — camp + us

这几个单词在进行拆分后，我们可以知道这几个词都和美国（US）有关，state + us 就是"美国状态地位"，所以 status 的含义就是"地位"；bonus 就是"美国的骨头"，含义为"奖金，红利"；camp + us 就是"美国的营地"，含义为"校园（很轻松，没有围墙）"。

这样的方法没有一定之规，考生可以根据自己的理解，形成记忆。

（四）口诀法

顾名思义，就是考生可以像编故事一样，将毫无关系的单词串联起来，例如：

绵羊（sheep） 走陡峭（steep） 哭泣（weep） 打扫（sweep） 再睡觉（sleep）

五、常用词根和词缀

↘ 词根

fer	带来	confer refer	offer transfer	differ suffer	infer	prefer
form	形状，形式	inform formal formation	perform former	platform information	transform format	uniform formula

（续）

pose	摆放	compose oppose	dispose propose	deposit purpose	expose suppose	impose
fin	结束，范围	define finite	refine finish	confine	infinite	
quire	寻求，得到	require	inquire	acquire		
vis	看	vision revise	visual devise	visible advise	television supervise	visit
scribe	写	describe	prescribe	script		
port	搬运	export passport	import portable	transport portion	opportunity proportion	support
pend	悬挂	expend	depend	suspend	expenditure	
sume	拿，取	assume	consume	presume	resume	
press	压，按	depress pressure	express	impress	compress	oppress
spect	看	aspect	respect	perspective	suspect	prospect
vail	强有力	available	prevail			
lect	选择	select dialect	elect reflect	collect	neglect	intellect
verse	转变	adverse	diverse	universe	reverse	converse
volve	转	revolve	involve	evolve		
mit	送，放出	commit summit	omit submit	transmit	permit	emit
tract	拉，拖	attract tractor	distract	contract	abstract	subtract
ceed	前行	exceed	succeed	proceed		
sist	站	assist	consist	resist	persist	insist
tain	拿住	attain entertain	contain retain	obtain maintain	stain	sustain
gress	前行	progress	regress	aggressive	congress	
dic	说话	contradiction indicate		dictation	predict	dictionary
tribute	给予	contribute	attribute	distribute		
lev	提高	elevator				
claim	大喊	exclaim	proclaim	declaim		

（续）

voc	叫喊	advocate	vocabulary	vocation	provoke	evoke
vac	空的	vacation	vacancy	vacant		
audi	听觉	audience audio auditorium		audit	auditor	audition
cent	百	percent	accent	innocent	decent	incentive
celer	快	accelerate				
cur	跑	current occur	currency excursion	curriculum		curtain
demo	人	demonstrate		democracy		demon
duct	带来	product	conduct			
dur	持续	endure	procedure	during		
fect	作用	perfect	effect	affect	infect	defect
fess	说	confess	professor	profession		
gene	出产，产生	gene generosity	generate generous	generation general		genius
ject	扔，投	object	subject	project	inject	reject
jud	判断	prejudice	judge	judicial		
manu	手	manufacture		manufacturer		manual
seque	跟随	subsequence		consequence		sequence
rupt	断裂	interrupt	bankrupt	corrupt	abrupt	erupt
sent	感觉	sentimental sensational		sensitive sense	sensible sensibility	
count	数字	account country	counter	encounter	discount	county
vey	看	survey	convey			
ply	重叠	apply supply	reply	imply	multiply	comply
prove	试验，验证	approve	improve			
tend	延伸，延展	attend tendency	contend tender	pretend	intend	extend
clude	关闭	conclude	include	exclude		
rect	正	correct	direct	erect		

↘ 前缀

anti-	反抗，反对	anti-corruption	anti-war
auto-	自己的，自动的	automation	autobiography
bi-	双的	bilingual	bilateral
dis-	相反	dishonest	disapprove
en-	使	enforce	encode
ex-	向外	export	external
im-	向内	import	implant
im-, in-	不	immortal	immature
inter-	相互，在内	interact	intertwine
mal-	坏，不良	malnutrition	maltreat
micro-	微小	microscope	microphone
mis-	错的	mislead	mischoice
out-	超过，过度	outweigh	outgrow
over-	过度	overweight	overdo
sub-	次的，亚于	submarine	subhealth
trans-	转换，横过	transform	transcontinental
tri-	三倍的	triangle	triagonal
un-	否定	unrest	unacceptable
under-	在下，不足	underabundant	underappreciated
uni-	单一的	uniform	unique
ab-	相反，变坏	abnormal	abuse
by-	副的，在旁的	byproduct	bypass
co-	共同	cooperate	coexist
cor-, col-	共同	collate	correspond
com-, con-	共同	combine	contemporary
de-	去掉	deforest	decode
em-, en-	包围；使……进入状态	embrace	empower
il-; ir-	不，否定	irregular	illegal

↘ 后缀

-ability -able	表能力	disability	capable
-er	动作执行者	examiner	employer
-ee	动作接受者	examinee	employee
-ality	性质，状态	personality	nationality
-ant	表示人	assistant	accountant
-ess	阴性的，雌性的	princess	hostess
-hood	表示身份，性质	neighborhood	childhood
-ify	使……化	simplify	purify
-ish	似……的	childish	selfish
-ism	主义，学说	capitalism	impressionism
-ize -ise -yze	……化	analyze	modernize
-less	不，没有	doubtless	valueless
-ogy	学科	biology	stomatology
-ness	性质，状态	carelessness	kindness
-ous -eous -ious	充满	hazardous	courteous
-ant	表示形容词	resistant	significant
-ance	表示名词	resistance	significance
-ary -ory	表示形容词	honorary	illusory
-tive	表示形容词	competitive	imaginative
-en	表动词，变成； 表形容词	quicken	wooden
-ence	表名词	existence	competence
-ial	表示形容词	beneficial	commercial
-ic	表示形容词	fantastic	cosmic
-ward	表示方向	upward	eastward
-ics	学科	physics	mathematics
-itude	性质，状态	solitude	fortitude
-ive	表示形容词	expensive	comprehensive
-ment	表示名词	encouragement	judgment
-or	表示人	actor	vendor

六、常用词组

↘ break

1. break away from

   The prisoner **broke away from** his guards. 犯人从看守者手中逃脱了。（挣脱，逃脱）

   This organization wished to **break away from** the committee and form a new one. 该组织想脱离委员会后自立门户。（脱离）

   She **broke away from** the others and opened up a two second lead. 她甩掉其他人，领先大约 2 秒的距离。[（尤指赛跑）甩掉]

2. break down

   Our car **broke down** on the highway. 我们的车子在高速公路上抛锚了。（出故障）

   Negotiations between the two sides have **broken down.** 双方谈判失败了。（失败）

   Her health **broke down** under the pressure of work. 在工作压力下，她的身体垮了。（垮掉）

   He **broke down** and wept when he heard the news. 他听到这个消息时不禁痛哭起来。（感情失去控制）

   Expenditure on the project **breaks down** as follows: raw materials $5,000, wages $4,000. 该项目开支如下：原材料 5000 美元，工资 4000 美元。（划分成部分）

   Firefighters had to **break** the door **down** to reach the people trapped inside. 消防员必须砸破这扇门才能营救困在里面的人。[打倒，砸破（某物）]

   He tried every means to **break down** her daughter's reserve, but in vain. 他竭尽所能去消除与她女儿之间的隔阂，但无济于事。（驱除，瓦解，消除）

   Break down your expenditure into bills, food and other. 将支出细分为现金、食物和其他。[将（金钱等）分类]

   Sugar and starch are **broken down** in the stomach. 糖和淀粉在胃里被分解。（使分解）

3. break for

   She had to hold him back as he tried to **break for** the door. 他突然冲着门跑去，她不得不拉住他。[（试图逃脱时）突然冲向]

4. break in

   Burglars **broke in** while we were away. 我们不在家时，盗贼闯入屋内行窃。（强行进入）

   Every April, the company will have a four-day orientation project to **break in** new recruits. 每年四月，公司会举办为期 4 天的新员工培训。（培训）

   She longed to **break in on** their conversation but didn't want to appear rude. 她想打断他们的谈话，但不想那么粗鲁。（打断）

5. break into

   As the professor stepped on the stage, all students **broke into** loud applause.

教授走上讲台时，所有学生爆发出热烈的掌声。（突然开始）

He **broke into** a run when he saw the police. 看见警察，他撒腿就跑。[撒腿就跑（突然开始快跑）]

I had to **break into** a $20 to pay the bus fare. 我不得不破开这张20美元的钞票付车票。（找开大面值钞票）

They had to **break into** the emergency food supplies because of the flood. 因为水灾，所以他们不得不动用应急储备的食物。（启用应急用品）

The company is having difficulty **breaking into** new markets. 公司打入新市场时遇到了困难。（顺利打入，成功参与）

6. break off

The back section of the plane **broke off**. 飞机座舱的后面脱落了。（折断，脱落）

He **broke off** in the middle of a sentence. 在句子中间他停顿了一下。（停顿，中断）

The country's government threatened to **break off** diplomatic relations. 该国政府以断绝外交关系相威胁。（断绝外交关系）

break off one's engagement 解除婚约

7. break out

She needed to **break out** of her daily routine and do something exciting. 她需要摆脱日常那些琐碎的工作，做一些有趣的事。[摆脱（状况），逃离（境地）]

Her face **broke out** in a rash. 她的脸突然长出皮疹。（突然布满某物）

He **broke out** in cold sweat. 他惊出了一身冷汗。（冒出）

8. break through（*n.* breakthrough）

The sun **broke through** at last in the afternoon. 下午，太阳终于从云层后面钻出来了。（冲破，突破）

a major **breakthrough** 重大突破

9. break up

The ship **broke up** on the rock. 船在礁石上撞得粉碎。（粉碎，破碎）

Their marriage has **broken up** / come to an end. 他们离婚了。（结束）

Sentences can be **broken up** into clauses. 句子可以分成从句。（分解，拆分）

↘ bring

1. bring about

What **brought about** the change in your attitude towards English study? 是什么原因导致你改变了学习英语的态度？（导致）

Most people are against **bringing about** the death penalty. 大多数人都反对恢复死刑。（恢复，重新使用）

2. bring back

Please **bring back** all library books by the end of the week. 请在本周末前归还所有从图书馆借的书。（归还）

The photo **brought back** many pleasant memories. 这张照片勾起许多美好的回忆。（使回忆起）

3. bring down

    The scandal may **bring down** the government. 这个丑闻可能导致政府垮台。（打垮，击败）

    We aim to **bring down** prices on all our computers. 我们打算降低我们所有计算机的价格。（降低，减少）

4. bring forth

    trees **bringing forth** fruit 结果的树

5. bring in

    Experts were **brought in** to advise the government. 让专家参与进来，为政府提建议。（让……参与）

    Two men were **brought in** for questioning. 两个男子被带到警察局问话。（逮捕）

    They want to **bring in** a bill to limit arms exports. 他们想提出限制武器出口的议案。（提出）

    His freelance work **brings** him **in** about $20,000 a year. 他做自由职业者，每年差不多有 2 万美元的收入。（挣得，获利）

6. bring off

    It was a difficult task but we **brought** it **off**. 任务很困难，不过我们顺利渡过了难关。（顺利渡过难关）

7. bring up

    We were **brought up** to respect authority. 我们受到的教育是要尊重权威。（抚养，养育）

↘ call

1. call for

    The government **called for** the immediate release of the hostages. 政府要求立即释放人质。（公开要求）

2. call forth

    His speech in public **called forth** an angry response. 他在公众场合的演讲引起了众怒。（引起，产生）

3. call in

    Cars with serious faults have been **called in** by the manufacturers. 厂家召回了有严重问题的车子。（召回）

4. call off

    The game was **called off** because of the bad weathers. 因为天气不好，所以比赛取消了。（取消）

5. call on / upon

    I now **call upon** the chairman to address the meeting. 现在我邀请主席为会议致辞。（邀请，恭请）

6. call up

The smell of the sea **called up** memories of her childhood. 海的味道让她回忆起童年时光。（使回忆起）

I **called** his address **up** on the computer. 我在电脑中调出他的地址。（调出地址/调用储存）

She **called up** her last reserves of strength. 她用尽最后一些力气。（使尽最后一点力气）

↘ **carry**

1. carry sb. back to = recall

The smell of the sea **carried her back to** the childhood. 海的味道让她回忆起童年时光。（回忆起）

2. carry off

Jean **carried off** all the prizes. 琼赢得了全部奖品。（赢得，获得）

3. carry out

Our planes **carried out** a bombing raid on enemy targets. 我们的飞机执行了一项轰炸敌方目标的任务。（执行，贯彻）

4. carry over

The confidence gained in remedial classes **carried over** into the children's regular school work. 孩子们在辅导班上获得的自信持续到他们正常的学校学习中去了。（延续）

5. carry sb./sth. through

His strong determination **carried him through** the ordeal. 他是靠自己坚强的决心渡过了难关。（帮助……渡过难关）

Despite powerful opposition, they managed to **carry their reforms through.** 尽管遇到了强大的阻力，他们还是设法进行了改革。（现实，完成）

↘ **come**

1. come about = happen

Can you tell me how the accident **came about**? 你能告诉我事故是如何发生的吗？（发生）

2. come across

Your speech **comes across** very well. 你的演讲相当受欢迎。（产生效果）

She **came across** some old photos in a drawer. 她在一个抽屉中偶然发现几张老照片。[（偶然）发现，遇见]

I hoped she would **come across with** some more information about the missing child. 我希望她会提供失踪孩子的一些信息。（提供，给予）

3. come along

When the right opportunity **comes along**, you should seize it. 当机遇出现时，你应该抓住。（到达，出现）

Your English has **come along** a lot recently because of your diligence. 因为你很勤奋，所以你的英语水平进步很大。（进步，进展）

4. come around / round

    Your mother hasn't yet **come round** from the anesthetic. 你母亲尚未从麻醉状态中苏醒过来。（恢复知觉）

5. come by

    Jobs are hard to **come by** now. 工作现在很难找。（得到，获得）

6. come out

    When will her new book **come out**? 她的新书什么时候出版？（出版，发行）

    The truth **came out** at the trial. 经过审讯，真相终于大白了。（真相大白）

7. come up

    The daffodils are just beginning to **come up**. 水仙花就要破土而出了。（破土而出，长出地面）

    I'm afraid something urgent has come up. 我想是发生了紧急事件。（发生）

    We'll let you know if any vacancies **come up**. 如果有空缺职位，我们会通知你。（出现）

    The question is bound to **come up** at the meeting. 会上一定会讨论这个问题。（被提及，被讨论）

    She **came up with** a new idea for increasing sales. 她想出了促进销售的新点子。（想出）

    His performance didn't really **come up to** his usual high standard. 他在表演中没有达到平时的高水平。（达到）

    We expect to **come up against** a lot of opposition to the plan. 我们预计这个计划会遭到很多人的反对。（面对，遭到反对）

↘ die

1. die away

    The sound of their laughter **died away**. 他们的笑声渐渐远去。（逐渐减弱，逐渐消失）

2. die back（植物）枝头枯萎（但根部仍活着）

3. die down

    The flames finally **died down**. 火焰终于熄灭了。（熄灭）

4. die off

    As she got older and older, her relatives all **died off**. 随着她越来越老，她的亲属都相继去世了。（相继死去）

5. die out

    This species has already **died out** because its habitat had been destroyed. 这一物种已经灭绝，因为它们的栖息地被毁掉了。（灭绝）

↘ fall

1. fall apart

    The deal **fell apart** when we failed to agree on the price. 由于我们双方没有就价格达成一致，生意没有做成。（破裂，告吹）

2. fall away

His supporters **fell away** as his popularity declined. 因为他的声望下降了，支持者的人数在减少。（减少）

The market for their products **fell away** to almost nothing. 他们产品的市场占有率几乎减到零。（消散）

3. fall behind

We can't afford to **fall behind** our competitors in using new technology. 我们再也不能在使用新技术方面掉在竞争对手的后面了。（落后）

4. fall down

That's where the theory **falls down**. 这便是该理论的不足之处。（失败，不起作用）

5. fall on / upon sb. or sth.

The children **fell on** the food and ate it greedily. 孩子们向食物扑去，贪婪地吃了起来。（扑向）

The full cost of the wedding **fell on** her parents. 婚礼的全部费用都落到她父母身上。（由……负担）

6. fall out

Jane and Paul **fell out** with each other. 简和保罗争吵不休。（争吵）

7. fall over

I rushed for the door and **fell over** the cat in the hallway. 我冲向门，在走廊时被猫绊倒了。（绊倒）

8. fall through

Our plan **fell through** because of lack of money. 我们的计划因缺钱而落空了。（失败）

↘ **give**

1. give away

He **gave away** most of his money to charity. 他把大部分钱都捐赠给了慈善机构。（捐赠）

The principal **gave away** the prizes at the school sports day. 校长在学校运动会上颁奖。（颁发）

They've **given away** two goals already. 他们已经白白送给对方两个球了。（白送）

She **gave away** state secrets to the enemy. 她向敌人泄露了国家机密。（泄露机密）

2. give in

give sth. in to sb. = hand over sth. to sb. 呈上，交上

3. give off

The flowers **gave off** a fragrant perfume. 花散发出香味。（散发，放出）

4. give out

After a month their food supplies **gave out**. 一个月后，他们的食物耗尽了。（用完，耗尽）

Her legs **gave out** and she collapsed. 她的腿残疾了，她整个人崩溃了。（坏掉）

The teacher **gave out** the exam papers. 老师发考试卷。（分发）

The radiator **gives out** a lot of heat. 暖气片散发出大量的热能。（散发）

5.　give up

After a week on the run, he **gave himself up to** the police. 逃亡一周之后，他向警方投案自首了。（投案自首）

I have **given up on** you. 我对你已不抱希望。（对……不抱希望）

➥ **go**

1.　go about

Despite the threat of war, people **went about** their business as usual. 尽管受到战争的威胁，人们还继续忙着自己的事，一如往常。（继续做，忙于某事）

How should I **go about** finding a job? 我该如何着手去找工作？（着手做）

2.　go after

She left the room in tears so I **went after** her. 她流着泪离开了房间，我追了出去。（追赶）

Unfortunately both my best friend and I are **going after** the same job. 不幸的是，我和我最好的朋友应聘的是同一份工作。（追求某人，谋求某事）

3.　go against sb.

He would not **go against** his parents' wishes so he went abroad for further study. 他不愿违背父母的意愿，于是他出国深造去了。（违背，不相符）

4.　go along

I'd **go along with** you there. 在那一点上我赞同你的意见。（赞成，支持）

5.　go at

John **went at** Bob when the class was over. 约翰一下课就扑向了鲍勃。（攻击某人）

He **went at** his breakfast as if he hadn't eaten for days. 他吃早餐时的样子就像多日没吃东西似的。（拼命干）

6.　go by

Things will get easier as time **goes by**. 随着时间的推移，事情会变得越发简单。（时间流逝）

He always **goes by** the rules. 他总是根据规则办事。（遵循，依照）

7.　go for

They have a high level of unemployment—but the same **goes for** many other countries. 该国失业率很高，不过其他很多国家也是这样。（适用于）

go for sth.

I hear you're **going for** that job. 我听说你准备争取那个职位。（争取获得）

8.　go in for

Several people **went in for** the race. 有几个人参加了赛跑。（参加考试或比赛等）

She doesn't **go in for** team games. 她对团队比赛项目不感兴趣。（对……感兴趣）

9. go through

He's amazingly cheerful considering all he's had to **go through**. 想到自己经历过的一切，他欣喜若狂。（经历）

Have you **gone through** all your money? 你把所有的钱都花光了吗？（用完，耗尽）

10. go with

Disease often **goes with** poverty. 疾病和贫穷常相伴而生。（与某物相伴而生）

It is very common that the color of green doesn't **go with** red. 一般说来，绿色与红色不相配。（与……相配）

11. go without

There wasn't time for breakfast, so I had to **go without**. 没时间吃早饭了，所以只好不吃了。（将就，没有……也行）

⤵ hand

1. hand down to sb.

These skills used to be **handed down** from father **to** son. 这些手艺在过去常常是父传子的方式。（传承）

2. hand in

Please **hand in** your papers. 请交卷。（上交，提交）

3. hand over

He resigned and **handed over** his work to his colleague. 他辞职了，并把工作移交给了同事。[（权力，责任）移交]

⤵ hold

1. hold back

The police were unable to **hold back** the crowd. 警察无法拦住人群。（拦阻）

You could become a good musician, but your lack of practice is **holding** you **back**. 你有可能成为一名优秀的音乐家，但是缺少练习正在妨碍你的发展。（妨碍发展）

hold back information 隐瞒信息

hold back one's anger 压住怒火

hold back tears 忍住泪水

hold sb. **back** from doing sth. 阻止某人做某事

2. hold down

It took three men to **hold** him **down**. 三个人才将他制服。（制服）

The people are **held down** by a repressive regime. 人民受到残酷政权的压迫。（压迫）

The rate of inflation must be **held down**. 通货膨胀率必须控制在较低的水平。（控制在低水平）

He was unable to **hold down** a job after the accident. 事故发生后他无法保住自己的工作了。（保住）

3. hold forth 喋喋不休，大发议论

4. hold on

They managed to **hold on** until help arrived. 他们一直坚持到救援到来。（坚持住，顶住）

These nuts and bolts **hold** the wheels **on**. 这些螺栓和螺母将车轮固定住。（固定住）

5. hold off

We could get a new computer now or **hold off** until prices are lower. 我们可以现在就买台新电脑或者推迟到价格低一些再买。（推迟）

He **held off** all the last-minute challengers and won the race in a new record time. 他与其他选手保持一定距离并赢得了比赛，创造了一项新纪录。（战胜，克服）

6. hold out

We can stay here as long as our supplies **hold out**.
只要给养充足，我们就留在这里。（维持，坚持）

The doctor **held out** little hope of her recovery. 医生对她康复不抱多大希望。（提供机会，给予希望，使有可能）

7. hold up

She is **holding up** well under the pressure. 她能很好地承受压力。（承受住）

An accident is **holding up** traffic. 事故阻碍了交通。（阻碍）

My application was **held up** by the postal strike. 邮政系统罢工把我的申请耽误了。（耽搁）

His idea was **held up** to ridicule. 他的想法被当成笑料。（举出例子；提出）

↘ keep

1. keep away from

His illness **kept** him **away from** work for several weeks. 他生病了，几周都无法工作。（阻止）

2. keep back

She was unable to **keep back** her tears. 她无法抑制住自己的泪水。（抑制或阻止感情等流露）

He **kept back** half the money for himself. 他将一半的钱留给自己。（保留或扣留某物一部分）

I'm sure they are **keeping** something **back** from me. 我确信他们有事瞒着我。（隐瞒）

3. keep down

The people have been **kept down** for years by a brutal regime. 人们已在暴政下被奴役多年。（压制，奴役）

The government is trying to **keep down** inflation. 政府正试图控制通货膨胀。（控制，防止）

4. keep off

I'm trying to **keep off** fatty foods. 我正在试着不吃脂肪多的食物。（回避，避免）

They lit a fire to **keep off** wild animals. 他们点燃火把以使野生动物无法靠近。（使某人／某物不接近）

5. keep on 继续

6. keep to sth.

He **kept to** his room for the first few days of term. 这个学期的头几天，他一直待在自己的房间里。（留在某个位置，不离开）

I'm resigning — but **keep** it **to** yourself! 我会辞职——但你自己知道就行了，不要说出来。（遵守，信守，对……保守秘密）

7. keep up

The rain **kept up** all afternoon. 整个下午都在下雨。（持续不变）

The high cost of raw materials is **keeping** prices **up**. 较高的原料价格使商品价格居高不下。（居高不下）

keep sb. up 使某人熬夜

➘ pay

1. pay back

I'll **pay** him **back** for making me look like a fool in front of everyone. 他让我在大家面前像个傻子，我要报复他。（报复）

2. pay in

Have you **paid** the cheque **in** yet? 你把支票存入银行了吗？（存入）

3. pay off

We **paid** him **off** at the end of the week. 我们周末给他算清工资后就把他解雇了。（付清工资解雇）

4. pay out

I **paid out** a lot of money for that car. 我为那辆车付出了一大笔钱。（付出大笔款项）

5. pay up 偿还（欠款），全部付清

➘ pick

1. pick at 磨蹭着吃；揪，扯

2. pick off

Snipers were **picking off** innocent civilians. 狙击手逐个瞄准无辜百姓射杀。（逐个瞄准射击）

3. pick out

She **picked out** a scarf to wear with the dress. 她挑选了一条围巾以配她穿的衣服。（精心挑选）

4. pick up

Sales have **picked up** 14% this year. 全年的销售增加了14%。（好转，改善）

All I seem to do is cook, wash and **pick up** after the kids. 我所做的全部工作是做饭、洗衣以及在孩子屁股后收拾。（收拾，整理）

The bus **picks up** passengers outside the airport. 公共汽车在机场外接旅客。（接载）

A lifeboat **picked up** survivors. 救生艇在营救生还者。（营救，搭救）

He was **picked up** by the police and taken to the station for questionings. 他被警察逮捕，并被带到派出所审问。（逮捕，抓捕）

He **picked up** the phone and dialed the number. 他拿起电话拨号。（拿起）

We were able to **pick up** the BBC World Service. 我们能收听到BBC World Service的节目。（接收信号、节目）

She **picked up** French when she was living in Paris. 她在巴黎生活期间学会了法语。（学到，得到）

Scientists can now **pick up** early symptoms of the disease. 科学家现在能辨认疾病的早期症状。（辨认）

I **picked up** my coat from the cleaner on the way home. 我在回家的路上到洗衣店取回衣服。（取回）

I seemed to have **picked up** a terrible cold from somewhere. 我好像从什么地方染上了重感冒。（感染）

pick up the trails of animals 追寻动物的踪迹

pick up the theme again 回到主题

I **picked up** the faint sound of a car in the distance. 我觉察到远处汽车微弱的声音。（察觉，发现）

⤵ pull

1. pull back

   Their sponsors **pulled back** at the last minutes. 他们的赞助人在最后一刻打了退堂鼓。（打退堂鼓）

   They **pulled back** a goal just before half-time. 下半场结束前他们扳回一球。（挽回局势）

2. pull down 拆毁

3. pull through

   The doctors think she will **pull through**. 医生认为她会痊愈的。（恢复，痊愈）

   It's going to be tough but we'll **pull through** it together. 这件事会很困难，不过我们会协力完成的。（完成，做成）

⤵ put

1. put sth. aside

   They decided to **put aside** their differences. 他们决定将分歧搁在一边。（搁置，不理睬）

2. put away

   She has a few thousand dollars **put away** for her retirement. 她攒了几千美元，留作退休后使用。（积攒）

   He must have **put away** a bottle of whisky last night. 他昨晚一定是喝了一瓶威士忌。（猛吃，喝）

3.   put back

Poor trading figures **put back** our plans for expansion. 贸易数据极差，我们扩张的计划因此推迟。（延迟，推迟）

Remember to **put** your clock **back** tonight because the time has officially changed. 记得把时钟拨慢，因为官方时间已更改。（拨慢时间）

4.   put down

The novel is so interesting that I couldn't **put it down**. 小说很精彩，我一看起来就无法释卷。（放下）

The meeting's on the 22nd. **Put it down** in your diary. 会议日期是 22 号，记在日记里。（写下）

The military government is determined to **put down** all opposition. 军人政府决定镇压所有反对者。（镇压，平定）

The cat is so miserable that we had to have it **put down**. 这只猫现在太痛苦了，我们不得不给它用药物结束生命。（用药物结束生命）

5.   put forward 拨快时钟；提出（建议）

6.   put off

The match had to be **put off** because of the heavy rain. 比赛因大雨而推迟。（推迟）

The sudden noise **put** me **off** my game. 突然的噪声让玩游戏的我分神了。（使分神）

7.   put on

Due to lack of regular exercise, I have **put on** several kilos. 因为缺乏锻炼，我增重了几公斤。（增加体重）

A foreign drama club is **putting on** a new drama in Beijing. 一个外国戏剧俱乐部在北京上演一场新戏剧。（举办，上演）

8.   put out

Firefighters soon **put** the fire **out**. 消防员很快扑灭了大火。（扑灭）

The plant **puts out** 500 new mobile phones a week. 工厂一周可以生产500部新手机。（生产，制造）

Police have **put out** a description of the man at large. 警察公布了这名在逃犯的情况。（公布）

➡ **take**

1.   take after （在外貌、性格等方面）与（父、母等）相像

2.   take apart 拆（机器）

3.   take away

I was given some pills to **take away** the pain on the back. 给我开了一些药，可以消除我的背痛。（解除，消除）

4.   take back

The picture **took** me **back** to my childhood. 这张图片让我回忆起童年时光。（使回想起）

5. take down 拆除；写下，记录

6. take in

The old woman **took in** those homeless children. 这位老妇人收留了那些无家可归的孩子。（收留）

He listened very attentively, **taking in** every word the professor said. 他听得十分认真，把教授的每一句话都领会了。（吸收）

7. take off 起飞，脱下，模仿

8. take on

The city has taken great changes recently and **takes on** a new look. 这座城市进来变化巨大，呈现出崭新的面貌。（呈现）

She was **taken on** as a trainee. 她被雇用了。（雇用）

9. take out

The fine will be **taken out** of your salary. 罚款将从你的工资中扣除。（扣除）

It is very awful for me to **take out** teeth. 拔牙真是太可怕了。（切除，摘除）

10. take over 接管

11. take to

I've **taken to** go to bed very early. 我养成了早睡的习惯。（养成……习惯）

He hasn't **taken to** his new school. 他还没有对这所新学校产生好感。（对……产生好感）

12. take up

Lap tops will not **take up** much room. 笔记本电脑占用空间较小。（占地方）

七、词汇专项练习及最新真题解析

Section A

Directions: *In this section all the sentences are incomplete. Four words or phrases, marked A, B, C and D, are given beneath each of them. You are to choose the word or phrase that best completes the sentence. Then, mark your answer on the **ANSWER SHEET**.*

1. He had always had a good opinion of himself, but after the publication of his best-selling novel he became unbearably _____.

   A. cordial   B. proud

   C. conceited   D. exaggerated

2. An enormous number of people in the world's poorest countries do not have clean water or adequate sanitation _____.

   A. capacities   B. facilities   C. authorities   D. warranties

3. Pleasure, or joy, is vital to _____ health.
   A. optimistic   B. optional   C. optimal   D. operational

4. I haven't met anyone _____ the new tax plan.
   A. in honor of   B. in search of   C. in place of   D. in favor of

5. At the party we found the shy girl _____ her mother all the time.
   A. harmonizing with   B. clinging to
   C. depending on   D. adjusting to

6. This software can be _____ to the needs of each customer.
   A. tailored   B. administrated   C. entailed   D. accustomed

7. If the cells cannot use sugar, the body begins to _____ its own tissues for food.
   A. break through   B. break down   C. break out   D. break over

8. If you are a member of the company, you must _____ to its rules.
   A. approach   B. conform   C. respond   D. abide

9. It is the only problem requiring special techniques and _____.
   A. qualification   B. therapies   C. specification   D. expertise

10. Some officials insist that something be done to _____ inflation.
    A. curb   B. sue   C. detoxify   D. condemn

11. Human beings are _____ creatures, designed to be on the move.
    A. distinctive   B. dynamic   C. intrinsic   D. mysterious

12. The fall in production over the past year has caused 200 workers to be made redundant and a further 500 have been _____ temporarily.
    A. laid off   B. laid down
    C. laid out   D. laid away

13. The black clouds and the lightning suggest that a big storm is _____.
    A. eminent   B. imminent   C. immense   D. immanent

14. Stories in this novel seem to have happened in the real world, however, all characters and plots are _____.
    A. imaginable   B. imaginative   C. imaginary   D. imaging

15. He has a very _____ plan: he wants to master three foreign languages and travel abroad in three years.
    A. arbitrary   B. aggressive   C. ambitious   D. abundant

16. The local government decided to gave the top _____ to education.
    A. authority   B. protection   C. profession   D. priority

17. When a psychologist does a general experiment about the human's attitudes towards pressure, he selects interviewees _____ and asks them questions.
    A. at random   B. in essence   C. at heart   D. in bulk

18. He was _____ of a crime he didn't commit. He fought for many years to prove his innocence.
    A. convicted   B. convinced   C. conceived   D. condemned

19. Finding out information about these universities has become easy for anyone with Internet _____.
    A. entrance   B. admission   C. access   D. entry

20. The disrespectful sons began to concern about the ultimate _____ of the family's property.
    A. proposal   B. disposal   C. removal   D. refusal

21. Two decades ago a woman who shook hands with others on her own _____ was usually viewed too forward.
    A. endeavor   B. initiative   C. motivation   D. preference

22. He wanted to stay at home, but at last he agreed, very _____ though, to go to the cinema.
    A. decisively   B. reluctantly   C. willingly   D. deliberately

23. His parents blamed his son for his _____ the younger children in school.
    A. imitating   B. intimating   C. intimidating   D. emigrating

24. Eating too much fat can _____ heart diseases and cause hypertension.
    A. distribute to   B. attribute to   C. devote to   D. contribute to

25. The soccer team has had five _____ victories in the last three years.
    A. successive   B. excessive   C. subsequent   D. eventual

26. The Car Club couldn't _____ to meet the demands of all its members.
    A. ensure   B. guarantee   C. insure   D. assure

27. In the Chinese household, grandparents and other relatives play _____ roles in raising children.
    A. incapable   B. insensible   C. indispensable   D. infinite

28. None of us expected the chairman to _____ at the party. We thought he was still in hospital.
    A. turn in   B. turn over   C. turn up   D. turn down

29. The European Union countries were once worried that they would not have _____

supplies of petroleum.

    A. proficient   B. efficient   C. potential   D. sufficient

30. His wife is constantly finding _____ with him, which makes him very angry.

    A. errors   B. weakness   C. fault   D. flaw

31. His neighbors became _____ of his behavior and contacted the police.

    A. suspicious   B. doubtful   C. susceptible   D. dubious

32. It is suggested that criticism without any tips for improvement is not _____ and should be avoided.

    A. constructive   B. destructive   C. productive   D. descriptive

33. It is _____ that the Internet is exerting a growing important influence on people's lives.

    A. indistinctive   B. indissoluble

    C. indispensable   D. indisputable

34. He _____ on her new dress without even looking at it.

    A. complemented   B. complimented

    C. praised   D. appraised

35. AIDS is becoming the top threat to people's health, and the _____ fatal disease claimed many lives.

    A. deceptively   B. invariably   C. imperatively   D. transiently

36. He is an extreme arbitrary leader, so everything must be done in _____ with his ideas.

    A. appliance   B. compliance   C. defiance   D. reliance

37. When he realized that he had been _____ to sign the contract, he threatened to take legal actions to cancel the agreement.

    A. adduced   B. induced   C. deduced   D. produced

38. Local people are encouraged to _____ their homes to save energy.

    A. insulate   B. insane   C. assault   D. insult

39. During the Olympics, the emergency services were _____ in the Olympic Village.

    A. by hand   B. in hand   C. at hand   D. on hand

40. In order to pursue the click rate, the Internet media reported _____ social news deliberately.

    A. sensitive   B. sensible   C. sensational   D. sensory

41. They set up a(n) _____ training schedule for the candidates for the final competition.

    A. ridiculous   B. rigorous   C. ambiguous   D. anonymous

42. The new traffic regulations of "even and odd-numbered license plates on alternate

days" will make a(n) _____ difference to most people.

A. appreciative

B. appreciable

C. comprehensive

D. comprehensible

43. At _____ Smith received a medal as a reward for his prominent achievements in research.

A. compliment

B. complement

C. commitment

D. commencement

44. As the most outstanding writer in the 20th century in America, Hemingway created lots of _____ works.

A. impartial   B. immortal   C. immemorial   D. immoral

45. We have arranged to go to the cinema on Friday, but we can be _____ and go another day.

A. probable   B. reliable   C. flexible   D. feasible

46. Some people apparently have an amazing ability to _____ the right answer.

A. come up with   B. look up to   C. put up with   D. clear up

47. On behalf of our school, I'm _____ to your generous help in the earthquake.

A. subject   B. inclined   C. liable   D. obliged

48. The appearance of this used car is quite _____, and it is much newer than it really is.

A. descriptive   B. impressive   C. deceptive   D. indicative

49. All the information we have collected in relation to that case _____ very little.

A. adds up to   B. comes up with   C. puts up with   D. keeps up with

50. We now obtain more than two-thirds of our protein from animal sources, while our grandparents _____ only one-half from animal sources.

A. originated   B. digested   C. deprived   D. derived

51. The new secretary has written a remarkably _____ report in a few pages but with all details.

A. concise   B. clear   C. precise   D. elaborate

52. Expected noises are usually more _____ than unexpected ones of the like magnitude.

A. manageable   B. controllable   C. tolerable   D. perceivable

53. With prices _____ so much, it's hard for the company to plan a budget.

A. fluctuating   B. waving   C. swinging   D. vibrating

54. Please do not be _____ by his bad manners since he is merely trying to attract attention.

A. disregarded   B. distorted   C. irritated   D. intervened

55. Sam assured his boss that he would _____ all his energies in doing this new job.
    A. call forth   B. call at   C. call on   D. call off

56. Care should be taken to decrease the length of time that one is _____ loud continuous noise.
    A. subjected to   B. filled with
    C. associated with   D. attached to

57. The news item about the earthquake is followed by a detailed report made _____.
    A. on the spot   B. on site
    C. on location   D. on the ground

58. Mother who takes care of everybody is usually the most _____ person in each family.
    A. considerate   B. considerable
    C. considering   D. constant

59. If you know what the trouble is, why don't you help them to _____ the situation?
    A. simplify   B. modify   C. verify   D. rectify

60. I tried very hard to persuade him to join our group but I met with a flat _____.
    A. disapproval   B. rejection   C. refusal   D. decline

61. He has failed me so many times that I no longer place any _____ on what he promises.
    A. faith   B. belief   C. credit   D. reliance

62. The wealth of a country should be measured _____ the health and happiness of its people as well as the material goods it can produce.
    A. in line with   B. in terms of
    C. regardless of   D. by means of

63. His _____ and unwillingness to learn from others prevent him from being an effective member of the team.
    A. arrogance   B. dignity   C. humility   D. solitude

64. An ambulance must have priority as it usually has to deal with some kind of _____.
    A. urgency   B. danger   C. emergency   D. crisis

65. The old man _____ defended the right of every citizen to freedom of choice in religion, which enabled him to win the respect of all people.
    A. peculiarly   B. indifferently   C. vigorously   D. inevitably

66. The _____ difference in Chinese dialect has become a problem in mutual communication among people.
    A. enormous   B. immense

C. imminent   D. eminent

67. In the family where the roles of men and women are not sharply separated and where many household tasks are shared to a greater or lesser extent, notions of male _____ are hard to maintain.
    A. privilege   B. predominance
    C. prevalence   D. priority

68. After years of being exposed to the sun and rain, the sign over the shop had become completely _____.
    A. illegal   B. eligible
    C. illegible   D. unreasonable

69. It's time you _____ some reading or the other students will leave you behind.
    A. got down to   B. adapted to
    C. held on to   D. attended to

70. Geologists maintain that a mountain is a mountain _____ its geological structure though it may not reach an altitude of 3,000 feet above sea level.
    A. by virtue of   B. in the way of
    C. by way of   D. for the sake of

71. Find out how researchers will inform you about the trial's progress or _____ you of any problem.
    A. denounce   B. secure   C. notify   D. ensure

72. America simply does not have enough prisons to _____ all its criminals.
    A. cope with   B. put up to   C. hold up   D. dispose of

73. Dying patients receive some small hope that the new treatment may _____ the course of disease but risk experiencing severe side effects.
    A. prolong   B. identify   C. alter   D. expose

74. The thief was caught because of the neighbors' _____.
    A. vigilance   B. aggregate   C. varnish   D. visage

75. A body that produces its own light waves, like the sun or an electric bulb, is said to be _____.
    A. illuminative   B. flashy   C. luminous   D. flaming

76. True, he couldn't see the tears, yet she was afraid that voice would _____ her emotion.
    A. give off   B. give away   C. give over   D. give out

77. Shops _____ the do-it-yourself craze by offering consumers bits and pieces which

they can assemble at home.

    A. ask for   B. send for   C. run for   D. cater for

78. A new technique, called electronic dental anaesthesia could soon _____ the need for the dreaded dentist's needle.

    A. amplify   B. decrease   C. stimulate   D. meet

79. Shortness of breath often goes hand in hand with _____, the kind that sweeps over the whole body and isn't confined to one area.

    A. infection   B. fatigue   C. syncope   D. suffocation

80. At the national level, the National Institutes of Health and especially the National Institute on Aging are _____ many types of research programs on aging.

    A. allocating   B. expanding   C. sponsoring   D. summing

81. HIV and AIDS may threaten the fundamental values of society, and any attempt to deal with them presents a _____ challenge.

    A. formidable   B. fatal   C. favorable   D. fantastic

82. Kelley's publicists abruptly _____ a planned seven-city publicity tour, announcing that their "publishing objectives have been accomplished".

    A. called off   B. called down   C. called up   D. called for

83. Crowding as an environmental variable is only beginning to be seriously examined and the data so far is _____.

    A. informative   B. inconclusive   C. inconspicuous   D. indisputable

84. During the sterilization process which follows, the cans are _____ to steam or boiling water with the temperature and duration varying according to the type of food.

    A. proportional   B. subjected   C. susceptible   D. liable

85. But research can have no economic impact if the new scientific discoveries are not _____ into marketable goods and services.

    A. launched   B. translated   C. dissected   D. conveyed

86. Nature never ceases to surprise us. Molecules with _____ structures and properties turn up in the laboratory all the time.

    A. bioactive   B. miniature   C. bizarre   D. invisible

87. Since patients cannot always tell the difference between psychologically induced chest pain and heart attack, the physician should _____ the possible causes of the pain.

    A. rule out   B. divide up   C. bring apart   D. sort out

88. David L. Rinion of School of Medicine, the University of California, Los Angeles says

that such a test, if it _____ expectations could usher in a new area of prenatal diagnosis.

    A. meets up with　B. comes up with　　C. sheds light on　　D. lives up to

89. Suffering from his leg illness, Tom is very _____ nowadays.

    A. emaciated　　B. eligible　　　C. elastic　　　　　D. exceptional

90. Today investigators are still far from _____ a master map of the vasculature of the heart.

    A. constituting　B. decoding　　　C. drafting　　　　D. encoding

91. I have never seen a more caring, _____ group of people in my life.

    A. emotional　　B. impersonal　　C. compulsory　　D. compassionate

92. As we need plain, _____ food for the body, we must have serious reading for the mind.

    A. wholesome　　B. diet　　　　　C. tasteful　　　　D. edible

93. The best exercise should require continuous _____, rather than frequent stops and starts.

    A. compassion　B. acceleration　C. frustration　　D. exertion

94. Salk won _____ as the scientist who developed the world's first effective vaccine against polio.

    A. accomplishment　　　　　　　B. qualification

    C. eminence　　　　　　　　　　　D. patent

95. A coronary disease is the widely-used term _____ insufficiency of blood supply to the heart.

    A. denoting　　B. donating　　　C. relating　　　　D. resorting

96. It is the builder's job to make sure that the house conforms to the architects' _____ in every way.

    A. regulations　B. specialities　　C. essentials　　D. specifications

97. I'm afraid that you'll have to _____ the deterioration of the condition.（2008 年真题）

    A. account for　B. call for　　　C. look for　　　　D. make for

98. Twelve hours a week seemed a generous _____ of your time to the nursing home.（2008 年真题）

    A. affliction　　B. alternative　　C. allocation　　D. alliance

99. Every product is _____ tested before being put into the market.（2008 年真题）

    A. expensively　B. exceptionally　C. exhaustively　D. exclusively

100. Having clean hands is one of the _____ rules when preparing food.（2008 年真题）

    A. potent　　　　B. conditional　　　　C. inseparable　　　　D. cardinal

101. The educators should try hard to develop the _____ abilities of children.（2008 年真题）

    A. cohesive　　　B. cognitive　　　C. collective　　　　D. comic

102. Mortgage _____ had risen in the last year because the number of low-income families was on the increase.（2008 年真题）

    A. defects　　　B. deficits　　　C. defaults　　　　D. deceptions

103. The symptoms may be _____ by certain drugs.（2008 年真题）

    A. exaggerated　B. exacerbated　　C. exceeded　　　D. exhibited

104. Her story was a complete _____ from start to finish, so nobody believed in her.（2008 年真题）

    A. facility　　　B. fascination　　　C. fabrication　　　D. faculty

105. The police investigating the traffic accident have not ruled out _____.（2008 年真题）

    A. salvage　　　B. safeguard　　　C. sabotage　　　D. sacrifice

106. The government always _____ on the background of employees who are hired for sensitive military projects.（2008 年真题）

    A. takes up　　　B. checks up　　　C. works out　　　D. looks into

107. The _____ conditions and places are likely to cause diseases.（2009 年真题）

    A. unsanitary　　B. insidious　　　C. insane　　　　D. inefficacious

108. The witness was _____ by the judge for failing to answer the question.（2009 年真题）

    A. abstained　　B. acquitted　　　C. admonished　　　D. adduced

109. He has _____ two cars this year because of traffic accidents.（2009 年真题）

    A. pulled of　　B. worn out　　　C. passed out　　　D. written off

110. People are much better informed since the _____ of the Internet.（2009 年真题）

    A. convenient　　B. advent　　　C. interface　　　D. aftermath

111. All instruments that come into contact with the patient must be _____ before being used by others.（2009 年真题）

    A. sterilized　　B. labeled　　　C. quarantined　　　D. retained

112. By adopting this cunning policy, the clinic risks _____ many of its patients.（2009 年真题）

    A. acquitting　　B. allocating　　　C. alleviating　　　D. alienating

113. Diabetes upsets the _____ of sugar, fat and protein.（2009 年真题）

    A. metastasis　　B. metabolism　　　C. malaise　　　D. maintenance

114. The muscular _____ can affect the way we feel mentally.（2009 年真题）

    A. potency   B. fiber   C. lethargy   D. synthesis

115. Evidence is widespread that HIV-infected persons show to _____ their unsafe behavior.（2009 年真题）

    A. respond to   B. reflect on   C. wipe out   D. put off

116. Publicly, they are trying to _____ this latest failure, but in private they are very worried.

    A. put off   B. laugh off   C. pay off   D. lay off

117. The poor nutrition in the early stages of infancy can _____ adult growth.

    A. degenerate   B. deteriorate   C. boost   D. retard

118. During rush hour, downtown streets are _____ with commuters.

    A. scattered   B. condensed   C. clogged   D. dotted

119. A number of black youths have complained of being _____ by the police.（2010 年真题）

    A. harassed   B. distracted   C. sentenced   D. released

120. Despite his doctor's note of caution, he never _____ from drinking and smoking.（2015 年真题）

    A. retained   B. dissuaded   C. alleviated   D. abstained

121. People with a history of recurrent infections are warned that the use of personal stereos with headsets is likely to _____ their hearing.（2015 年真题）

    A. rehabilitate   B. jeopardize   C. tranquilize   D. supplement

122. Impartial observers had to acknowledge that lack of formal education did not seem to _____ Larry in any way in his success.（2015 年真题）

    A. refute   B. ratify   C. facilitate   D. impede

123. When the supporting finds were reduced, they should have revised their plan _____ .（2015 年真题）

    A. accordingly   B. alternatively   C. considerably   D. relatively

124. It is increasingly believed among the expectant parents that prenatal education of classical music can _____ future adults with appreciation of music.（2015 年真题）

    A. acquaint   B. familiarize   C. endow   D. amuse

125. If the gain of profit is solely due to rising energy prices, then inflation should be subsided when energy prices _____ .（2015 年真题）

    A. level out   B. stand out   C. come off   D. wear off

126. Heat stroke is a medical emergency that demands immediate _____ from qualified medical personnel. (2015 年真题)

    A. prescription   B. palpation   C. intervention   D. interposition

127. Asbestos exposure results in Mesothelioma, asbestosis and internal organ cancers, and _____ of these diseases is often decades after the initial exposure. (2015 年真题)

    A. offset   B. intake   C. outlet   D. onset

128. Ebola, which spreads through body fluid or secretions such as urine, _____ and semen, can kill up to 90% of those infected. (2015 年真题)

    A. saline   B. saliva   C. scabies   D. scrapes

129. The newly designed system is _____ to genetic transfection, and enables an incubation period for studying various genes. (2015 年真题)

    A. comparable   B. transmissible   C. translatable   D. amenable

130. Employers have a legal obligation to pay _____ to their workers for injuries. (2016 年真题)

    A. compensation   B. compromise   C. commodity   D. consumption

131. The argument between the two patients became so fierce that the doctor had to _____. (2016 年真题)

    A. alleviate   B. aggravate   C. extinguish   D. intervene

132. But despite all the legal hustle and bustle, they don't actually expect to _____ death sentences to life terms without parole. (2016 年真题)

    A. induce   B. convert   C. revive   D. swerve

133. To maintain physical well-being, a person should eat _____ food and get sufficient exercise. (2016 年真题)

    A. integral   B. gross   C. wholesome   D. intact

134. The Central Government's pledge to maintain the _____ and stability of Hong Kong at all costs is a great encouragement to the local finance. (2016 年真题)

    A. provision   B. prosperity   C. privilege   D. preference

135. It is pointed out that patients must be reassured that "their lives will not be _____ as a result of bed shortages". (2016 年真题)

    A. facilitated   B. forfeited   C. fulfilled   D. furnished

136. The cause of his death has been a mystery and _____ unknown so far. (2016 年真题)

    A. exclusively   B. superficially   C. utterly   D. doubtfully

137. It is known that some ways of using resources _____ can destroy the environment as

well as the people living in it. （2016 年真题）

    A. recklessly   B. sparingly   C. sensibly   D. incredibly

138. Cholera is a preventable waterborne bacterial infection that is spread through _____ water. （2016 年真题）

    A. filtered   B. distilled   C. contaminated   D. purified

139. We welcome him not _____ as a new broom but rather as a very old friend. （2016 年真题）

    A. by the way   B. at all events   C. by no means   D. in any sense

140. Chronic high-dose intake of vitamin A has been shown to have _____ effects on bones. （2017 年真题）

    A. adverse   B. prevalent   C. instant   D. purposeful

141. Drinking more water is good for the rest of your body, helping to lubricate joints and _____ toxins and impurities. （2017 年真题）

    A. screen out   B. knock out   C. flush out   D. rule out

142. Rheumatologist advises that those with ongoing aches and pains first seek medical help to _____ the problem. （2017 年真题）

    A. affiliate   B. alleviate   C. aggravate   D. accelerate

143. Generally, vaccine makers _____ the virus in fertilized chicken eggs in a process that can take four to six months. （2017 年真题）

    A. penetrate   B. designate   C. generate   D. exaggerate

144. Danish research shows that the increase in obese people in Denmark is roughly _____ to the increase of carbon dioxide in the atmosphere. （2017 年真题）

    A. equivalent   B. temporary   C. permanent   D. relevant

145. Ted was felled by a massive stroke that affected his balance and left him barely able to speak _____. （2017 年真题）

    A. bluntly   B. intelligibly   C. reluctantly   D. ironically

146. In a technology-intensive enterprise, computers _____ all processes of the production and management. （2017 年真题）

    A. dominate   B. overwhelm   C. substitute   D. imitate

147. Although most dreams apparently happen _____, dream activity may be provided by external influences. （2017 年真题）

    A. homogeneously   B. instantaneously

    C. spontaneously   D. simultaneously

148. We are much quicker to respond, and we respond far too quickly by giving _____ to

our anger.（2017 年真题）

A. vent   B. impulse   C. temper   D. offence

149. By maintaining a strong family _____, they are also maintaining the infrastructure of society.（2017 年真题）

A. bias   B. honor   C. estate   D. bond

150. The medical team discussed their shared _____ to eliminating this curable disease.（2017 年真题）

A. obedience   B. susceptibility   C. inclination   D. dedication

答案及解析

1. **【答案】C**

   【解析】 此题考点为备选词是否符合句意。cordial 热诚的，衷心的；proud 自豪的；conceited 自负的；exaggerated 夸张的，夸大的。此题解题的关键在于题干中所给的信息。have a good opinion of oneself 意思是"自视过高"。unbearably 意思是"不堪忍受的"。只有 C 符合句意。

   题干译文：他一向自视过高，但在他最畅销的小说出版后，他又开始变得自负，让人无法忍受。

2. **【答案】B**

   【解析】 此题考点为备选词是否符合句意。capacity 容量，能力，才能；facility 设施，设备；authority 权威；warranty 正当理由，保证。此题解题的关键在于题干中所给的信息。enormous 庞大的；adequate 适当的，足够的；sanitation 卫生。故只有 B 符合句意。

   题干译文：在那些世界上最穷困的国家里有许多人没有清洁的水或者足够的卫生设施。

3. **【答案】C**

   【解析】 此题考点为形近词辨析。optimistic 乐观的；optional 可选择的；optimal 最佳的，最理想的；operational 操作的，运作的。只有 C 符合句意。

   题干译文：愉悦或快乐，是保持理想健康状态的关键。

4. **【答案】D**

   【解析】 此题考点为词组辨析。in honor of 的含义是"为纪念……"，例如：The monument is in honor of soldiers losing lives for the country. 这个纪念碑是为了纪念为国家牺牲的士兵们。in search of 的含义是"寻找"，例如：He went in search of a doctor for his sick son. 他为他生病的儿子寻找医生。in place of 的含义是"替代"，例如：Nothing can be used in place of love of mother. 没有什么可以用来替代母爱。in favor of 的含义是"赞同，支持"，例如：Those who are in favor of my suggestion nodded. 那些支持我的建议的人们点着头。只有 D 符合句意。

题干译文：我还没遇到一个支持新税计划的人。

5. 【答案】B

【解析】此题考点就是备选词组的含义是否符合句意。harmonize with 的含义是"与……和谐，协调"，例如：The colors harmonize well with the decorations on the wall. 这个颜色和墙上的装饰很协调。cling to 的含义是"依附，依靠，坚持"，例如：I was caught in the heavy rain and wet clothes clung to my body. 我淋了雨，湿衣服紧贴在身上。depend on 的含义是"依靠，依赖"，例如：He hasn't found a job so he has to depend on his parents. 他还没找到工作，所以他依靠父母生活。adjust to 的含义是"适应，调节"，例如：You should adjust yourself to the new environment as soon as possible. 你应该尽快适应新环境。

题干译文：在聚会上我们发现这个害羞的女孩一直黏着她妈妈。

6. 【答案】A

【解析】此题考点为备选词是否符合句意。tailor 做名词时的含义是"裁缝"，做动词时的含义是"定做，专门制作"，例如：Special courses are tailored to the needs of specific groups. 制定特殊课程，以满足特殊群体的需要。administrate 管理，支配；entail 使必要，使承担；accustom 使习惯于，固定搭配是 be accustomed to。此题解题的关键在于题干中的介词 to，根据固定搭配可以排除 B 和 C，再根据题干句意要求排除 D。

题干译文：这个软件可以为顾客量身定做。

7. 【答案】B

【解析】此题考点为词组辨析。break through "突破，克服"，例如：They have broken through in the fight against AIDS. 他们在抗击艾滋病方面已经有所突破。In front of the platform, he managed to break through his reserve. 在讲台前，他试图克服拘谨。break down "使……分解，出故障"，例如：Sugar and starch are broken down in the stomach. 糖和淀粉在胃里被分解。Our car broke down on the way home. 我们的车在回家路上抛锚了。break out 的含义是"爆发"，例如：Fire broke out last night. 昨晚上发生了火灾。break over 这个搭配极为少见，意思是"破例"。

题干译文：如果细胞不能使用糖，身体就开始分解自身的组织来提供养分。

8. 【答案】B

【解析】此题解题的关键在于题干中的介词 to，根据四个备选单词各自的含义以及介词搭配就可以解题。approach 做动词的含义是"临近"，例如：The winter is approaching. 冬季即将来临。做名词，且与介词 to 连用，含义是"方式，方法"，例如：I support his approach to the problem. 我支持他解决这个问题的方法。conform "顺应，遵守（法律、规则等），相符合"，例如：You should conform to the local customs when you are in foreign countries. 在外国你应该遵从当地风俗。Every driver is required to conform to traffic laws. 每一个驾驶员都必须遵守交通法规。This building doesn't conform to the style of this city. 这座建筑物与这个城市的风格不一致。respond 的含义是"回答"，例如：He hasn't responded to my letter. 他还没给我回信。abide 的含义是"忍受，容忍"，常与 by 连用，意为"遵守"，例如：It is the students' responsibility to abide by regulations in school. 遵守学校规章制度是学生的责任。故本题选 B。

题干译文：如果你是公司成员，就必须遵守公司的规章。

9. **【答案】D**

【解析】 此题解题的关键在于题干所给的信息。qualification 资格；therapy 治疗；specification 规格，说明书；expertise 专门的知识或技能。

题干译文：这是唯一一个要求特殊技巧和技能的问题。

10. **【答案】A**

【解析】 此题解题的关键在于题干中的动宾搭配。curb 控制，遏制；sue 起诉，控告；detoxify 使解毒；condemn 谴责，判刑。

题干译文：一些官员建议要采取措施遏制通货膨胀。

11. **【答案】B**

【解析】 此题解题的关键在于题干所给的信息。题干中 on the move 的含义是"在活动中，在进行中"，例如：Science is always on the move. 科学总是在进步。根据这个词组的含义就可以解题。四个选项含义如下：distinctive 有特色的；dynamic 动态的，有活力的；intrinsic 本质的，本身的；mysterious 神秘的。

题干译文：人类是富有活力的生物，总是在前进。

12. **【答案】A**

【解析】 此题的考点是固定搭配的辨析，解题的关键在于题干所给予的信息。题干中 redundant 的含义是"多余的"。to be made redundant 的含义就是"冗员而被裁减"。lay off 的含义是"解雇"，例如：Many workers were laid off last year. 去年许多工人被解雇了。lay down 的含义是"放下"，例如：The killer surrendered and laid down his arms. 凶手投降，放下了武器。lay out 的含义是"布局，安排，展示"，例如：The living room is poorly laid out. 客厅布局很差。lay away 的含义是"储备"，例如：Many animals always lay away food for winter. 许多动物都会为冬天储存食物。

题干译文：去年生产力下降使得 200 名工人被裁员还有 500 名工人被暂时解雇。

13. **【答案】B**

【解析】 此题考点为形近词辨析。四个选项含义如下：eminent 著名的，卓越的；imminent 即将发生的；immense 广大的，无边无际的；immanent 内在的，固有的。

题干译文：乌云和闪电说明暴风雨即将来临。

14. **【答案】C**

【解析】 此题考点为形近词辨析。四个选项含义如下：imaginable 可以想象的，可能的；imaginative 富有想象力的；imaginary 虚构的，想象的；imaging 为名词，意为"使成像"。

题干译文: 这本小说里面的故事似乎在现实世界发生过,但所有人物和情节都是虚构的。

15. 【答案】C

【解析】此题解题关键在于题干提供的信息。四个选项含义如下:arbitrary 专横的；aggressive 侵略的；ambitious 有野心的，雄心勃勃的；abundant 丰富的，充裕的。

题干译文: 他有一个很雄心勃勃的计划:三年中要掌握三门外语,以及出国旅行。

16. 【答案】D

【解析】此题考点是固定搭配。各选项含义如下:authority 权威,威信；protection 保护；profession 职业,表白,宣布；priority 优先权。give the top priority to 给予······最优先权。

题干译文: 当地政府决定优先发展教育。

17. 【答案】A

【解析】此题考点是词组含义。各选项含义如下: at random 随意地；in essence 本质上；at heart 本质上；in bulk 大批地。

题干译文: 当一个心理学家要就人类对压力的态度进行试验时,他会随意选择被访问者问他们一些问题。

18. 【答案】A

【解析】此题解题关键在于题干中的介词 of 以及句意。be convicted of 的含义是"被控······罪",例如:The young man was convicted of theft. 这个年轻人被控盗窃罪。be convinced of 的含义是"确信",例如:I am fully convinced of his honesty. 我完全相信他的诚实。conceive of 的含义是"构思,想到",例如:Unfortunately, he didn't conceive of the possibility of any difficulty. 不幸的是,他没能想到任何困难的可能性。condemn 的含义是"谴责,判刑"。

题干译文: 他被判刑,但其实他并没有犯罪。他多年来一直为证明自己的清白而斗争。

19. 【答案】C

【解析】此题考点为近义词辨析。entrance 的含义是广义的"入口"；admission 的含义是"允许进入"；access 符合句意的"互联网入口"；entry 的含义是"入口,通道"。

题干译文: 对于能上网的人来说,找到这些大学信息很容易。

20. 【答案】B

【解析】此题考点为形近词辨析,解题的关键在于题干所提供的信息。四个选项含义如下:proposal 提议,建议；disposal 处置,安排；removal 移动,切除；refusal 拒绝。题干中 disrespectful 的含义是"无礼的"。

题干译文: 不孝之子开始关注家产如何处置了。

21. 【答案】B

【解析】此题考点为固定搭配。on one's own initiative 的含义是"主动地",例如:I felt very surprised that he came to help on his own initiative. 他主动来帮忙,我感到很意外。其他三项:endeavor 努力；motivation 动机；preference

偏爱。题干中的 decade 指"十年"。

题干译文：二十年前主动握手的女士通常被认为太超前了。

22. 【答案】B

【解析】此题解题的关键在于题干提供的信息。四个选项的含义为：decisively 果断地；reluctantly 不情愿地；willingly 自愿地；deliberately 故意地。题干中的转折词是解题的信号词。

题干译文：他想待在家里，但最终还是不情愿地同意去看电影。

23. 【答案】C

【解析】此题考点为形近词辨析。imitate 模仿；intimate 形容词的含义是"亲密"，动词的含义为"提示，通告"；intimidate 威胁，恐吓；emigrate 移民。

题干译文：因为儿子在学校威胁年龄较小的孩子，父母批评了他。

24. 【答案】D

【解析】此题考点为形近词组辨析。distribute to 的含义是"分发，分配"，例如：They distributed new clothes to those orphans. 他们把新衣服分发给那些孤儿。attribute to 的含义是"归因于"，例如：He attributed his success to diligence. 他把成功归功于勤奋。devote to 的含义是"致力于"，例如：The scientist devoted himself to his research. 这位科学家致力于他的研究。contribute to 的含义是"贡献，造成，导致"，例如：His living habits contributed to his poor health. 他的生活习惯导致他健康不佳。

题干译文：吃太多脂肪能导致心脏病和高血压。

25. 【答案】A

【解析】此题考点为四个备选单词的含义与题干句意。四个选项含义如下：successive 连续的，继承的；excessive 过多的，过分的；subsequent 后来的，并发的；eventual 最终的。

题干译文：这个足球队在过去三年里连续取得了五场胜利。

26. 【答案】B

【解析】此题考点为形近词辨析。ensure 的含义是"保证，担保"，例如：The pills ensure that you can have a good sleep tonight. 这药片保证你今晚能睡个好觉。guarantee 的含义是"保证"，例如：We guarantee to deliver the goods in three weeks. 我们保证三周后交货。insure 的含义是"为……投保险"，例如：He insured himself against illness. 他为自己投保了病险；assure 的含义是"向……保证"，例如：I assure you that I didn't mean to hurt you. 我向你保证我没打算要伤害你。

题干译文：汽车俱乐部不能保证满足所有会员的需求。

27. 【答案】C

【解析】此题考点为四个备选单词的含义与题干句意。四个选项含义如下：incapable 无能的；insensible 无知觉的；indispensable 不可缺少的；infinite 无限的，无穷的。

题干译文：在中国家庭里，祖父母以及其他亲戚在抚养孩子上起着不可或缺的作用。

28. 【答案】C

【解析】此题考点是词组辨析。turn in 的含义是"归还"，例如：You are required to turn in your pass when you leave here. 你离开这里的时候要交还通行证。turn over 的含义是"翻转"，例如：She turned over in the bed and couldn't fall asleep. 她在床上辗转反侧无法入睡。turn up 的含义是"到来，出现"，例如：She is still hoping that good luck will turn up. 她仍旧希望好运出现。turn down 的含义有：①拒绝，例如：She turned down his invitation politely. 她礼貌地谢绝了他的邀请。②把……调小，例如：He turned the lights down in the room. 他把房间里的灯光调暗了。

题干译文：我们没人料到主席出现在聚会上，我们以为他还在住院。

29. 【答案】D

【解析】此题考点为形近词辨析。四个选项含义如下：proficient 精通的；efficient 有效率的；potential 潜在的；sufficient 充足的。

题干译文：欧盟国家曾担心他们不会有充足的石油供应了。

30. 【答案】C

【解析】此题考点为固定搭配，find fault with sb. 的含义是"挑某人的毛病"。

题干译文：他妻子总是在挑他的毛病，这让他很生气。

31. 【答案】A

【解析】此题考点为固定搭配。根据提干信息可以推断，所填词的含义为"可疑"。A 项 suspicious 的含义为"感觉可疑的，令人怀疑的"，通常与介词 of 或者 about 连用，例如：I am suspicious of his intention. 我怀疑他的用意。B 项 doubtful 不确定"，例如：I am doubtful about accepting extra work. 我对接受额外的工作不确定。C 项 susceptible 的含义是"易受影响的"，与介词 to 连用，例如：These plants are susceptible to frost damage. 这些植物易受霜冻危害。D 项 dubious 的含义是"不可信的，没把握的"，通常与介词 about 连用。例如：I am dubious about the whole idea. 我对整个想法持怀疑态度。

题干译文：他的邻居对他的行为感到可疑，因此通知了警察。

32. 【答案】A

【解析】此题考点为形近词辨析。四个选项的含义如下：constructive 有建设性的；destructive 破坏性的；productive 生产的；descriptive 描述性的。此题解题的关键在于题干空白处所需的含义。备选项可以通过词根，如 construct，destroy，produce，describe 了解含义。

题干译文：没有任何改进建议的批评是没有建设性的，应该避免。

33. 【答案】D

【解析】此题考点为形近词辨析。四个选项的含义如下：instinctive 没有特色的；indissoluble 不能分解的；indispensable 不可或缺的；indisputable 无可争辩的。

题干译文：毋庸置疑，互联网对人们生活的影响越来越大。

34. 【答案】B

【解析】此题考点为形近词辨析。解题的关键在于动词和介词搭配。complement 是名词也是动词，做动词时含义为"补充（使完美）"，例如：The couple should complement each other. 夫妇应该相互互补（达到完美）。做名词时含义有：①补充物，与介词 to 连用，例如：a complement to your diet 饮食上的补充。②足数，足额，例如：We've taken our full complement of employees this year. 今年我们招入的职员已经满员了。compliment 可以做动词和名词，含义为"称赞"。做动词时要与介词 on 连用，例如：The teacher complimented him on his diligence. 老师称赞了他的勤奋。praise 表示"表扬"，词组为 praise sb. for sth.。appraise 是及物动词，含义为"评价"。

题干译文：他甚至都没看一眼就称赞了她的新衣服。

35. 【答案】B

【解析】此题考点为四个备选单词的含义与题干句意。deceptively 的含义是"迷惑地，虚伪地"；invariably 的含义是"总是，始终如一"，例如：This acute infection of the brain is almost invariably fatal. 这种急性大脑传染病几乎总是致命的。imperatively 的含义是"命令式地"；transiently 的含义是"瞬时地，短暂地"。只有 B 符合句意。在题干中，claim 的含义是"导致死亡"，而不是"索取或宣称"，例如：The car crash claimed three lives. 撞车事故夺走三条生命。

题干译文：艾滋病成为人类健康的最大威胁，这个一贯致命性的疾病夺去很多人的生命。

36. 【答案】B

【解析】此题考点为形近词辨析，解题的关键在于题干中的 arbitrary。这个单词的含义为"专断的，独裁的"，因而可以推断空白处的含义。appliance 的含义是"器具，用具"；compliance 的含义为"顺从，遵从"，与介词 with 连用，例如：Compliance with the regulations is expected of all students. 所有学生都要遵守规章制度。defiance 的含义是"违抗"；reliance 的含义是"依靠，信任"，与介词 on 或者 upon 连用，例如：Too much reliance on the teacher is not beneficial to students. 过分依赖老师对学生不利。

题干译文：他是一个极其独断专行的领导，所以任何事情都必须遵从他的想法。

37. 【答案】B

【解析】此题考点形近词辨析。adduce 的含义是"引证，举出例证"；induce 的含义是"劝诱，引诱，诱发"，例如：These pills will induce sleep. 这些药片会引起困意。deduce 的含义是"推论，演绎出"；produce 的含义是"生产，产生"。

题干译文：当他意识到被诱使签署合同的时候，他威胁要采取法律手段取消协议。

38. 【答案】A

【解析】此题考点为四个备选单词的含义与题干句意。insulate 的含义是"使隔热，使绝缘"，常用词组为 insulate sth. from / against sth.，例如：The room is insulated against noise. 这个房间隔音。insane 的含义是"患精神病的"；

assault 的含义是"攻击"；insult 的含义是"侮辱"。

题干译文：当地居民被鼓励去给房屋加隔热装置以节约能源。

39. 【答案】D

【解析】此题考点为形近词组辨析。by hand "手工的，亲手送递"，例如：The fabric is painted by hand. 这个织品是手工制作的。in hand 的含义是"在手头，在进行中"；at hand 的含义是"（时间或距离上）接近"，例如：Winter is close at hand. 冬天就要到了；on hand 的含义是"（尤指服务）现有"。

题干译文：奥运会期间，在奥运村随时都有急诊服务。

40. 【答案】C

【解析】此题考点为形近词辨析。sensitive 是形容词，意为"敏感的，对……过敏"，与介词 to 连用，例如：I am sensitive to sea food. 我对海鲜过敏。sensible 意为"明智的"，例如：It is sensible for you to buy a relatively cheap house. 对你来说买一个相对便宜的房子是明智的。sensational 意为"轰动性的"；sensory 意为"感官的，感觉的"，sensory organs 意为"感官"。

题干译文：为了追求点击率，网络媒体故意报道轰动性的社会新闻。

41. 【答案】B

【解析】此题考点为形近词辨析。四个选项含义如下：ridiculous 荒谬可笑的；rigorous 严格的；ambiguous 不明确的，模棱两可的；anonymous 匿名的。

题干译文：他们为参加决赛的选手制订了很严格的训练计划。

42. 【答案】B

【解析】此题考点为形近词辨析。四个选项含义如下：appreciative 有欣赏力的，感激的；appreciable 相当于 considerable, 含义为"相当多的，相当大的"；comprehensive 全面广泛的；comprehensible 可以理解的。根据题干信息，空白处需要一个表示量多少的形容词。故 B 正确。

题干译文：对大多数人而言，新的"单双号限行"交通法规作用很大。

43. 【答案】D

【解析】此题考点为形近词辨析。compliment 的含义是"称赞，恭维"；complement 的含义是"补足"；commitment 的含义有：①许诺，承担义务，与介词 to 连用，例如：make a commitment to providing best service 提供最佳服务的承诺。②奉献，投入，与介词 to 连用，例如：Whatever you do, you are required 100% commitment to your career. 无论你做什么，都应该百分之百地投入工作中。commencement ①开始；②毕业典礼。

题干译文：在毕业典礼上，史密斯因为他在研究方面的卓越贡献获得一枚奖章，以示奖励。

44. 【答案】B

【解析】此题考点为形近词辨析。impartial（根据构词法可以得知 im + partial）意为"公平的，不偏不倚的"；immortal 意为"不朽的"；immemorial 可以联想到 memory，因而意为"古老的，远古的"；immoral（根据构词法可以得知 im +

moral）意为"不道德的"。

题干译文：作为美国 20 世纪最杰出的作家，海明威创作了许多不朽之作。

45. 【答案】C

【解析】此题考点为形近词辨析。各选项含义如下：probable 很可能的，大概的；reliable 可信赖的，可靠的；flexible 灵活的；feasible 切实可行的。

题干译文：我们已经定好了周五去看电影，但我们可以灵活一点，改天去。

46. 【答案】A

【解析】此题考点为词组辨析。come up with 的含义是"找到（答案），拿出（一笔钱）"，例如：The young man finally came up with a good idea of increasing sales. 这个年轻人最终找到增加销量的好主意。look up to sb. 的含义是"钦佩，仰慕某人"；put up with 的含义是"忍受，容忍"，例如：I can't put up with his bad temper any more. 我再也忍受不了他的坏脾气了。clear up 是指"天气放晴；（疾病）痊愈；清理，打扫；解决，解释，解答"，例如：clear up the mystery 揭开谜团。

题干译文：显然，有些人有一种惊人的能力，很快能得到正确答案。

47. 【答案】D

【解析】此题考点为固定搭配以及词组辨析。be subject to 的含义有：①易遭受，例如：Flights are subject to delay because of fog. 飞机因大雾可能延误。②取决于，例如：The article is subject to your approval. 这篇文章等你的批准。③服从于，例如：He is not subject to discipline. 他不守纪律。incline 的含义是"有……趋势，倾向于"，例如：I incline to the view that we should be more careful now. 我倾向于我们现在应该更小心谨慎的观点。be liable to 的含义有：①可能受……影响，例如：You are more liable to injury if you don't take regular exercise. 如果你没能定期锻炼，你更容易受伤。②负有责任，例如：People with high income are liable to high tax. 高收入者必须纳高税。be obliged to sb. for sth. 的含义是"感激，感谢"，例如：I'm much obliged to you for helping us. 承蒙相助，本人不胜感激。

题干译文：我代表学校感谢你在地震中的慷慨相助。

48. 【答案】C

【解析】此题考点为形近词辨析。四个选项含义如下：descriptive 描述性的；impressive 印象深刻的；deceptive 欺骗性的；indicative 指示的。

题干译文：这辆旧车的外表相当具有欺骗性，比实际要新很多。

49. 【答案】A

【解析】此题考点为词组辨析。题干中的词组 in relation to 的含义是"和……有关的"。四个选项含义为：add up to 合计；come up with 找出答案；put up with 忍受，容忍；keep up with 跟上。

题干译文：我们收集的所有和那个案子有关的信息太少了。

50. 【答案】D

【解析】此题考点为备选单词是否与句意符合。解题的关键在于：while 表示对比，因而空白处应该为 obtain 的同义词。originate from 的含义是"起源于"，例如：The hot dog did not originate in the United States, but in Germany. 热狗不是起源于美国，而是起源于德国。digest 的含义是"消化"；deprive 的含义是"剥夺"，与介词 of 连用，例如：If you don't drive carefully, I will deprive you of your license. 如果你不谨慎驾驶的话，我就要没收你的驾照了。derive from 的含义是"从……获得"，例如：You can derive great pleasure from travel. 你可以从旅行中获得很多乐趣。

题干译文：现在我们从动物身上获得三分之二之多的蛋白质，而我们的祖父母们只能从动物身上获得一半。

51. 【答案】A
【解析】此题考点为备选单词含义是否符合句意。解题的关键在题干，题干是个由 but 连接的转折并列句，根据转折关系就可以推断空白处单词的含义。各选项含义为：concise 简明的；clear 清楚的；precise 精确的；elaborate 精心制作的，详细阐述的。

题干译文：这个新的秘书写了一份相当简洁，仅几页的报告，但却包含了所有信息。

52. 【答案】C
【解析】此题考点为备选单词含义是否符合句意。解题的关键在题干，题干是由两个互为反义的单词构成的对比。各选项含义为：manageable 易管理的，易处理的；controllable 可以控制的；tolerable 忍受的；perceivable 可以知觉的。

题干译文：预料之中的噪声通常比预料之外的同等强度的噪声更容易忍受。

53. 【答案】A
【解析】此题考点为近义词辨析。各选项含义为：fluctuate 一般指价格上下波动；wave 挥舞，摇曳；swing 摇摆，如钟摆的摆动；vibrate 震动（如汽车经过，房屋震动）。

题干译文：由于价格波动较大，这个公司很难做预算。

54. 【答案】C
【解析】此题考点为备选单词是否与句意搭配。四个选项含义如下：disregard 漠视，不理；distort 歪曲，曲解；irritate 恼怒；intervene 干涉，介入。

题干译文：请不要因为他的不礼貌而恼怒，因为他只是试图引起注意。

55. 【答案】A
【解析】此题考点为词组辨析。call forth 的含义是"唤起，引起"，例如：The song called forth sad memories. 这首歌唤起了伤心的回忆。call at 的含义是"停靠，停留"，例如：This train called at the small village. 这辆火车停靠在这个小山村。call on 的含义是"请求，要求"，例如：The government called on citizens to save energies as possible as they could. 政府要求公民们尽可能地节约能源。call off 的含义是"取消"，例如：The game was called off because of bad weather. 比赛因恶劣天气而取消了。

题干译文：山姆向老板保证他会尽全力做好这份新工作。

56. 【答案】A

【解析】此题考点为词组辨析。四个选项的含义是：be subjected to 遭受……影响；fill with 装满；associate with 联系；attach to 把……系上，例如：Please attach the dog to the tree. 请把狗拴到树上。I attach importance to the education. 我认为教育很重要。

题干译文：要注意减少受持续噪声影响的时间。

57. 【答案】A

【解析】此题考点为词组辨析。on the spot 的含义是"当场，现场，立即，马上"，例如：Certain decisions had to be taken by the man on the spot. 某些决定必须由现场人员做出。on site 的含义是"在现场，临场"，例如：Since all the materials are on site so that work can start immediately. 既然所有材料都到了，立即开工。on location 的含义是"（电影）外景拍摄地"，例如：The movie was shot entirely on location in Rome. 这部电影的外景完全是在罗马拍摄的。on the ground 在地上。

题干译文：地震新闻报道后，紧接着就出现一份详细的现场报道。

58. 【答案】A

【解析】此题考点为形近词辨析。considerate 表示"细心周到的"；considerable 表示"数量上相当可观的"；considering 可以用作介词，表示"考虑到，鉴于"，例如：Considering that he is only a beginner, he did pretty well. 鉴于他只是一个初学者，他做得非常好了。constant 表示"持续的，不断的"。题干需要一个形容词修饰人。

题干译文：母亲要照顾家里的每个人，她们通常是每个家庭里最细心周到的人。

59. 【答案】D

【解析】此题考点为形近词辨析。simplify 这个单词的词根是 simple，词缀 -ify 表示"使……化"，因而单词的含义就是"使……简单化"；modify 表示"对……稍加修改使更适合，缓和"；verify 表示"核实，校验"；rectify 表示"矫正，改正"。

题干译文：如果你知道问题是什么，为什么你不帮助他们整顿局面呢？

60. 【答案】C

【解析】此题考点为近义词辨析。disapproval 是名词，其动词形式为 disapprove，含义为"不赞成"，通常与介词 of 连用，例如：I disapprove of your plan. 我不赞成你的计划。rejection 的含义为"否决，回绝"，用于拒绝提议等。例如：Her proposal met with unanimous rejection. 她的建议遭到了一致否决。refusal 的含义为"拒绝，回绝"，但通常表示 to say that you will not do sth. that sb. has asked you to do 拒绝别人请你做的事情，例如：the refusal of a request / an invitation 拒绝请求 / 邀请。decline 作为名词，含义为"（数量、价值上）减少，下降"，例如：economic decline 经济衰退；decline 作为动词，有"婉言谢绝"的含义，但题干上需要一个名词。题干中，前半句话已经给出了解题信息，劝说加入，因而 refusal 最合适。

题干译文：尽管我努力地劝说他加入我们集团，却遭到了他的断然拒绝。

61. 【答案】D

【解析】此题考点为近义词辨析，而解题关键在于固定搭配。四个备选单词均有"信任"的含义，但各自的用法不同。faith 的含义为"信仰，信任"，固定搭配为 have faith in sb. or sth.，例如：We have faith in the government's promises. 我们对政府的承诺有信心。belief 的用法与 faith 相同；credit 表示"相信"的含义时，作为动词主要用于疑问句或者否定句；reliance 的含义是"依赖，依靠，信任"，固定搭配为 place reliance on / upon sth.，例如：Students should not be encouraged too much reliance on their teachers. 不应鼓励学生过多依赖老师。

题干译文：他让我失望多次，以至于我不再相信他的承诺。

62. 【答案】B

【解析】此题考点为词组辨析。in line with 的含义如下：①与……成一排，例如：An eclipse happens when the earth and moon are in line with the sun. 地球、月亮、太阳成一条直线，日食就发生了。②与……一致，例如：Annual pay increases will be in line with inflation. 每年加薪将与通货膨胀挂钩。in terms of 的含义是"依据，根据"，例如：In terms of my view, I disapprove of the plan. 就我的观点看，我不同意这个计划。regardless of 的含义是"不管，不顾"，例如：He is always expressing his own views regardless of others' feeling. 他总是表达自己观点，不顾别人的感受。by means of 的含义是"借助……手段"，例如：The load was lifted by means of a crane. 重物是借助起重机吊起来的。

题干译文：衡量一个国家的财富，应该依据国民生活健康和幸福的状况，以及能够生产的物质财富。

63. 【答案】A

【解析】此题考点为四个备选词是否符合句意。解题的关键在于题干所提供的信息。unwillingness to learn from others 为解题线索。四个选项的含义如下：arrogance 傲慢，自大；dignity 尊严；humility 谦卑；solitude 孤独。

题干译文：他傲慢自大，不愿意向他人学习，这使得他不能成为一个团队的有效成员。

64. 【答案】C

【解析】此题考点为近义词辨析。首先，题干中的关键词为 ambulance，含义为"急救车"，因而 B 项 danger 与 D 项 crisis（危机）就不适合题干语境。urgency 的含义是"时间紧迫，某事必须得到处理"，例如：The attack added a new urgency to the peace talk. 这个袭击事件使得和平谈判越发紧迫。emergency 指的是"突发事件"。

题干译文：救护车必须享有优先权，因为它通常被用于处理一些突发事件。

65. 【答案】C

【解析】此题考点为四个备选词是否符合句意。根据题干所提供的信息，空白处应该为修饰谓语动词 defend 的副词。根据题干中的后半句我们可以推断出这位长者应该是积极维护。peculiarly 表示"奇特地"；indifferently 表示"冷漠、漠不关心地"；inevitably 表示"不可避免地"；vigorously 表示"精力充沛地"，在题干中表示"积极地"。

题干译文：这位老者积极维护每个公民自由选择宗教的权利，他因此赢得了人们的尊重。

66. 【答案】A

【解析】此题考点为近义词、形近词辨析。根据题干的信息，空白处应该是一个表示"大"的形容词来修饰名词difference。四个选项含义分别为：enormous巨大的，immense是指体积或者数量大到无法衡量的地步。Imminent"即将到来的，逼近的"，例如：No one has given out a warning of the imminent danger. 没人为即将到来的危险发出警告。eminent 卓越的，杰出的。

题干译文：汉语方言之间的巨大差异成为人们互相交流的一个问题。

67. 【答案】B

【解析】此题考点为备选单词是否符合句意。根据题干所提供的信息，可以推断出空白处的含义为"主导地位"。notion 的含义是"观念"；四个选项含义为：privilege 特权，特别待遇；predominance（数量上）占优势或者占主导地位；prevalence 流行；priority 优先权。

题干译文：在男女角色没有明显划分，家务事由双方共同承担的家庭中，男尊女卑的观点是很难维持的。

68. 【答案】C

【解析】此题考点为形近词辨析。各选项含义如下：illegal 非法的；eligible 符合条件的；illegible 字迹模糊，无法辨认的；unreasonable 不合理的。

题干译文：经过多年日晒雨淋，这个商店的招牌已经完全无法辨认。

69. 【答案】A

【解析】此题考点为词组辨析。get down to 的含义是"开始认真做某事"，例如：It's high time I got down to thinking about my essay. 我该认真思考我的论文了。adapt to 的含义是"适应"，例如：When freshmen enter the university, they should adapt themselves to the new environment soon. 大一新生入校后应该尽快适应新环境。hold on to 的含义是"保住（优势），不送，不卖（某物）"，例如：You should hold on to your oil shares. 你应该保留你的石油股份。attend to 的含义是"处理，应付"，例如：I have some urgent business to attend to. 我有些急事需要处理。只有 A 项符合句意。另外，It's time that 句型里，从句动词要用动词的过去式。

题干译文：该是你静下心读书的时候了，否则你会落在其他同学的后面。

70. 【答案】A

【解析】此题考点为词组辨析。by virtue of 的含义是"由于，凭借"，例如：He was exempt from charges by virtue of being so young. 他因为年龄小而免费。in the way of 的含义是"关于，就……而言"，用于疑问句或否定句，例如：There isn't much in the way of entertainment here. 这里没有什么娱乐活动。by way of 的含义是"经由，路过"，例如：I arrived in Paris by way of London. 我途经伦敦到达巴黎。for the sake of 的含义是"为了……某人起见"，例如：The couple still stayed together for the sake of children. 这对夫妇因为孩子还是住在一起。只有 A 符合句意。

题干译文：地质学家认为山是因其地质结构特点才被称为山，即使它的海拔高度不足 3000 英尺。

71. 【答案】C

【解析】此题解题关键在于题干中的 or，or 表示前后两个句子为并列关系，所以空白处需要和 inform 近义的词。denounce 的含义是"告发，公然抨击"，例如：The minister's bribery was denounced in the newspapers. 这位部长的受贿行为在报纸上受到谴责。The passer-by denounced the offenders to the police. 这个路人向警察告发了肇事者。secure 的含义是"获得，使安全"，例如：To secure the major arms deal contract, he has put substantial sum of money into the bank account of the party in power. 为了获得大宗武器交易合同，他向执政党的银行账户存入数量可观的现金。ensure 的含义是"确保"，例如：We must ensure the purity of drinking water in the flooded area. 我们必须保证洪灾地区饮用水的纯净。notify 的含义是"通知"，是题干中 inform 的近义词，故 C 项为正确答案。

题干译文：你会发现研究者们会通知你试验的进程，或者通知你出现的问题。

72. 【答案】C

【解析】此题考点为词组。cope with 的含义是"应付，处理"。dispose of 的含义是"处理，解决"，例如：His high debts forced him to dispose of his art treasures. 高额债务迫使他处理掉他的艺术珍品。hold up 的含义是"承受住，拦劫，举起"，例如：The young man was accused of holding up a pedestrian. 这个小伙子被控拦劫一个行人。All I can do is to try to hold up two of us so well. 我所能做的就是让我们两个人的感情继续发展下去。put up to 词组不存在。

题干译文：美国没有足够的监狱容纳所有的罪犯。

73. 【答案】A

【解析】此题解题关键在于题干中的"dying patients""course of disease"等信息，意思分别为"即将死去的病人""患病期"。prolong 的含义是"延长，拖延"；identify 的含义是"辨认"；alter 的含义是"改变"；expose 的含义是"揭穿，使暴露"。

题干译文：临终的病人有了一线希望，新的治疗可以延长患病期，但要冒着严重副作用的危险。

74. 【答案】A

【解析】vigilance 的含义是"警惕，警觉"；aggregate 的含义是"聚集，集合"；varnish 的含义是"粉饰，装饰"；visage 的含义是"容貌"。

题干译文：因为邻里的警觉，这个小偷被抓住了。

75. 【答案】C

【解析】此题解题关键在于 produces its own light wave。illuminative 的含义是"照明的"；flashy 的含义是"闪光的，一瞬间的，浮华的"；luminous 的含义是"发光的"；flaming 的含义是"火焰般的"。

题干译文：像太阳和灯泡那样自身产生光波的物体被认为是发光的。

76. 【答案】B

【解析】此题考点为形近词组辨析。选项词组解释参见"常用词组"中 give 的解释。

题干译文：的确，他没能看见她的眼泪，然而她担心声音会暴露她的情感。

77. 【答案】D

【解析】此题考点为形近词组辨析。这道题的解题关键在于题干中适合 craze 的动词搭配。ask for 的含义是"请求，要求"，例如：As the boss of this company, I have the right to ask for an explanation. 作为公司老板，我有权利要求一个解释。send for 的含义是"派人去请，召唤"，例如：He is so ill that we have to send for a doctor. 他病得太重了，我们必须派人去请个大夫了。run for 的含义是"竞选"；cater for 的含义是"迎合"，例如：TV programmes couldn't cater for different tastes. 电视节目不能迎合不同的爱好。

题干译文：商店通过给消费者提供能回家自己组装的零部件来迎合他们 DIY 的狂热追求。

78. 【答案】B

【解析】解此题要依靠语境。amplify 的含义是"放大"；decrease 的含义是"减少"；stimulate 的含义是"刺激"；meet 如果与 need 搭配含义为"满足……的需要"。题干语境是"减少需求"，故 B 正确。

题干译文：一种称为牙科电子麻醉的新技术将很快能减少对可怕的牙医针的需求。

79. 【答案】B

【解析】解此题要依靠语境。infection 的含义是"感染"；fatigue 的含义是"疲劳"；syncope 的含义是"昏厥"；suffocation 的含义是"窒息"。shortness of breath 的含义是"气短"，go hand in hand with 的含义是"共同行动，紧密联系"。sweep 的含义是"横扫，席卷"。be confined to 的含义是"局限于……"。

题干译文：气短经常与疲劳紧密联系，这种情况遍布全身并且不局限于某一个部位。

80. 【答案】C

【解析】此题解题关键在于与 types of research programs 的搭配。allocate 的含义是"分派"；expand 的含义为"扩张"；sponsor 的含义是"发起，赞助，倡议"；sum 的含义是"总计，概括"。

题干译文：从国家层面上看，国家健康研究所尤其是国家老年研究所正主办许多形式的有关老年的研究项目。

81. 【答案】A

【解析】此题解题要依靠语境，尤其是句中 "threaten the fundamental values of society" "challenge" 等词语的提示。formidable 的含义是"强大的，可怕的，难以对付的"，例如：The task is formidable and impossible to achieve without international cooperation. 这项任务很艰巨，没有国际合作不可能实现。fatal 的含义是"致命的"。favorable 的含义是"有利的"，例如：Spring is favorable to fly a kite. 春天适合放风筝。fantastic 的含义是"极好的，难以置信的"，

例如：He made fantastic progress on English in the short period. 在这么短时间内他英语进步神速。题干中 fundamental 的含义是"基本的"。

题干译文：HIV 和 AIDS 可能威胁到社会的基本价值观，任何针对两者的尝试都是可怕的挑战。

82. 【答案】A

【解析】此题考点为形近词组辨析。其他选项的含义和例句参见"常用词组"。abrupt 的含义是"突然"。

题干译文：Kelley 的公关人员突然取消七个城市的宣传巡回计划，宣布他们的"宣传目标已经完成"。

83. 【答案】B

【解析】此题解题关键在于语境，尤其是题干中"is only beginning to be seriously examined"的提示。informative 的含义是"见多识广的"；inconclusive 的含义是"无确定结果的"；inconspicuous 的含义是"不明显的"；indisputable 的含义是"无可争议的"。variable 的含义是"变量"。

题干译文：将拥挤作为一个环境变量来研究才刚刚开始，至今尚无结论性的数据。

84. 【答案】B

【解析】此题考点为词组含义。be proportional to 的含义是"与……成比例"，例如：The result of the exam is always proportional to your efforts. 考试结果总是和你的努力成比例。be subjected to 的含义是"使经历，使遭受"，例如：Your wages will be subjected to changes based on your performance. 你的薪水会因你的表现而有变化。be susceptible to 的含义是"易受……的感染或影响"，例如：This kind of plant is susceptible to disease. 这种植物容易受病害的侵袭。be liable to 的含义是"有……的倾向"，例如：Your silly attempt is liable to failure. 你愚蠢的尝试多半是要失败的。

题干译文：在紧接着的杀菌过程中，罐头被放入水蒸气或者沸腾的水中，温度和持续时间因食物的类别而不同。

85. 【答案】B

【解析】此题解题关键在于语境。launch 的含义是"发射，发起"，例如：The recruitment of new members has been launched this afternoon. 招募新会员的工作今天下午已经启动了。translate 的含义除了"翻译"以外，还有"转移，调动"。dissect 的含义是"解剖，详细分析"，例如：Commentators are still dissecting the result of the election. 评论家们还在详细分析选举的结果。convey 的含义是"传达"。

题干译文：但是如果新的研究发现不能转化为市场商品和服务，研究就没有经济影响。

86. 【答案】A

【解析】此题考点为语境搭配。bioactive 的含义是"生物活性的"；miniature 的含义是"小型的"；bizarre 的含义是"奇异的，怪诞的"；invisible 的含义是"看不见的"。题干中 property 的含义是"财产，性质"。all the time 的含义是"总是，一直”。

题干译文：大自然给我们的惊奇从未停止。实验室中不断发现拥有生物活性结构和特性的分子。

87. 【答案】D

【解析】此题考点为词组含义。rule out 的含义是"消除，排除"，例如：He didn't rule out the possibility to change his mind. 他没有排除改变想法的可能性。divide up 的含义是"瓜分"；bring apart 的搭配不成立；sort out 的含义是"选出，分类"，例如：She is sorting out the good apples from bad ones. 她正在把好的苹果和坏的分开。

题干译文：由于病人不能总是辨别心理诱发的胸痛和心脏病发作引起的胸痛，医生应该挑选出疼痛的可能原因。

88. 【答案】D

【解析】此题考点为固定搭配。meet up with 的含义是"意外碰到"。come up with 的含义是"提出，想出"，例如：They are beating their brains to come up with a solution to the sticky problem. 他们正绞尽脑汁想出这个棘手问题的解决办法。shed light on 的含义是"阐明"。live up to 的含义是"符合，达到预期标准"，例如：They will do their utmost to live up to their parents' expectations. 他们会竭尽全力，不辜负父母的期望。usher 的含义是"引导"。

题干译文：洛杉矶的加利福尼亚大学医学院的 David L. Rinion 说，如果符合预期，这样的测试能够开辟一个产前诊断的新领域。

89. 【答案】A

【解析】此题考点为单词词义。emaciated 的含义为"瘦弱的，憔悴的"。eligible 的含义是"有资格的，合格的"，例如：Everyone with an annual income of $ 100,000 may be eligible to apply for the membership of this club. 任何年收入 10 万元的人都有资格申请成为这个俱乐部的会员。elastic 的含义是"有弹性的"。exceptional 的含义是"例外的"，例如：Forestry has advanced with exceptional speed. 植树造林以罕见的速度得到了发展。

题干译文：深受腿病折磨，汤姆最近非常憔悴。

90. 【答案】C

【解析】此题考点为固定搭配。constitute 的含义是"构成，建立"；decode 的含义是"解码"；draft 的含义是"绘制，起草"；encode 的含义是"编码，译码"。只有 draft 与 map 搭配。master 的含义是"主要的"，vasculature 的含义是"脉管系统"。

题干译文：如今调查者仍旧没能绘制出心脏脉管系统的精确图。

91. 【答案】D

【解析】此题解题关键在于 caring "关怀的"，空白处需要一个与这个词近义的词。emotional 情感的；impersonal 非个人的；compulsory 必需的，义务的；compassionate 有同情心的（与 caring 近义）。

题干译文：他们是我见过的最关心人、具有同情心的一群人。

92. 【答案】A

【解析】wholesome 的含义是"有益健康的"；diet 的含义是"饮食"；tasteful 的含义是"有滋味的，有品位的"；edible 的含义是"可食用的"。

题干译文：正如为了身体我们需要简单健康的食物一样，我们的心智发展也需要严肃的阅读。

93. 【答案】D

【解析】此题通过 rather than frequent stops and starts 可以解题。compassion 的含义是"同情心"；acceleration 的含义是"加速"；frustration 的含义是"挫败"；exertion 的含义是"努力，运用，发挥"，例如：He failed to lift the rock in spite of all his exertions. 他虽竭尽全力，但仍然未能将那石头搬起来。

题干译文：最好的锻炼要求持久的努力，而不是频繁的做做停停。

94. 【答案】C

【解析】accomplishment 的含义是"成就，完成"。qualification 的含义是"资格"。eminence 的含义是"显赫，崇高"，例如：He reached eminence as a doctor. 他已成为名医。patent 的含义是"专利权"。

题干译文：Salk 作为发明世界上第一个有效的小儿麻痹疫苗的科学家赢得了显赫的声誉。

95. 【答案】A

【解析】denote 的含义是"象征，表示"，例如：A smile often denotes pleasure and friendship. 微笑常常表示高兴和友善。donate 的含义是"捐赠"；relate 的含义是"有关联"，通常与介词 to 连用；resort 的含义是"求助，诉诸"，通常与介词 to 连用。coronary disease 的含义是"冠心病"。

题干译文：冠心病是一个广泛使用的术语，表示对心脏的供血不足。

96. 【答案】D

【解析】本题考查词义辨析。regulation 意为"规定，规矩"，speciality 意为"专业"，essential 意为"重要，关键"，specification 意为"规格，尺寸"。满足建筑设计师的"规格"符合上下文语义。regulation 侧重于约束行为的规范，放这里不合适。

题干译文：修建者的工作是使房子在所有方面都符合设计师的规格要求。

97. 【答案】A

【解析】此题考点为形近词组辨析。account for 的含义是"解释，（在数量方面）占"；call for 的含义是"要求，接人"；look for 的含义是"寻找"；make for 的含义是"移向，攻击，造成"。

题干译文：恐怕你得就状况的恶化做出解释。

98. 【答案】C

【解析】此题考点为意思搭配。affliction 的含义是"痛苦"；alternative 的含义是"选择，备选"；allocation 的含义是"派发，分配"；alliance 的含义是"结盟，联姻"。generous 的含义是"慷慨大方的"。此题空白处的选项应该和 time 搭配，故 C 项为正确答案。

题干译文：你每周有 12 小时都在养老院，这种时间分配似乎挺慷慨。

99. 【答案】C

【解析】此题解题关键在于语境。expensively 的含义是"昂贵地"；exceptionally 的含义是"例外地"；exhaustively 的含义是"彻底地，无遗漏地"；exclusively 的含义是"排外地，独占地"。

题干译文：每个产品在投入市场前都是经过彻底检验的。

100. 【答案】D

【解析】此题解题关键在于语境。potent 的含义是"有效的，强有力的"，例如：I was eventually convinced by his potent arguments. 最终我被他有力的论述说服了。conditional 的含义是"有条件的"；inseparable 的含义是"不可分开的"；cardinal 的含义是"主要的"，例如：The cardinal idea of this party for the election is that everybody should enjoy equality. 这个政党竞选的主要思想就是人人享有平等。

题干译文：烹调前洗手是主要规定之一。

101. 【答案】B

【解析】此题考点为形近词辨析。cohesive 的含义是"黏性的"；cognitive 的含义是"认知的"；collective 的含义是"集体的"；comic 的含义是"喜剧的"。

题干译文：教育者应该努力发展孩子的认知能力。

102. 【答案】C

【解析】此题考点为形近词辨析。defect 的含义是"缺陷"，例如：The type of cars has been withdrawn from the market because of mechanical defects. 这款车因为机械缺陷撤市了。deficit 的含义是"赤字，亏损"，例如：The current trade deficit indicates a serious imbalance between our import and export trade. 当前的贸易赤字表明我们的进出口贸易严重失调。default 的含义是"默认值，缺席，拖欠，违约"；deception 的含义是"欺诈，骗局"；mortgage 的含义是"抵押"。

题干译文：按揭借款违约在近一年里呈上升趋势,这是因为低收入家庭的数目一直上涨。

103. 【答案】B

【解析】此题考点为单词含义。exaggerate 的含义是"夸大"。exacerbate 的含义是"加重，恶化"，例如：Scratching exacerbates a skin rash. 皮疹挠后会恶化。exceed 的含义是"超过，领先"；exhibit 的含义是"展览"。

题干译文：症状可能会因某些药物加重。

104. 【答案】C

【解析】此题解题关键在于语境的提示。facility 的含义是"设施"；fascination 的含义是"魔力，魅力"；fabrication 的含义是"捏造"；faculty 的含义是"才能，全体教职员工，（大学）系"。

题干译文：她的故事彻头彻尾是捏造的，所以没人相信她。

105. 【答案】C

【解析】此题考点为单词含义。salvage 的含义是"海上救助，打捞"；safeguard 的含义是"保卫，保护"；sabotage 的含义是"蓄意破坏"，例如：Owing to the sabotage, the train jumped the rails. 由于破坏，火车出轨了。sacrifice 的含义是"牺牲，祭品"，例如：Success in the job is not worth the sacrifice of health. 以牺牲健康而来的工作上的成功不值得。rule out 在这里的含义为"排除"。

题干译文：调查交通事故的警察没排除蓄意破坏的可能性。

106. 【答案】B

【解析】此题考点为词组含义，语境中介词 on 是解题关键。take up 的含义为"占地方"；check up 的含义是"检查，调查，核查"，例如：He was careful enough to check up every detail. 他非常仔细，把每一个细节都核对过了。The police are checking up on him. 警方正在调查他。work out 的含义是"解决，算出"；look into 的含义为"调查，观察"。

题干译文：政府总是会对受雇于敏感军事项目的员工的背景进行调查。

107. 【答案】A

【解析】此题解题关键在于语境，尤其是短语 cause disease 的提示。unsanitary 的含义是"不洁净的"。insidious 的含义是"阴险的，隐伏的"，例如：That insidious man bad-mouthed me to almost everyone else. 那个阴险的家伙几乎见人便说我的坏话。Bleeding may be chronic and insidious or brisk and life-threatening. 出血可以是慢性的、隐伏的或者是活跃的、危及生命的。insane 的含义是"精神错乱的"；inefficacious 的含义是"无效力的"。

题干译文：不卫生的条件和环境可能引起疾病。

108. 【答案】C

【解析】此题考点为单词含义。abstain 的含义是"放弃，戒除"，例如：The doctor asked the patient to abstain from smoking. 医生让这个病人戒烟。acquit 的含义是"释放，开释"，例如：He was acquitted of the crime. 他被宣告无罪。admonish 的含义是"训诫，提醒"，例如：His wife admonished him not to drive too fast. 他妻子警告他不要开快车。adduce 的含义是"引证，举出"，例如：I can adduce several reasons for his strange behavior. 我可以列举出几个他行为古怪的原因。根据词义以及语境，我们可以判断 C 项正确。

题干译文：证人因为没能回答问题而受到法官的警告。

109. 【答案】D

【解析】此题考点为词组含义。pull of 的搭配不成立；wear out 的含义是"穿破，磨损，耗尽"；pass out 的含义是"昏倒，失去知觉"。write off 的含义是"注销，报废"，例如：He wrote off three cars in a year because of his dreadful driving. 因他可怕的驾车技术，他一年内报废了三辆车。根据 because of traffic accidents 我们可以推断他的车不是用坏了，而是报废了，故答案 D 正确。

题干译文：因为交通事故，今年他已经报废了两辆车。

110. 【答案】B

【解析】此题考点为固定搭配。advent 的含义是"到来"，因而 advent of the Internet

的含义就是"互联网的到来"。convenient 是形容词，含义是"便利的"；interface 的含义是"界面，接口"；aftermath 的含义是"（不幸事件的）后果"。

题干译文：自从有了互联网，人们信息更灵通了。

111. 【答案】A

【解析】此题根据已知语境我们可以知道空白处的含义应该是消毒。sterilize 的含义是"消毒"；label 的含义是"贴标签"；quarantine 的含义是"隔离，检疫"，例如：This is a highly infectious disease. All the patients must be put under quarantine. 这种病的传染性极大，病人必须采取隔离措施。retain 的含义是"保留"，例如：You have to retain your ticket for inspection. 你应该留票以备验票。

题干译文：所有病人接触过的器具必须在他人使用前进行消毒。

112. 【答案】D

【解析】此题解题关键在于题干中 risk 的提示，表示"诊所冒着……的风险"，所以空白处应该选取贬义的词。acquit 的含义是"释放，开释"；allocate 的含义是"分配"；alleviate 的含义是"缓解，减轻（疼痛或痛苦）"；alienate 的含义是"疏远"。cunning 的含义是"狡猾的"。

题干译文：诊所采取了这个狡猾的政策，这样做的风险是可能会减少患者资源。

113. 【答案】B

【解析】此题考点为单词词义。metastasis 的含义是"转移"；metabolism 的含义是"新陈代谢"；malaise 的含义是"身体不适"；maintenance 的含义是"维护，保持"。upset 的含义是"推翻，反倒，颠覆"。

题干译文：糖尿病破坏了糖、脂肪和蛋白质的代谢机制。

114. 【答案】C

【解析】此题解题关键在于 affect，这个词通常表示产生不好的影响。potency 的含义是"效力，力量"，例如：The doctor says that he will not wake until the anesthetic loses potency. 医生说要等麻醉剂的药劲过了他才能醒。fiber 的含义是"纤维"；lethargy 的含义是"没精打采，昏睡"；synthesis 的含义是"合成"。只有选项 C 可以产生不好的影响，故答案是 C。

题干译文：肌肉无力会影响我们的精神感知方式。

115. 【答案】B

【解析】respond to 的含义是"对……回应"，例如：I will respond to your message when I return. 我回来后会回复你的信息。reflect on 的含义是"反思，仔细思考"；wipe out 的含义是"消除"，例如：Medical experts are trying to wipe out the malaria in some countries. 医学专家正设法消除一些国家的疟疾。put off 的含义是"推迟"。

题干译文：大量事实表明，HIV 病毒感染者在反思他们不安全的行为。

116. 【答案】B

【解析】此题解题关键在于 but 和 worry，转折结构提示空白处需要一个与它意思相反的词。put off 的含义是"推迟"；laugh off 的含义是"一笑置之"，例如：An actor has to learn to laugh off bad reviews. 演员须学会对贬斥性评论一笑置之的本事。pay off 的含义是"还清（债务）"；lay off 的含义是"解雇"。只有 B 项与 worry 互为反义词。

题干译文：在公开场合，他们对最近一次的失败一笑置之，但私下里他们很是担心。

117.【答案】D

【解析】此题解题关键在于语境，尤其是短语 poor nutrition 和 adult growth，由此可知应该选择贬义的词填入空白处。degenerate 的含义是"衰退，退化"；deteriorate 的含义是"恶化"；boost 的含义是"促进，推动"；retard 的含义是"阻止，妨碍"。infancy 的含义是"婴儿期"。

题干译文：婴儿期早期阶段营养不良可阻碍成年发育。

118.【答案】C

【解析】此题解题要注意题干中的限定成分"during rush hour"。scatter 的含义是"分散"，例如：When the tree falls, the monkeys scatter. 树倒猢狲散。condense 的含义是"浓缩，凝结，归纳"；clog 的含义是"阻塞，阻碍"；dot 的含义是"点缀"。commuter 的含义是"每日往返上班者"。

题干译文：高峰期，市区街道挤满了上下班的人。

119.【答案】A

【解析】此题解题关键在于语境提示，complain of 的含义是"抱怨，控诉"，所以空白处需要表示贬义的词。harass 的含义是"骚扰"，例如：The court ordered him to stop harassing his ex-wife. 法庭命令他停止骚扰他的前妻。distract 的含义是"使分心"，常与介词 from 连用，例如：The noise outside distracted me from my work. 门外的噪声使我分心，不能集中精力工作。sentenced 的含义是"宣判，判决"；release 的含义是"释放"。

题干译文：很多黑人年轻人抱怨曾被警察骚扰过。

120.【答案】D

【解析】选项 A 为"滞留"；选项 B 为"劝阻"；选项 C 为"减轻"；选项 D"戒除，远离"。根据题意，本题答案为 D。

题干译文：尽管医生有警示，但他从未戒烟戒酒。

121.【答案】B

【解析】选项 A 为"康复"；选项 B 为"伤害，使……危险"；选项 C 为"安静"；选项 D 为"补充"。根据题意，本题答案为 B。

题干译文：医生警告，有感染复发病史的人使用戴在头上的耳机随身听可能会伤害他们的听力。

122.【答案】D

【解析】选项 A 为"驳斥"；选项 B 为"批准"；选项 C 为"促进"；选项 D 为"妨碍"。根据题意，本题答案为 D。

题干译文：公正的观察者不得不承认，正规教育的欠缺似乎并未妨碍 Larry 取得成功。

123.【答案】A

【解析】选项 A 为"相应地";选项 B 为"有选择地";选项 C 为"巨大地";选项 D 为"相关地"。根据题意，本题答案为 A。

题干译文：支持性的成果减少了，他们应该随之修改计划。

124.【答案】C

【解析】选项 A 为"使……认识"；选项 B 为"使……熟悉"；选项 C 为"赋予"；选项 D 为"娱乐"。根据题意，本题答案为 C。

题干译文：期望值很高的父母们越来越相信，古典音乐的胎教会赋予未来成年人对音乐的欣赏能力。

125.【答案】D

【解析】选项 A 为"平坦，达到平衡"；选项 B 为"突出"；选项 C 为"成功"；选项 D 为"磨损，逐渐消失"。根据题意，本题答案为 D。

题干译文：如果收益仅仅来自于上升的能源价格，那么当能源价格下调时，通货膨胀应该会下降。

126.【答案】C

【解析】选项 A 为"处方"；选项 B 为"触诊"；选项 C 为"干预"；选项 D 为"插嘴，提出异议"。根据题意，本题答案为 C。

题干译文：热中风是一种医学紧急情况，需要合格的医疗人员立刻干预。

127.【答案】D

【解析】选项 A 为"抵消，补偿"；选项 B 为"吸入"；选项 C 为"发泄"；选项 D 为"启动，发病"。根据题意，本题答案为 D。

题干译文：接触石棉能导致间皮瘤、石棉沉滞症和内脏癌症，并且这些疾病的发病都是在首次感染的几十年后。

128【答案】B

【解析】选项 A 为"盐溶液"；选项 B 为"唾液"；选项 C 为"疖疮"；选项 D 为"摩擦"。根据题意，本题答案为 B。

题干译文：埃博拉病毒通过体液、尿液、精液等排泄物运行，可以杀死多达 90% 的感染者。

129.【答案】D

【解析】选项 A 为"可比拟的"；选项 B 为"可传递的"；选项 C 为"可转换的，可翻译的"；选项 D 为"易控制的，经得起检验的"。根据题意，本题答案为 D。

题干译文：新设计的系统能经受基因传染的抗击，还能留出潜伏期，以便研究各种基因。

130.【答案】A

【解析】compensation 赔偿；compromise 折中，妥协；commodity 商品；consumption 消耗，消费。

题干译文：雇主在法律上有义务支付给工人工伤赔偿金。

131.【答案】D

【解析】alleviate 减轻，缓和（痛苦或困难）；aggravate 使加重，使恶化；extinguish

熄灭（火或光），使消亡，使（想法或希望）破灭；intervene 干预，介入，例如：The army will have to intervene to prevent further fighting. 部队不得不介入以阻止战争继续。The police don't usually like to intervene in disputes between husbands and wives. 警察通常不喜欢介入夫妻之间的争吵。

题干译文：两位患者的争吵很激烈，医生不得不出面干涉。

132.【答案】B

【解析】induce 劝诱，诱导；引产，催生；诱发（身体反应）。convert 与 to 连用，意思是"转变为"；revive 使复兴、复原、复苏。swerve ①突然转向，例如：The car swerved sharply to avoid the dog. 汽车突然改变方向以避开狗。②改变，背离（主意、做法、目的等），例如：swerve from the truth 违背真理。hustle and bustle 的含义为"熙熙攘攘，喧闹繁忙"，例如：He wants a cottage far away from the hustle and bustle of city life. 他想要一座远离尘嚣的小屋。

题干译文：尽管法律上仍有争论，但他们并不期望死刑改为不可假释的无期徒刑。

133.【答案】C

【解析】integral 不可缺少的，例如：Vegetables are an integral part of our diet. 蔬菜是我们饮食中不可缺少的部分。（用于名词前，作为组成部分的，内置的）。gross ①总共的，例如：gross income 总收入；②（仅用于名词前）恶劣的，糟糕的，例如：gross violation。wholesome 对健康有益的；intact 完好无损的。

题干译文：为了保持身体健康，人应该吃对健康有益的食物并且保证足够的锻炼。

134.【答案】B

【解析】provision 条款，规定，粮食；prosperity 繁荣；privilege 特权，特殊待遇；preference 偏好；优待。

题干译文：中央政府不惜一切代价保证香港的繁荣和稳定大大刺激了当地金融业。

135.【答案】B

【解析】facilitate 促进，使便利；forfeit 没收；丧失；fulfill 实现（希望、目标等）；履行，执行；furnish 配备家具；提供，供应。

题干译文：必须向患者保证他们不会因为床位紧张而丧命。

136.【答案】C

【解析】exclusively 仅仅，唯独；superficially 表面地，不重要地；utterly 完全地；doubtfully 不确定地。

题干译文：他的死因一直以来都是谜，至今全然未知。

137.【答案】A

【解析】recklessly 不计后果地；sparingly 节省地；sensibly 明智地；incredibly 不可思议地。

题干译文：众所周知，一些不计后果地利用资源的方式会破坏环境，影响人们的生活。

138.【答案】C

【解析】filtered 过滤的；distilled 蒸馏的；contaminated 被污染的；purified 纯净的。

题干译文：霍乱是一种可预防的、经水传播的细菌性感染疾病，细菌通过污水得以传播。

139.【答案】D

【解析】by the way 顺便说一下；at all events 无论如何；by no means 决不；in any sense 从任何意义上说。

题干译文：从任何意义上说，我们欢迎他，不是把他当作新成员，而是一个老朋友。

140.【答案】A

【解析】维生素 A 的慢性高剂量摄入已证明对骨骼有不利影响。adverse "不利的"，prevalent "流行的"，instant "立刻的，即时的"，purposeful "有目的的，故意的"。根据题意，本题选择 adverse。

141.【答案】C

【解析】多喝水对身体是有益的，有助于润滑关节并冲洗掉毒素和杂质。screen out "筛查"，knock out "击倒"，flush out "冲刷掉"，rule out "排除"。根据题意，本题正确答案为 C。

142.【答案】B

【解析】风湿病学家建议，那些持续疼痛和痛苦的人首先应该借助医疗来缓解问题。affiliate "加入，为……工作"，alleviate "减少，减缓"，aggravate "使严重，使恶化"，accelerate "使加速"。根据题意，正确答案为 B。

143.【答案】C

【解析】一般来说，疫苗制造者可以在受精的鸡蛋中生产病毒，这个过程会持续四到六个月。penetrate "穿透"，designate "指定"，generate "生产，产生"，exaggerate "夸张"。根据题意，正确答案为 C。

144.【答案】A

【解析】A。丹麦的研究表明，丹麦肥胖人数的增加大致相当于大气中二氧化碳的增加。equivalent to "相当于，等同于"，temporary "暂时的"，permanent "永恒的"，relevant "相关的"。根据题意，本题正确答案为 A。

145.【答案】B

【解析】泰德得了一次严重的中风，平衡受到影响，连话都难以说清楚了。bluntly "直言地"，intelligibly "清晰地"，reluctantly "不情愿地"，ironically "讽刺地"。根据题意，正确答案为 B。

146.【答案】A

【解析】在技术密集型企业中，计算机控制着生产和管理的所有过程。dominate "主导，控制"，overwhelm "压倒，淹没"，substitute "代替"，imitate "模仿"。根据题意，正确答案为 A。

147.【答案】C

【解析】虽然大多数梦是明显的自发行为，但梦境可能是由外部影响造成的。homogeneously "同质地"，instantaneously "立即地"，spontaneously "自发地"，simultaneously "同时地"。根据题意，正确答案为 C。

148. 【答案】A

【解析】我们更快地做出了回应，通过发泄愤怒而做出的这种回应方式过于迅速了。give vent to sth "发泄（愤怒）"，impulse "脉搏"，temper "脾性"，offence "防卫"。根据题意，正确答案为 A。

149. 【答案】D

【解析】通过维持强有力的家族联结，同时也维持了社会的基层结构。bias "偏见"，honor "荣誉"，estate "财产"，bond "联系，联结"。根据句意，正确答案为 D。

150. 【答案】D

【解析】句意：医疗队讨论了他们对消除这种可治愈疾病的共同贡献。obedience "顺从"，susceptibility "易受影响（或伤害）的特性"，inclination "倾向于"，dedication "贡献"。根据句意，此题选择 D。

Section B

Directions: *Each of the following sentences has a word or phrase underlined. There are four other words or phrases beneath each sentence. Choose the word or phrase which would best keep the meaning of the original sentence if it were substituted for the underlined part. Mark your answer on the* ***ANSWER SHEET***.

1. It would be wildly optimistic to believe that these advances offset such a large reduction in farmland.

   A. take in   B. make up   C. cut down   D. bring about

2. To study the distribution of disease within an area, it is useful to plot the cases on the map.

   A. mark   B. allocate   C. erase   D. pose

3. The temperature of the atmosphere becomes colder as elevation increases.

   A. altitude   B. aptitude   C. latitude   D. longitude

4. I have no idea of fashion, so my choice of clothes seems quite arbitrary.

   A. assertive   B. decisive   C. optional   D. tasteful

5. This child was so obstinate that he refused to admit to his mistakes.

   A. obsessive   B. furious   C. stubborn   D. rebellious

6. The indomitable spirit displayed by athletes embodies the new look of this nation.

   A. brave   B. unsubdued   C. determined   D. industrious

7. The two sides had an in-depth exchange of views on how to enhance their further cooperation.

   A. specific   B. shallow   C. profound   D. thorough

8. Children should be carefully <u>insulated</u> from harmful experiences.
   A. isolated   B. seceded   C. absent   D. distinguished

9. <u>In the light of</u> the current situation, I have to review my plans.
   A. Throwing light on   B. In line with
   C. In accordance with   D. In terms of

10. In today's competitive job market, people, especially young men are required to be <u>aggressive</u> and industrious.
    A. invasive   B. belligerent   C. progressive   D. enterprising

11. <u>Assimilating</u> the report in computing requires much time, for I'm not specialized in this field.
    A. Digesting   B. Incorporating   C. Imitating   D. Compiling

12. As a member of the society, a person should <u>be responsible for</u> and dedicate to the society.
    A. answer for   B. account for   C. charge for   D. compensate for

13. To my surprise, the young man was <u>resourceful</u> enough to find infinite ways to express his emotions with gestures.
    A. imaginary   B. imaginative   C. plentiful   D. versatile

14. To lower the risk of <u>secondary diseases</u> of pregnancy, it may be required that you have a change in your lifestyle as soon as you confirm you are pregnant.
    A. complication   B. complexity   C. knottiness   D. hindrance

15. This treaty gave an <u>impetus</u> to the trade between the two countries and the respective development in industry.
    A. impetuous   B. impulse   C. hindrance   D. impasse

16. He suffered a <u>hideous</u> torment when the enemy caught him, but he didn't surrender himself at all.
    A. painful   B. inhumane   C. horrid   D. brutal

17. The average commercial business can shut down in such an emergency but a hospital doesn't dare, for lives are <u>at stake</u>.
    A. on hand   B. in circulation
    C. under consideration   D. at risk

18. We never wondered whether some other dish might be an equally tasty <u>substitute</u> for dumplings on the eve of Spring Festival.
    A. alternative   B. allusion   C. alteration   D. altercation

19. The sales representative was dismissed as he <u>was accused of</u> cheating customers.
    A. was accustomed to   B. adhered to

C. was charge with   D. stuck to

20. The middle-aged man killed his wife and his children in person. Nothing can extenuate such <u>appalling</u> behavior.
    A. appealing   B. dreadful
    C. imprudent   D. displeasing

21. Don't trust the speaker any more, since his deeds are never <u>compatible with</u> his ideology.
    A. suitable for   B. consistent with
    C. in harmony with   D. in favor of

22. Juveniles are more <u>vulnerable to</u> negative influences and outside pressures, including peer pressure.
    A. susceptible to   B. favorable to
    C. relevant to   D. capable of

23. Is there anything at work that might subject you to <u>dangerous</u> chemicals?
    A. vicious   B. insidious   C. hazardous   D. notorious

24. Ginger tea may also help <u>alleviate</u> the misery of colds by increasing circulation.
    A. expel   B. diminish   C. endure   D. chop

25. Thousands of people became victims and many children became orphans in the <u>deadly</u> quake.
    A. brutal   B. terrible   C. horrible   D. lethal

26. When she thought no one was looking at she opened the cupboard and took a few sweets <u>on the sly</u>.
    A. secretly   B. punctiliously   C. dilatorily   D. cunningly

27. We no longer keep up the close friendship of few years ago, though we still visit each other <u>on occasion</u>.
    A. at times   B. at a time
    C. at all times   D. at one time

28. The British people belong to one of the <u>wealthy</u> countries of Europe and enjoy a high standard of living compared to the rest of the world.
    A. powerful   B. affluent
    C. promising   D. almighty

29. <u>Without question</u>, people's lives here have improved dramatically in the past twenty years.
    A. Out of the question   B. Apparently

C. Undoubtedly　　　　　　　　D. Naturally

30. Workers were <u>indignant</u> at the unfair treatment and the indifferent attitudes of their boss.
 A. imprudent　　B. wrathful　　　C. tenacious　　　D. impatient

31. He was unwilling to press her with questions about her health, since she seemed to make light of the <u>indisposition</u>.
 A. aliment
 B. situation
 C. ailment
 D. incompetence

32. It is an important responsibility for the government to provide safe and <u>wholesome</u> food to the society and the public.
 A. decent　　B. wholesale　　　C. moral　　　D. salubrious

33. It is <u>absurd</u> that women must be paid less than men for doing the same work.
 A. unreasonable
 B. immoral
 C. ridiculous
 D. abnormal

34. It is believed that this taxi driver is <u>upright</u> and he has never charged extra money for services.
 A. vertical　　B. honest　　　C. modest　　　D. incorruptible

35. Safety officials have <u>earnestly</u> questioned whether the increased use of synthetic materials heightens the risk of fire.
 A. cautiously　　B. severely　　　C. accurately　　　D. seriously

36. The senator agreed that his support of the measure would <u>jeopardize</u> his chances for reelection.
 A. benefit　　B. endanger　　　C. hinder　　　D. disturb

37. We were very angry with his <u>ambiguous</u> views on how to tackle the problem completely.
 A. obscure　　B. ambitious　　　C. indifferent　　　D. explicit

38. In the Han Dynasty, the royal government sent special envoys to the Western countries to <u>disseminate</u> the Chinese culture.
 A. disclose　　B. spread　　　C. analyze　　　D. deliver

39. I shall never forget the look of intense <u>anguish</u> on the face of his parents when they knew his death.
 A. surprise　　B. stress　　　C. dilemma　　　D. misery

40. Wives tend to believe that their husbands are infinitely <u>resourceful</u> and versatile.
 A. diligent　　B. clever　　　C. capable　　　D. perfect

41. There is no denial that in the tropical areas there is a high <u>incidence</u> of malaria.
    A. morbidity
    B. precedent
    C. mobility
    D. proficiency

42. We want you to report all the events of that morning <u>in sequence</u> without any delay.
    A. at length
    B. in order
    C. in advance
    D. in earnest

43. Most lecturers find it <u>expedient</u> to use notes when addressing to the public.
    A. beneficent
    B. contributive
    C. advantageous
    D. profitable

44. Some people prefer to remain <u>anonymous</u> when they call the police to report a crime.
    A. undisturbed
    B. unnoticed
    C. unrecorded
    D. unnamed

45. Young children may show a relatively precocious pattern of movement at one age and an <u>immature</u> pattern at a subsequent age.
    A. puerile
    B. sophisticated
    C. crude
    D. worldly

46. The soldiers swore <u>allegiance</u> to their motherland before the war.
    A. truthfulness
    B. loyalty
    C. faith
    D. endurance

47. Don't drive the car if you are drunk, because death was <u>instantaneous</u> in a fatal accident.
    A. instance
    B. spontaneous
    C. homogenous
    D. immediate

48. Workaholics tend to have a(n) <u>compulsive</u> and unrelenting need to work at any time.
    A. compulsory
    B. obstructive
    C. constructive
    D. impulsive

49. We've made great efforts to <u>exterminate</u> mosquitoes and flies in the tropical areas.
    A. erase
    B. eliminate
    C. demolish
    D. ruin

50. Poor eyesight will <u>exempt</u> you <u>from</u> military service.
    A. prevent from
    B. deprive from
    C. free from
    D. hinder from

51. The 19th-century physiology was <u>dominated</u> by the study of the transformation of food energy into body mass and activity.
    A. boosted
    B. governed
    C. clarified
    D. pioneered

52. Surely, it would be <u>sensible</u> to get a second opinion before taking any further action.
    A. realistic
    B. sensitive
    C. reasonable
    D. sensational

53. The Chinese people hold their ancestors in great <u>veneration</u>.
    A. recognition
    B. sincerity
    C. heritage
    D. honor

54. I worked to develop the <u>requisite</u> skill for a managerial.
    A. perfect
    B. exquisite
    C. unique
    D. necessary

55. If exercise is a bodily maintenance activity and an <u>index</u> of physiological age, the lack of sufficient exercise may either cause or hasten aging.
    A. instance　　　B. indicator　　　　C. appearance　　　D. option

56. The doctor advised Ken to avoid <u>strenuous</u> exercise.
    A. arduous　　　B. demanding　　　C. potent　　　　　D. continuous

57. The hospital should be held <u>accountable</u> for the quality of care it delivers.
    A. practicable　B. reliable　　　　C. flexible　　　　　D. responsible

58. Greenpeace has been invited to <u>appraise</u> the environment costs of such an operation.
    A. esteem　　　B. appreciate　　　C. evaluate　　　　D. approve

59. The company still hopes to find a buyer, but the future looks <u>bleak</u>.
    A. chilly　　　　B. dismal　　　　　C. promising　　　　D. fanatic

60. These were vital decisions that <u>bore upon</u> the happiness of everybody.
    A. ensured　　　B. ruined　　　　　C. achieved　　　　D. influenced

61. Memory can be both enhanced and <u>impaired</u> by use of drugs.
    A. inhibited　　B. injured　　　　C. induced　　　　　D. intervened

62. Is it true that this is the major <u>drawback</u> of the new medical plan?
    A. defect　　　　B. assistance　　　C. culprit　　　　　D. triumph

63. The physician was becoming <u>exasperated</u> with all the questions they were asking.
    A. frustrated　　B. perplexed　　　C. irritated　　　　D. crippled

64. We were shocked at the physician's <u>callous</u> disregard for the human dimension of medicine.
    A. involuntary　B. apparent　　　C. deliberate　　　　D. indifferent

65. For years, biologists have known that chimpanzees and even some monkeys produce a <u>panting</u> sound akin to human laughter.
    A. rocking　　　B. gasping　　　　C. vibrating　　　　D. resonating

66. Everybody at the party was in a very relaxed and <u>jolly</u> mood.
    A. rejoicing　　B. reconciling　　　C. refreshing　　　　D. resenting

67. The bacterial infection is curable with <u>judicious</u> use of antibiotics.
    A. impudent　　B. imprudent　　　C. purulent　　　　D. prudent

68. He tried to run, but he was <u>hampered</u> by his broken leg.
    A. endangered　B. endured　　　C. encountered　　　D. encumbered

69. The whole holiday was a <u>colossal</u> waste of money.
    A. consecutive　B. conductive　　C. considerate　　　D. considerable

70. The idea of correcting defective genes is not particularly underlined controversial in the scientific community.

    A. inevitable   B. applicable   C. disputable   D. incredible

2010 年真题

1. The chemical was found to be detrimental to human health.

   A. toxic   B. immune   C. sensitive   D. allergic

2. It will be a devastating blow for the patient, if the clinic closes.

   A. permanent   B. desperate   C. destructive   D. sudden

3. He kept telling us about his operation in the most graphic detail.

   A. verifiable   B. explicit   C. precise   D. ambiguous

4. The difficult case tested the ingenuity of even the most skillful physician.

   A. credibility   B. commitment   C. honesty   D. talent

5. He left immediately on the pretext that he had to catch a train.

   A. claim   B. clue   C. excuse   D. talent

6. The nurse was filled with remorse of not believing her.

   A. anguish   B. regret   C. apology   D. grief

7. The doctor tried to find a tactful way of telling her the truth.

   A. delicate   B. communicative   C. skillful   D. considerate

8. Whether a person likes a routine office job or not depends largely on temperament.

   A. disposition   B. qualification   C. temptation   D. endorsement

9. The doctor ruled out Friday's surgery for the patient's unexpected complications.

   A. confirmed   B. facilitated   C. postponed   D. cancelled

10. It is not easy to remain tranquil when events suddenly change your life.

    A. cautious   B. motionless   C. calm   D. alert

2011 年真题

1. She fell awkwardly and broke her leg.

   A. embarrassingly   B. reluctantly
   C. clumsily   D. dizzily

2. Throughout most of the recorded history, medicine was anything but scientific.

   A. more or less   B. by and large   C. more often than not   D. by no means

3. The students were captivated by the way the physician presented the case.

   A. illuminated   B. fascinated   C. alienated   D. hallucinated

4. We demand some <u>tangible</u> proof of our hard work in the form of statistical data, a product or a financial reward.

    A. intelligible   B. infinitive   C. substantial   D. deficient

5. But diets that restrict certain food groups or promise unrealistic results are difficult or unhealthy to <u>sustain</u> over time.

    A. maintain   B. reserve   C. conceive   D. empower

6. The molecular influence pervades all the traditional <u>disciplines</u> underlying clinical medicine.

    A. specialties   B. principles   C. rationales   D. doctrines

7. One usually becomes aware of the onset of puberty through <u>somatic</u> manifestations.

    A. juvenile   B. potent   C. physical   D. matured

8. His surgical procedure should succeed, for it seems quite <u>feasible</u>.

    A. rational   B. reciprocal   C. versatile   D. viable

9. These are <u>intensely</u> important questions about quality and the benefits of special care and experience.

    A. irresistibly   B. vitally   C. potentially   D. intriguingly

10. This guide gives you information on the best self-care <u>strategies</u> and the latest medical advances.

    A. tends   B. techniques   C. notions   D. breakthroughs

2012 年真题

1. She, a crazy fan, felt a <u>tingle</u> of excitement at the sight of Michael Jackson.

    A. glimpse   B. gust   C. panic   D. pack

2. She could never <u>transcend</u> her resentments against her mother's partiality for her brother.

    A. discipline   B. complain   C. conquer   D. defy

3. One could neither <u>trifle with</u> a terror of this kind, nor compromise with it.

    A. belittle   B. exaggerate   C. ponder   D. eliminate

4. <u>In light of</u> his good record, the police accepted defense.

    A. In place of   B. In view of   C. In spite of   D. In search of

5. City officials stated that workers who lied on their employment applications may be <u>terminated</u>.

    A. accused   B. punished   C. dismissed   D. suspended

6. An outbreak of swine flu outside of Mexico City was <u>blamed for</u> the deaths of more

than a hundred people in April 2009.

A. attached to　　B. ascribed to　　　　C. composed of　　　　D. related to

7. When a forest goes ablaze, it <u>discharges</u> hundreds of chemical compounds, including carbon monoxide.

A. puts out　　　B. passes off　　　　C. pulls out　　　　D. sends out

8. Unfortunately, the bridge under construction clasped in the earthquake, so they had to do the whole thing again <u>from scratch</u>.

A. from the beginning　　　　　　　　B. from now on
C. from time to time　　　　　　　　D. from the bottom

9. Identical twin sisters have led British scientists to a breakthrough in leukemia research that <u>promises</u> more effective therapies with fewer harmful side-effects.

A. administers　　B. nurtures　　　　C. inspires　　　　D. ensures

10. Radical environmentalists have blamed pollutants and synthetic chemicals in pesticides for the <u>disruption</u> of human hormones.

A. disturbance　　B. distraction　　　　C. intersection　　　　D. interpretation

2013 年真题

1. Christmas shoppers should be aware of the possible <u>defects</u> of the products sold at a discount.

A. deficits　　　B. deviations　　　　C. drawbacks　　　　D. discrepancies

2. The goal of this training program is to raise children with a sense of responsibility and necessary courage to be willing to <u>take on</u> challenges in life.

A. despise　　　B. evade　　　　C. demand　　　　D. undertake

3. After "9.11", the Olympic Games severely <u>taxed</u> the security services of the host country.

A. improved　　B. burdened　　　　C. inspected　　　　D. tariffed

4. The clown's performance was so funny that the audience, adults and children alike, were all thrown into <u>convulsions</u>.

A. a fit of enthusiasm　　　　　　　B. a scream of fright
C. a burst of laughter　　　　　　　D. a cry of anguish

5. We raised a <u>mortgage</u> from Bank of China and were informed to pay it off by the end of this year.

A. loan　　　　B. payment　　　　C. withdrawal　　　　D. retrieval

6. The advocates highly value the "sport spirit", while the opponents devalue it, asserting

that it's a(n) sheer hypocrisy and self-deception.

    A. fine   B. sudden   C. finite   D. absolute

7. Whenever a rattlesnake is agitated, it begins to move its tail and make a rattling noise.

    A. irritated   B. tamed   C. stamped   D. probed

8. The detective had an unusual insight into criminal's tricks and knew clearly how to track them.

    A. induction   B. perception   C. interpretation   D. penetration

9. My little brother practices the speech repeatedly until his delivery and timing were perfect.

    A. presentation   B. gesture   C. rhythm   D. pronunciation

10. In recent weeks both housing and stock prices have started to retreat from their irrationally amazing highs.

    A. untimely   B. unexpectedly

    C. unreasonably   D. unconventionally

2014 年真题

1. All Nobel Prize winners' success is a process of long-term accumulation, in which lasting efforts are indispensable.

    A. irresistible   B. cherished   C. inseparable   D. requisite

2. The Queen's presence imparted an air of elegance to the drinks reception at Buckingham Palace of London.

    A. bestowed   B. exhibited   C. imposed   D. emitted

3. Physicians are clear that thyroid dysfunction is manifest in growing children in the form of mental and physical retardation.

    A. intensified   B. apparent   C. representative   D. insidious

4. The mechanism that the eye can accommodate itself to different distances has been applied to automatic camera, which makes a revolutionary technique advance.

    A. yield   B. amplify   C. adapt   D. cast

5. Differences among believers are common; however, it was the pressure of religious persecution that exacerbated their conflicts and created the split of the union.

    A. eradicated   B. deteriorated   C. vanquished   D. averted

6. When Picasso was particularly poor, he might have tried to obliterate the original composition by painting over it on canvases.

    A. duplicate   B. eliminate   C. substitute   D. compile

7. For the sake of animal protection, environmentalists <u>deplored</u> the construction program of a nuclear power station.
   A. disapproved　B. despised　　　C. demolished　　　D. decomposed

8. Political figures in particular are held to very strict standards of moral <u>fidelity</u>.
   A. loyalty　　　B. morality　　　C. quality　　　D. stability

9. The patient complained that his doctor had been <u>negligent</u> in not giving him a full examination.
   A. fury　　　B. ardent　　　C. careless　　　D. brutal

10. She has been handling all the complaints without <u>wrath</u> for a whole morning.
    A. fury　　　B. chaos　　　C. despair　　　D. agony

2015 年真题

1. Every year more than 1,000 patients in Britain die on transplant waiting lists, <u>prompting</u> scientists to consider other ways to produce organs.
   A. propelling　B. prolonging　　C. puzzling　　　D. promising

2. Improved treatment has changed the outlook of HIV patients, but there is still a serious <u>stigma</u> attached to AIDS.
   A. disgrace　B. discrimination　C. harassment　　D. segregation

3. Survivors of the shipwreck were finally rescued after their courage of persistence lowered to zero by their physical <u>lassitude</u>.
   A. depletion　B. dehydration　　C. exhaustion　　D. handicap

4. Scientists have invented a 3D scan technology to read the otherwise <u>illegible</u> wood-carved stone, a method that may apply to other areas such as medicine.
   A. negative　B. confusing　　C. eloquent　　　D. indistinct

5. Top athletes <u>scrutinize</u> both success and failure with their coach to extract lessons from them, but they are never distracted from long-term goals.
   A. anticipate　B. clarify　　C. examine　　　D. verify

6. His <u>imperative</u> tone of voice reveals his arrogance and arbitrariness.
   A. challenging　B. solemn　　C. hostile　　　D. demanding

7. The discussion on the economic collaboration between the United States and the European Union may be <u>eclipsed</u> by the recent growing trade friction.
   A. erased　B. triggered　　C. shadowed　　　D. suspended

8. Faster increases in prices <u>foster</u> the belief that the future increases will be also stronger, so that higher prices fuel demand rather than quench it.

A. nurture　　　B. eliminate　　　C. assimilate　　　D. puncture

9. Some recent developments in photography allow animals to be studied in previously inaccessible places and in <u>unprecedented</u> detail.
 A. unpredictable
 B. unconventional
 C. unparalleled
 D. unexpected

10. A veteran negotiation specialist should be skillful at <u>manipulating</u> touchy situation.
 A. estimating　　B. handling　　C. rectifying　　D. anticipating

2016 年真题

1. In any event, lethal injections are under federal <u>scrutiny</u>.
 A. sanction　　B. restriction　　C. census　　D. examination

2. The humble tomato could become a(n) <u>potent</u> weapon in the fight against prostate cancer.
 A. inexpensive　　B. powerful　　C. conventional　　D. lethal

3. Men's perception of the amount of caregiving they do is completely <u>at odds with</u> women's.
 A. in tune with
 B. in favor of
 C. for the sake of
 D. in disagreement with

4. Huangshan Mountain is <u>eminent</u> for its natural scenery and deserves a visit.
 A. renowned　　B. notorious　　C. popular　　D. mysterious

5. Obesity is a condition perpetuated by a <u>diversity</u> of factors.
 A. severity　　B. reliability　　C. variety　　D. specificity

6. He is usually well-behaved; this rudeness is only a(n) <u>lapse</u>.
 A. error　　B. sin　　C. guilt　　D. offense

7. Did you detect a touch of <u>jaundice</u> in her remark?
 A. grievance　　B. sympathy　　C. jealousy　　D. indignation

8. In 1912, German doctors attempted to treat children who had underactive thyroids with normal thyroid cells, but <u>to little avail</u>.
 A. by no means　　B. in vain　　C. of no account　　D. at stake

9. To many observers, he spent his wealth <u>lavishly</u>.
 A. fearlessly　　B. conspicuously　　C. wastefully　　D. ferociously

10. At present, no medical therapy is known to affect <u>progressions</u> of rheumatic mitral stenosis.
 A. deterioration　　B. accumulation　　C. expansion　　D. promotion

2017 年真题

1. Inform the manager if you are on medication that makes you drowsy.
   A. uneasy　　　　B. sleepy　　　　　C. guilty　　　　　D. fiery

2. Diabetes is one of the most prevalent and potentially dangerous diseases in the world.
   A. crucial　　　　B. virulent　　　　C. colossal　　　　D. widespread

3. Likewise, soot and smoke from fire contain a multitude of carcinogens.
   A. a matter of　　B. a body of　　　C. plenty of　　　D. sort of

4. Many questions about estrogen's effects remain to be elucidated, and investigations are seeking answers through ongoing laboratory and clinical studies.
   A. implicated　　B. implied　　　　C. illuminated　　　D. initiated

5. A network chatting is a limp substitute for meeting friends over coffee.
   A. accomplishment　　　　　　B. refreshment
   C. complement　　　　　　　　D. replacement

6. When patients spend extended periods in hospital, they tend to become overly dependent and　lose interest in taking care of themselves.
   A. extremely　　B. exclusively　　C. exactly　　　D. explicitly

7. Attempts to restrict parking in the city centre have further aggravated the problem of traffic congestion.
   A. ameliorated　　B. aggregated　　C. deteriorated　　　D. duplicated

8. It was reported that bacteria contaminated up to 80% of domestic retail raw chicken in the United States.
   A. inflamed　　　B. inflicted　　　C. infected　　　　D. infiltrated

9. Researchers recently ran the numbers on gun violence in the United States and reported that right-to-carry-gun laws do not inhibit violent crime.
   A. curb　　　　　B. induce　　　　C. lessen　　　　D. impel

10. Regardless of our uneasiness about stereotypes, numerous studies have shown clear difference between Chinese and western parenting.
    A. specifications　　　　　　B. sensations
    C. conventions　　　　　　　D. conservations

2018 年真题

1. The truly competent physician is the one who sits down, senses the "mystery" of another human beings, and offers the simple gifts of personal interest and

understanding.

A．imaginable　　B．capable　　C．sensible　　D．humble

2. The physician often <u>perceived</u> that treatment was initiated by the patient.

A．conserved　　B．theorized　　C．realized　　D．persisted

3. Large community meals might have served to <u>lubricate</u> social connections and alleviated tensions.

A．facilitate　　B．intimidate　　C．terminate　　D．mediate

4. Catalase activity reduced glutathione and Vitamin E levels were decreased <u>exclusively</u> in subjects with active disease.

A．definitely　　B．truly　　C．simply　　D．solely

5. Ocular anomalies were frequently observed in this cohort of <u>offspring</u> born after in vitro fertilization.

A．fetuses　　B．descendants　　C．seeds　　D．orphans

6. Childhood poverty should be regarded as the single greatest public health <u>menace</u> facing our children.

A．breach　　B．grief　　C．threat　　D．abuse

7. A distant dream would be to <u>deliberately</u> set off quakes to release tectonic stress in a controlled way.

A．definitely　　B．desperately　　C．intentionally　　D．identically

8. Big challenges still await companies <u>converting</u> carbon dioxide to petrol.

A．applying　　B．relating　　C．relaying　　D．transforming

9. Concerns have recently been voiced that the drugs <u>elicit</u> unexpected cognitive side effects, such as memory loss, fuzzy thinking and learning difficulties.

A．ensue　　B．encounter　　C．impede　　D．induce

10. A leaf before the eye shuts out Mount Tai, which means having one's view of the important overshadowed by the <u>trivial</u>.

A．insignificant　　B．insufficient　　C．substantial　　D．unexpected

答案及解析

1. 【答案】B

【解析】offset 意为"补偿，抵消"；四个选项含义如下：take in ①吞入，吸入；例如：Fish can take in oxygen through their gills. 鱼用鳃吸入氧气。②欺骗，例如：I was taken in by his story. 我被他的故事给骗了。③留宿，例如：The old man took in these homeless people. 这个老人收留了这些无家可归的人。

make up ①弥补，例如：Saying sorry to me couldn't make up my damage. 对我说对不起不能弥补对我的伤害。②形成，构成；例如：Female students make up only one third of the student numbers in this university. 女学生仅占这所大学学生人数的三分之一。③编造，例如：The student made up an excuse for being late. 这个学生为迟到编造了一个借口。cut down 削减，例如：This company had to cut down its expenses in this project. 公司不得不削减这个项目的开支。bring about 导致，例如：What brought about the change in his attitude? 什么使得他改变了主意？

题干译文：可以很乐观地相信这些进步弥补了农业的大幅度减产。

2. 【答案】A

　　【解析】plot 意为"绘制，划分，策划"；四个选项含义为：mark 标注，注明；allocate 分派，分配；erase 抹去；pose 摆姿势。

　　题干译文：为了研究这个区域内病情的分布，在地图上标明情况很有用。

3. 【答案】A

　　【解析】elevation 的含义是"海拔"。四个选项含义为：altitude 高度，海拔；aptitude 才能，能力；latitude 纬度；longitude 经度。

　　题干译文：随着海拔升高，大气温度会降低。

4. 【答案】C

　　【解析】arbitrary 的含义是"任意的，专制的，武断的"。assertive 的含义是"断定的，过分自信的"，例如：He is an assertive boy, always insisting on his own rights and opinions. 他是个过分自信的男孩，总是坚持自己的权利和观点。decisive 的含义是"决定性"；tasteful 的含义是"高雅的，雅致的"。根据句意可以知道 arbitrary 的含义不是"武断专制的"，而是"不加选择的，随意的"，故只有 C 符合句意。

　　题干译文：我不了解时尚，所以我对衣服的选择很随意。

5. 【答案】C

　　【解析】根据句意所提供的信息：不肯承认错误，可以判断画线词的含义为"倔强的，固执的"。四个选项含义如下：obsessive 着迷的，迷恋的；例如：an obsessive attention to details 十分注重细节。furious 狂怒的，暴怒的；固定搭配是 be furious with sb. at sth. 例如：He was furious with himself for the failure in the exam. 他生自己的气，怪自己考试不及格。stubborn 固执的，倔强的；例如：He is as stubborn as a donkey. 他倔得像头驴；rebellious 反抗的，叛逆的。

　　题干译文：这个孩子很倔强不肯承认错误。

6. 【答案】B

　　【解析】题干画线词 indomitable 的含义为"不屈不挠的"，display 的含义为"呈现"，embody 的含义为"体现"。unsubdued 的含义为"不屈服的"；determined 的含义为"坚决的"；industrious 的含义是"勤勉刻苦的"。通过题干中的 athlete（运动员）可以推断出画线词的大概含义，只有 B 项符合句意。

题干译文：运动员所展现的不屈不挠的精神体现了这个国家的新风貌。

7. 【答案】D
　　【解析】根据画线部分的主要词汇 depth 可以知道 in-depth 的含义为"深入的"。specific 的含义是"明确的，具体的"，例如：specific instructions 明确的指示。shallow 的含义为"浅薄的"，不符合句意。profound 的含义为"深切的，深刻的，严重的"，例如：have a profound effect on 对……起到深远影响；profound insights 深刻的见解；profound disability 严重残疾。thorough 的含义为"深入的，细致的，彻底的"，例如：a thorough investigation 全面调查；a thorough cleaning 大扫除。只有 D 项与题干画线部分意思最接近。

　　题干译文：双方就如何加强进一步的合作深入交换了意见。

8. 【答案】A
　　【解析】题干中画线词 insulate 的含义为"绝缘，隔热"。这里 insulate sb. / sth. from / against 含义是"免受……的（不良影响）"。四个选项含义为：isolate from "使隔离，使孤立"，例如：He was isolated from other prisoners. 他被与其他犯人隔离起来。secede 脱离，退出；be absent from 缺席，不在，例如：be absent from school 缺课。distinguish from "区分，区别"，例如：He can distinguish a genuine antique from a reproduction. 他能区分真古董和仿制品。由此可知 A 项最适合。

　　题干译文：孩子应注意避免受到不良经验的影响。

9. 【答案】C
　　【解析】in the light of 的含义为"根据，按照"。四个选项含义为：throw light on 解释，阐明；例如：As the time went by, all the unsettled questions were thrown light on in the end. 随着时间的推移，所有未解决的问题都最终得到了解释。in line with 和……站成一排，与……相似或符合，例如：Your plan is in line with my ideas. 你的计划与我的想法一致。in accordance with 依照；例如：In accordance with his father's wish he gave the money to the school. 依照他父亲的愿望，他把钱捐给了学校。in terms of 就……而言；例如：In terms of learning strategies, I don't think this teaching method is beneficial to students. 就学习策略而言，我认为这个教学方法对学生不利。

　　题干译文：根据目前的状况，我必须重新审视我的计划了。

10. 【答案】D
　　【解析】题干画线词 aggressive 的含义是"侵略的，进取的"。根据题干的信息，aggressive 的含义应该是褒义的。四个选项含义为：invasive 侵略的，在医学上含义为"侵袭的"；例如：invasive cancer 扩散性肿瘤。belligerent 好斗的，挑衅的；progressive 进步的，逐步的；例如：a progressive muscular disease 逐渐严重的肌肉病症。enterprising 有进取心的，与画线词意思相同。

　　题干译文：在当今激烈的就业市场，人们尤其是年轻人要有进取心、要勤奋。

11. 【答案】A

【解析】题干画线词 assimilate 的含义为"吸收，消化"。四个选项含义为：digest 的含义是"消化，吸收"，与题干画线词意义相同；incorporate 的含义为"包含，纳入"，例如：The new design incorporates all the latest fashionable elements. 这个新设计包含所有最新的时尚元素。imitate 模仿；compile 编纂。

题干译文：消化这篇有关计算技术的报告很费时，因为我不是这一专业的。

12. 【答案】A

【解析】题干画线词组 be responsible for 的含义为"对……负责"。四个选项含义为：answer for 的含义为"对……负责"，例如：Everyone should answer for his or her action. 每个人都应该对自己的行为负责。account for 的含义有：①解释，说明，例如：He didn't account for his absence. 他没有解释缺席的原因。②占……时间、空间，例如：Girls account for two thirds of students in this college. 这所大学女生占三分之二。charge for 索价，例如：We won't charge you for delivery. 我们免费送货。compensate for 赔偿，补偿，例如：Nothing can compensate for my loss. 什么也不能补偿我的损失。

题干译文：作为社会一分子，人人应该对社会负责，为社会做贡献。

13. 【答案】B

【解析】画线词 resourceful 含义为"足智多谋的，机智的"；四个选项含义为：imaginary 虚构的，不真实的。imaginative 有创造性的，与画线词意义相近；plentiful 丰富的；versatile 多面手，多才多艺的。

题干译文：令我惊奇的是，这个年轻人非常机智，可以找到很多方式用肢体语言表达他的情感。

14. 【答案】A

【解析】画线词组的含义为"并发症"。complication 的含义就是"并发症"；其他三项的含义为：complexity 复杂性；knottiness 困难，难题，纠纷；hindrance 障碍。

题干译文：为了降低怀孕的并发症，要求你在确定自己怀孕后改变生活方式。

15. 【答案】B

【解析】题干画线词 impetus 的含义是"推动力，促进"。四个选项含义为：impetuous 是形容词，含义为"冲动的，轻率的"，例如：She regretted her impetuous decision. 她后悔做出轻率的决定。impulse 为名词，含义为"推动"，例如：On impulse, I bought the expensive antique. 我一心血来潮就买下了这个昂贵的古董。hindrance 障碍；impasse 僵局，例如：They reached an impasse in the negotiations. 他们在谈判过程中陷入僵局。

题干译文：这个条约给两国间贸易以及各自工业发展提供了推动力。

16. 【答案】C

【解析】题干画线词 hideous 是形容词，含义是"骇人听闻的，可怕的"。torment 含义是"痛苦，折磨"，surrender oneself 含义是"自首，投降"。四个选项含义为：painful（身心）痛苦的；inhumane 残忍的，不人道的；horrid 可怕的，恐怖的；brutal 残忍的。只有 C 项与画线词义接近。

题干译文：当敌人抓到他的时候，他受尽折磨，但他根本就没屈服。

17. 【答案】D

【解析】题干中的画线词组 at stake 的含义可以通过语境信息推断出来，即"危险中"。on hand 的含义为"现有的"，相当于 available，例如：Medical service is on hand. 提供医疗服务。in circulation 含义是：①流通中，例如：A number of forged banknotes are in circulation. 大量假币在流通中。②社交，交际，例如：After a month in hospital, she is back in circulation. 住了一个月的医院后，她又活跃起来了。under consideration 的含义为"考虑中"，例如：The proposal is currently under consideration. 这个提议目前正在考虑中。at risk 含义为"在危险中"，与画线词组意思相同。

题干译文：在紧急情况下商业部门可以关门，但医院不可以，因为性命攸关。

18. 【答案】A

【解析】题干画线词 substitute 含义为"替代品"，常与介词 for 连用。题干中，on the eve of Spring Festival 含义为"春节的除夕"。四个选项含义为：alternative 选择物，替代品；allusion 提及，暗示，例如：His writings are full of classical allusions. 他的作品里有许多典故。alteration 变更，改造；altercation 争论，口角。

题干译文：我们从来就没想过是否其他事物可以成为除夕饺子的替代品，并且一样好吃。

19. 【答案】C

【解析】题干画线词组的含义为"被控告"，be dismissed 被开除，sales representative 销售代表。四个选项含义为：be accustomed to 相当于 be used to doing，即"习惯于"，例如：I am accustomed to taking a walk after super. 我习惯于晚饭后散步。adhere to 坚持，遵循，例如：She adheres to teaching methods she learned over 20 years ago. 她还在遵循 20 年前她所学到的教学方法。be charged with 被控告，例如：He was charged with murder. 他被控谋杀。stick to 坚持，例如：He promised to help us, but he didn't stick to his word. 他答应帮助我们，但他失言了。

题干译文：这个销售代理被开除了，因为他被控欺骗顾客。

20. 【答案】B

【解析】题干画线词 appalling 含义为"骇人听闻的，可怕的"。in person 含义为"亲手，亲自"，extenuate 含义为"减轻，使人原谅"，例如：Because of extenuating circumstances, the court acquitted him of the crime. 因考虑到情有可原，法庭判他无罪。各选项含义为：appealing 与画线词形似，但含义为：①吸引人的，有感染力的；②可怜的，恳求的。dreadful 可怕的，与画线词含义相同；imprudent 轻率的，鲁莽的；displeasing 不愉快的。

题干译文：这个中年男子亲手杀害了他的妻子和孩子，这种骇人听闻的行为罪不可恕。

21. 【答案】B

【解析】题干画线词组 compatible with 的含义为"与……一致"。四个选项含义如下：be suitable for 适合，例如：No one in the applicants is suitable for the job. 申请者中无人适合这个工作。be consistent with 与……一致，例如：The results are entirely consistent with our earlier research. 结果与我们先前的研究完全一致。be in harmony with 融洽，和睦，例如：People should be in harmony with the environment. 人们要与环境相和谐。be in favor of 的含义是：①赞同，例如：He was in favor of the proposal. 他赞同这个提议。②看中，选择，例如：He abandoned teaching in favor of a career as a musician. 他弃教从事音乐。

题干译文：别再相信这个发言人了，因为他的行为从来就与他的观念不一致。

22. 【答案】A

【解析】题干画线词组 be vulnerable to sth. 意为"易受……伤害"，例如：In case of food poisoning, young children are easily vulnerable. 在食物中毒的问题上，年龄小的孩子容易受危害。juvenile 意为"青少年"。各选项含义为：be susceptible to 容易受……的影响。be favorable to 对……有利、有帮助，例如：The terms of this agreement are favorable to both sides. 协议中的条款对双方都有利。be relevant to 与……紧密相关，例如：The evidence they found is relevant to the case. 他们找到的证据与这个案件相关。be capable of 有能力做。

题干译文：青少年更容易受消极影响和外部压力的影响，包括同龄人的压力。

23. 【答案】C

【解析】题干中 subject sb. to 的含义是"使经受"，例如：The essay subjected him to criticism. 这篇论文让他受到批评。vicious 恶毒的；insidious 阴险的；hazardous 危险的；notorious 声名狼藉的。故 C 正确。

题干译文：工作中有让你接触有害化学物质的东西吗？

24. 【答案】B

【解析】题干画线词 alleviate 的含义为"减轻，缓解"。四个选项含义如下：expel 驱散，消除；diminish 减少；endure 忍耐；chop 砍，剁。B 项符合画线词的含义。

题干译文：姜也可以通过促进血液循环有助于减轻感冒的痛苦。

25. 【答案】D

【解析】题干画线词 deadly 的含义为"致命的"，victim 的含义为"受害者"，orphan 的含义为"孤儿"。四个选项含义如下：brutal 残忍的；terrible 可怕的；horrible 恐怖的；lethal 致命的。

题干译文：上千人成为受害者，许多孩子在这场致命的地震中成为孤儿。

26. 【答案】A

【解析】题干画线词组 on the sly 含义为"秘密地，偷偷地"，例如：He has to visit his children on the sly. 他必须偷偷地去看他的孩子。选项中只有 A 项 secretly 符合这个词组的含义。其他三项：punctiliously 谨小慎微地；dilatorily 慢吞吞地，迟缓地；cunningly 狡猾地。

题干译文：她认为没人在看的时候，打开了橱柜，偷偷地拿出了一些糖果。

27. 【答案】A

【解析】题干画线词组 on occasion 的含义为"偶尔，有时"。四个选项含义为：at times 偶尔；at a time 每次，一次，例如：take three pills at a time 一次服三粒。at all times 始终（无论什么时候），例如：You should have a cool head at all times. 无论什么时候你都应该保持清醒的头脑。at one time 曾经，一度，例如：She was my best friend at one time. 曾经她是我最好的朋友。

题干译文：我们在几年前就没再保持深厚的友谊，尽管我们偶尔互相拜访。

28. 【答案】B

【解析】题干画线词含义为"富有的"。各选项含义如下：powerful 强大的；affluent 丰富的，富裕的；promising 有希望的，有前途的；almighty 全能的。可知只有选项 B 符合画线词含义。

题干译文：英国人属于欧洲富有国家之一，和其他国家相比，他们享有很高的生活水平。

29. 【答案】C

【解析】题干画线词组 without question 含义为"毫无疑问"。各选项含义如下：out of the question 不可能，例如：Another trip abroad this year is out of the question. 今年再次出国旅行是不可能的。apparently 显然地，相当于 obviously；undoubtedly 的含义即为"毋庸置疑地"；naturally 自然地。

题干译文：毫无疑问，这里人们的生活在过去的二十年间发生了翻天覆地的变化。

30. 【答案】B

【解析】题干画线词 indignant 的含义为"愤怒的"，常与介词 at 或者 about 连用，例如：They were indignant at the way they had been treated. 他们对自己受到的待遇很愤怒。各选项含义如下：imprudent 轻率的，鲁莽的；wrathful 愤怒的；tenacious 顽强的；impatient 不耐烦的。

题干译文：工人们对不公待遇和老板漠然的态度很愤恨。

31. 【答案】C

【解析】题干画线单词 indisposition 的含义为"小病，微恙"。各选项含义如下：aliment 滋养品；situation 状况；ailment 疾病（尤指微恙）；incompetence 无能力。

题干译文：他不想老是问起她的健康情况，因为她对自己的病好像不很在乎。

32. 【答案】D

【解析】题干画线词 wholesome 的含义为"有益健康的"。各选项含义如下：decent 端庄的，得体的；wholesale 批发的，大规模的；moral 有道德的；salubrious 的含义即为"有益健康的"。

题干译文：提供给社会和大众安全、有益健康的食品是政府十分重要的责任。

33. 【答案】C

【解析】题干画线词 absurd 的含义为"荒谬的"。四个选项含义为：unreasonable 不合情合理的；immoral 不道德的；ridiculous 荒谬的；abnormal 不正常的。

题干译文：做同样的工作，女性的工资要比男性的低，太荒谬了。

34. 【答案】B

【解析】题干画线单词 upright 的含义为"正直的"。四个选项含义为：vertical 垂直的；honest 诚实的，正直的；modest 谦虚的；incorruptible 清廉的。

题干译文：这个出租车司机很正直，从来不多要钱。

35. 【答案】D

【解析】题干画线单词 earnestly 的含义为"认真地"；各选项含义如下：cautiously 谨慎地；severely 严重地；accurately 精确地；seriously 认真地，符合题干画线词含义。

题干译文：安全官员很认真地置疑是否合成材料使用越多，火灾的隐患就会越大。

36. 【答案】B

【解析】题干画线单词 jeopardize 的含义为"危害"，例如：If you are impolite to your boss, it may jeopardize your chance of success. 如果你对老板不礼貌，也许会危及你事业的成功。四个选项含义为：benefit 对……有利；endanger 危及，危害；hinder 阻碍；disturb 扰乱。只有 B 项符合题干画线单词的含义。

题干译文：参议员认为支持这项措施将会危及改选。

37. 【答案】A

【解析】题干画线词 ambiguous 的含义为"模棱两可的，模糊不清的"。各选项含义如下：obscure 朦胧的，模糊的，与题干画线词含义相同。ambitious 有野心的，雄心勃勃的；indifferent 漠然的；explicit 清楚的。

题干译文：我们对他在如何彻底解决这个问题上模棱两可的态度很是生气。

38. 【答案】B

【解析】题干画线单词 disseminate 的含义为"传播，散布"，例如：disseminate rumors 散布谣言；disseminate Buddhism 传播佛教。题干 envoy 的含义为"特使，外交使节"。四个选项含义为：disclose 揭露，暴露；spread 传播；analyze 分析；deliver 递送。

题干译文：在汉代，皇室派遣特使前往西方国家传播中国文化。

39. 【答案】D

【解析】题干画线词 anguish 的含义为"痛苦"。各选项含义如下：surprise 惊奇；stress 压力；dilemma 进退两难的困境；misery 痛苦，可知 D 符合画线词含义。

题干译文：我永远不会忘记当他父母得知他死亡的消息时，脸上极其痛苦的表情。

40. 【答案】B

【解析】题干画线词 resourceful 的含义为"机智的"，四个选项含义为：versatile 多才多艺的。diligent 勤劳的，勤勉的；capable 有能力的；perfect 完美的，只有选项 clever 符合题干画线词含义。

题干译文：妻子们总是认为她们的丈夫一定是足智多谋、多才多艺的。

41. 【答案】A

【解析】题干画线单词 incidence 的含义为"发病率"，malaria 意思为"疟疾"，tropical 意思为"热带的"，句型 there is no denial that 意为"不可否认的是……"。各选项含义如下：morbidity 发病率，与画线单词含义相同；precedent 先例；mobility 活动性，灵活性；proficiency 熟练，精通程度。

题干译文：不可否认，在热带地区，疟疾的发病率很高。

42. 【答案】B

【解析】题干画线词组 in sequence 含义为"依次，顺次"；四个选项含义为：at length 详细地，相当于 in details；in order 依次，与题干画线词组含义相同；in advance 提前；in earnest 认真地。

题干译文：我们想让你依次报告那天早上发生的所有事情，不得延误。

43. 【答案】C

【解析】题干画线单词 expedient 的含义为"有利的"。各选项含义如下：beneficent 仁慈的，慈善的；contributive 贡献的，资助的；advantageous 有利的，为正确答案；profitable 有利可图的。

题干译文：大多数演讲者发现对公众发表演讲的时候使用笔记提示是有利的。

44. 【答案】D

【解析】题干画线单词 anonymous 的含义为"匿名的"。四个选项的含义为：undisturbed 不受干扰的；unnoticed 不被注意的；unrecorded 不被记录的；unnamed 匿名的，与题干画线单词含义相同。

题干译文：一些人打电话报警的时候更愿意匿名。

45. 【答案】A

【解析】题干画线单词 immature 的含义为"不成熟的"。各选项的含义如下：puerile 未成熟的，孩子气的，幼稚的，与画线单词词义相同。sophisticated 久经世故的；crude 天然的，未加工的；worldly 世间的。

题干译文：小孩子可能在某一年龄显示出相对早熟的行为模式，并且在后面的年龄段显现出相对不成熟的行为模式。

46. 【答案】B

【解析】题干画线单词 allegiance 的含义为"忠贞，效忠"，与介词 to 连用，固定搭配为：to pledge / swear allegiance to sb. 宣誓 / 发誓效忠某人。四个选项的含义为：truthfulness 真实，坦率；loyalty 忠诚，与介词 to 连用，如：remain loyal to the principles 信守原则；faith 信仰，信任，与介词 in 连用；endurance 忍耐力。

题干译文：战前，战士们发誓效忠祖国。

47. 【答案】D

【解析】题干画线单词 instantaneous 的含义为"瞬间的，刹那的"。各选项含义如下：instance 实例，情况；spontaneous 自发的，自然产生的；homogenous 同质的；immediate 立即的，即刻的。

题干译文：如果你喝醉了，不要驾车，因为在致命的车祸中死亡就发生在一瞬间。

48. 【答案】A

【解析】题干画线单词 compulsive 的含义为"强迫性的，必需的"。workaholic 的含义是"工作狂"，unrelenting 的含义是"不宽恕的，不缓和、不松懈的"。

各选项含义如下：compulsory 必需的，如 compulsory courses 必修课；obstructive 妨碍的；constructive 有建设性的；impulsive 冲动的。

题干译文：工作狂总是在任何时候都有难以抑制、不松懈想要工作的需求。

49. 【答案】B

【解析】题干画线单词 exterminate 的含义为"消除"，mosquitoes 意为"蚊子"，flies 意为"苍蝇"。各选项含义为：erase 擦除，抹去；eliminate 消除，符合画线单词含义；demolish 毁坏，推翻；ruin 毁坏。

题干译文：我们尽力消除热带地区的蚊蝇。

50. 【答案】C

【解析】题干画线词组 exempt from 的含义为"使……免除"，eyesight 意为"视力"，military service 指的是"服兵役"。各选项含义为：prevent from 防止；deprive from 剥夺，使丧失；free from 免予；hinder from 阻碍，例如：A former injury was hindering him from playing his best. 旧伤使他无法发挥出最好水平。

题干译文：你视力不佳，可以免兵役。

51. 【答案】B

【解析】画线词 dominate 的含义是"支配"。boost 的含义是"促进"；govern 的含义是"统治，掌管"；clarify 的含义是"澄清"；pioneer 的含义是"做先驱，开辟"。只有 B 项接近画线词的含义。physiology 的含义是"生理学"，body mass 的含义是"体重"。

题干译文：19 世纪的生理学是以食物能量转化为体重和身体活动的研究为主导的。

52. 【答案】C

【解析】画线词 sensible 的含义是"明智的，合情理的"。realistic 的含义是"现实的"；sensitive 虽然形似画线词，但其含义是"敏感的"；reasonable 的含义是"合情合理的"；sensational 的含义是"轰动的，耸人听闻的"。此题值得注意的形似画线词的选项很可能不是答案。

题干译文：当然，在实施任何行动前听听别人的意见是明智的。

53. 【答案】D

【解析】画线词 veneration 的含义是"崇敬"。recognition 的含义是"承认"；sincerity 的含义是"真诚"；heritage 的含义是"遗产"；honor 的含义是"荣誉，荣幸"。只有选项 D 与画线词意思接近。ancestor 的含义是"祖先"。

题干译文：中国人极其尊敬他们的祖先。

54. 【答案】D

【解析】画线词 requisite 的含义是"必要的"，例如：He hasn't got the requisite qualifications for this job. 他不具备这项工作所需的资格。perfect 的含义是"极好的，优秀的"；exquisite 与画线词形似，但其含义是"精致的"，例如：Her skirt has very exquisite lace. 她的裙子有非常精致的花边。unique 的含义是"独特的，唯一的"；necessary 与画线词近义。managerial 的含义是"管理者"。

题干译文：我努力培养自己管理者必要的技能。

55. 【答案】B

【解析】画线词 index 的含义是"指标"；instance 的含义是"事例"；indicator 的含义是"指示"；appearance 的含义是"外表"；option 的含义是"选择"。maintenance 的含义是"保养，维护"。hasten 的含义是"催促"。

题干译文：如果锻炼是身体维护活动和生理年龄的一项指标，那么缺乏足够锻炼可能会导致或者加速衰老。

56. 【答案】A

【解析】画线词 strenuous 的含义是"费力的"，例如：He made strenuous attempts to stop her. 他为阻止她做出了极大的努力。arduous 的含义是"费力的，辛勤的"，例如：Although the work was arduous, he finished it in a short time. 虽然这项工作很费力，他仍然很快就做完了。demanding 的含义是"要求多的"，例如：Teaching is a demanding profession. 教学工作是个要求很高的职业。potent 的含义是"有效力的"；continuous 的含义是"连续不断的"。

题干译文：医生建议 Ken 避免强度大的运动。

57. 【答案】D

【解析】画线词 accountable 的含义是"负有责任的"，例如：I am not accountable to you for my actions. 我没有义务要对你说明我的行动。reliable 的含义是"可靠的"；flexible 的含义是"灵活的，有弹性的"；responsible 通常与介词 for 连用，与画线词近义。

题干译文：这个医院应该有必要就提供的服务质量进行说明。

58. 【答案】C

【解析】画线词 appraise 的含义是"评价，估价"。esteem 的含义是"尊敬"；appreciate 的含义是"感激，欣赏"；evaluate 与画线词近义，意思是"评价"；approve 的含义是"赞成"，通常与介词 of 连用，例如：Her father didn't approve of her marriage to the poor guy. 她父亲不同意她嫁给一个穷小子。

题干译文：绿色和平组织被邀请参加评估这样的经营活动对环境产生的代价。

59. 【答案】B

【解析】画线词 bleak 的含义是"阴郁的，严寒的，黯淡的"，例如：The future of this firm will be very bleak indeed if we keep losing money. 要是我们继续亏本的话，这家公司的前途会非常黯淡。chilly 的含义是"寒冷的，冷淡的"，例如：chilly welcome 冷淡的迎接；dismal 的含义是"阴沉的，凄凉的"，例如：take a dismal view of economy 对经济不抱乐观态度。promising 的含义是"有希望的，有前途的"；fanatic 的含义是"狂热的"，例如：be fanatic about pop music 痴迷于流行音乐。根据题干语境提示，可以得知 bleak 的含义是"渺茫的"。故 B 正确。

题干译文：公司仍旧希望找到买家，但未来看上去希望渺茫。

60. 【答案】D

【解析】画线词组 bear upon 的含义是"与……有关，影响"；ensure 的含义是"保证，确保"；ruin 的含义是"毁坏"；achieve 的含义是"达成"；influence

的含义是"影响"。vital 的含义是"至关重要的，生死攸关的，有活力的"，例如：The heart is a vital organ. 心脏是维持生命必需的器官。

题干译文：这些是关系到每个人幸福的重要决定。

61. 【答案】B

【解析】画线词 impair 的含义是"损害"。inhibit 的含义是"禁止，抑制"；injure 的含义是"受伤"；induce 的含义是"引诱，导致"，例如：Too much food probably induces sleepiness. 吃得太多可能引起困意。intervene 的含义是"干涉，干预"。

题干译文：吃药可以增强记忆，也可能损害记忆。

62. 【答案】A

【解析】画线词 drawback 的含义是"缺点"；defect 的含义是"缺陷"；assistance 的含义是"帮助"；culprit 的含义是"犯人"；triumph 的含义是"胜利"。

题干译文：这个就是新医疗计划中的严重缺陷吗？

63. 【答案】C

【解析】画线词 exasperate 的含义是"恼怒"。frustrate 的含义是"挫败"；perplex 的含义是"困惑，糊涂"；irritate 的含义是"激怒"；cripple 的含义是"使……跛"。

题干译文：他们正在问的这些问题激怒了这个医生。

64. 【答案】D

【解析】画线词 callous 的含义是"麻木的，无情的"。involuntary 的含义是"非自愿的"；apparent 的含义是"明显的"；deliberate 的含义是"故意的"；indifferent 的含义是"冷漠的"；disregard 的含义是"漠视，忽视"。

题干译文：我们惊讶于这个医生对医学人文层面的无情漠视。

65. 【答案】B

【解析】画线词 panting 的含义是"喘息"。rocking 的含义是"摇动的"；gasping 的含义是"气喘的"；vibrating 的含义是"震动的"；resonating 的含义是"共鸣的，共振的"。akin to 的含义是"类似，近于"，例如：Pity is often akin to love. 怜悯经常类似于爱。

题干译文：多年以来，生物学家已经得知黑猩猩甚至一些猴子能够发出类似于人笑的气喘声。

66. 【答案】A

【解析】画线词 jolly 的含义是"愉快的"。rejoicing 的含义是"高兴的"；reconciling 的含义是"和解，妥协"；refreshing 的含义是"有精神的"；resenting 的含义是"仇恨，生气"。此题根据 relaxed 的含义，可以得知 jolly 的含义与 relaxed 近义。

题干译文：晚会上每个人都很放松，心情愉快。

67. 【答案】D

【解析】画线词 judicious 的含义是"明智的，审慎的"。四个选项是形近词，要注意辨析。impudent 的含义是"鲁莽的"；imprudent 的含义是"轻率的"；purulent 的含义是"化脓的，脓性的"；prudent 的含义是"审慎的"。antibiotics 的含义是"抗生素"。

题干译文：谨慎地使用抗生素可以治愈细菌感染。

68. 【答案】D

【解析】画线词 hamper 的含义是"妨碍"。endanger 的含义是"受到……的危险"；endure 的含义是"忍耐，持续"；encounter 的含义是"意外遭遇"；encumber 的含义是"阻碍"，例如：The girl's long skirt encumbered her while running. 这女孩子的长裙在她跑的时候阻碍她的行动。

题干译文：他试着跑，但他的断腿阻碍了他。

69. 【答案】D

【解析】画线词 colossal 的含义是"巨大的"。consecutive 的含义是"连续的"；conductive 的含义是"传导性的"；considerate 的含义是"体贴周到的"；considerable 的含义是"相当大的"。

题干译文：整个假期太浪费钱了。

70. 【答案】C

【解析】画线词 controversial 的含义是"有争议的"。inevitable 的含义是"必然的，不可避免的"；applicable 的含义是"可适用的"；disputable 的含义是"有争议的"；incredible 的含义是"不可思议的"。

题干译文：修正有缺陷基因的想法在科学领域不是特别有争议。

2010 年真题

1. 【答案】A

【解析】画线词 detrimental 的含义是"有害的"，与介词 to 连用，例如：Lack of sleep is detrimental to one's health. 睡眠不足有害健康。toxic 的含义是"有毒的"；immune 的含义是"免疫的"，与介词 to 连用，例如：He has made a firm decision, so he was immune to all persuasions. 他决定已下，对所有劝说都无动于衷。sensitive 意思是"敏感的"；allergic 的含义是"过敏的"，与介词 to 连用，例如：I am highly allergic to the pollen. 我对花粉高度过敏。

题干译文：这个化学物质被发现对人体健康有危害。

2. 【答案】C

【解析】画线词 devastating 的含义是"毁灭的"；permanent 的含义是"永久的"；desperate 的含义是"绝望的，不顾一切的"，例如：He is so thirsty that he is desperate for a glass of water. 他渴极了，极想喝一杯水。destructive 的含义是"破坏性的"；sudden 的含义是"突然的"。

题干译文：这个诊所如果关闭将会是对病人毁灭性的打击。

3. 【答案】B

【解析】画线词 graphic 的含义是"图案的，形象生动的（尤指令人不快的事物）"；verifiable 的含义是"可核实的"；explicit 的含义是"清楚明白的"；precise 的含义是"精准的"；ambiguous 的含义是"模棱两可的"。可知与画线词含义最接近的是 B。

题干译文：他一直在绘声绘色地向我们讲述他动手术的详细情况。

4. 【答案】D

【解析】画线词 ingenuity 的含义是"聪明才智，独创力"。credibility 的含义是可靠性；commitment 的含义是"承诺，保证"；honesty 的含义是"诚实"；talent 的含义是"才能"，与画线词近义。

题干译文：这个疑难病例即使对最有经验的医生也是一个考验。

5. 【答案】C

【解析】画线词 pretext 的含义是"借口，托词"，与介词 for 或者不定式 to do 连用。claim 的含义是"宣称"；clue 的含义是"提示"；excuse 的含义是"借口"；circumstance 的含义是"环境，事件"。

题干译文：他借口必须赶火车，立即离开了。

6. 【答案】B

【解析】画线词 remorse 的含义是"遗憾，内疚，自责"，与介词 for 连用。anguish 的含义是"苦闷，痛苦"；regret 的含义是"遗憾"；apology 的含义是"抱歉"；grief 的含义是"悲痛"。

题干译文：这个护士因为不被信任而感到内疚自责。

7. 【答案】D

【解析】本题题意是："医生尽量用妥善的方式告诉她真相。" tactful 是"机智的，得体的，圆滑的"的意思。从本句的场景看，应该选 D。干扰项是 C。医生告诉病人不好的消息应该谨慎、考虑周到，是要照顾到病人的心里感受的。这些含义是 skillful 没有的。各选项含义如下：A．精巧的；B．无隐晦的，畅谈的；C．灵巧的，熟练的；D．考虑周到的。

题干译文：这个医生设法找一个妥善的方式告诉她实情。

8. 【答案】A

【解析】画线词 temperament 的含义是"气质，性情"。disposition 的含义是"性格，性情"；qualification 的含义是"资格"；temptation 的含义是"诱惑"；endorsement 的含义是"赞同，支持，宣传"。

题干译文：一个人是否喜欢日常办公室工作很大程度上取决于他的性情。

9. 【答案】D

【解析】画线词组 rule out 的含义是"消除，排除"；confirm 的含义是"确认"；facilitate 的含义是"促进，帮助"；postpone 的含义是"推迟"；cancel 的含义是"取消"；complication 的含义是"并发症"。

题干译文：因为病人突发并发症，医生取消了周五的手术。

10. 【答案】C

【解析】画线词 tranquil 的含义是"平静的"；cautious 的含义是"谨慎小心的"；motionless 的含义是"一动不动的"；calm 的含义是"平静的，镇定的"；alert 的含义是"警觉的，灵敏的"。

题干译文：当有事儿突然改变你的生活，保持平静其实很难。

2011 年真题

1. 【答案】C

   【解析】本题考查语义和词汇辨析。画线词 awkwardly 意为 "笨拙地"。embarrassingly 意为 "尴尬地"，reluctantly 意为 "不情愿地"，clumsily 意为 "笨拙地"，dizzily 意为 "眩晕地"。故 C 为正确选项。

   题干译文：她很笨拙地摔倒了，腿摔折了。

2. 【答案】D

   【解析】本题考查固定搭配。anything but 意为 "不是……"，与 by no means 同义。more or less 意为 "或多或少"，by and large 意为 "总的说来"，more often than not 意为 "多半"。故选 D。

   题干译文：在历史记录中，药学绝对算不上科学。

3. 【答案】B

   【解析】本题考查语义。只有 fascinated 表示 "被吸引"。illuminate 意为 "照亮"，alienate 意为 "异化"，hallucinate 意为 "出现幻觉"。故选 B。

   题干译文：学生被医生举例的方式所吸引。

4. 【答案】C

   【解析】本题考查语义与词汇辨析。tangible 意为 "实际的，有形的，确凿的"，与 substantial 含义相同。intelligible 意为 "可理解的"，infinitive 意为 "无限的，不定的"，deficient 意为 "不足的"。故选 C。

   题干译文：我们需要以数据统计、产品或是金钱回报等有形的方式来证明我们辛勤的工作。

5. 【答案】A

   【解析】本题考查近义词辨析。sustain 意为 "坚持，维持"，与 maintain 同义。reserve 意为 "保留"，conceive 意为 "察觉"，empower 意为 "赋权"。故本题选 A。

   题干译文：限制某些食物种类或是承诺不切实际效果的饮食很难长时间维持，或者说长时间坚持会对健康不利。

6. 【答案】A

   【解析】discipline 意为 "纪律，学科"，与 specialties 意思相同。principle 意为 "原则"，rationale 意为 "基本原理"，doctrine 意为 "教义"。故 A 为正确答案。

   题干译文：临床药学的传统学科中处处可见分子学的影响。

7. 【答案】C

   【解析】somatic 意为 "身体的"，与 physical 含义相同。juvenile 意为 "未成年的"，potent 意为 "强有力的"，mature 意为 "成熟的"，故选 C。

   题干译文：一个人往往通过身体体征意识到青春期的开始。

8. 【答案】D

   【解析】feasible 意为 "可能的，可实行的"，与 viable 同义。rational 意为 "合理的，理性的"，reciprocal 意为 "互惠的，彼此相反的"，versatile 意为 "多才多艺的"，故本题选 D。

   题干译文：他的手术应该能成功，因为看上去是可行的。

9. 【答案】B

【解析】intensely 意为"强烈地"，与 vitally 近义。irresistibly 意为"无法抵抗地"，potentially 意为"潜在地，可能地"，intriguingly 意为"有魅力地"。故本题选 B。

题干译文：这些有关质量、特殊护理和经验的益处的问题是极其重要的。

10. 【答案】B

【解析】strategy 意为"策略，技巧"，与 technique 近义。tend 意为"趋势"，notion 意为"理念"，breakthrough 意为"突破"。故本题应选 B。

题干译文：这份指南给出了最佳自我护理的策略和最新医疗发展的信息。

2012 年真题

1. 【答案】B

【解析】画线词 a tingle of 的含义是"一丝丝，一阵阵"，这里指的是一阵激动。A 项 glimpse 的含义是"匆匆一瞥"，因而不能和 excitement 连用；C 项 panic 的含义是"恐慌"；D 项 pack 的含义是"包装，一包"，这两个词都不能和 excitement 连用。B 项 gust 表示"一阵（风）"。

题干译文：她是个疯狂的歌迷，见到迈克尔·杰克逊的时候她感到很激动。

2. 【答案】C

【解析】画线词 transcend 的含义是"超越"；A 项 discipline 的含义是"训练"；B 项 complain 的含义是"抱怨"，常与 about 连用；C 项 conquer 的含义是"克服，征服"；D 项 defy 的含义是"藐视，公然对抗"。

题干译文：母亲对弟弟的偏心使他心生怨恨，无法释怀。

3. 【答案】A

【解析】画线单词 trifle with 是"玩弄，轻视"的含义，与 belittle 同义。exaggerate 意为"夸张"；ponder 意为"思考"；eliminate 意为"删除，清除"。故本题选 A。

题干译文：任何人都不能小看这种恐惧，也不能向它妥协。

4. 【答案】B

【解析】画线单词 in light of 意思是"从……的方面，考虑到……"，与 in view of 同义。in place of 意为"反而，然而"，与 instead of 同义；in spite of 意为"尽管"；in search of 意为"寻找"。故本题选 B。

题干译文：考虑到他的良好记录，警察接受了他的辩护。

5. 【答案】D

【解析】画线单词 terminate 意思是"终止，停止"，与 suspend "延迟，停止"同义。accuse 意为"控诉"；punish 意为"惩罚"；dismiss 意为"解散"。故选 D。

题干译文：市政府官员说，在应聘申请中有撒谎嫌疑的人会被终止聘用。

6. 【答案】D

【解析】画线单词 be blamed for 意思是"承担……责任"，与 ascribe to 意思相近。attach to 意为"与……联系"；compose of 意为"由……组成"；relate to 意为"与……联系"。故本题选 D。

题干译文：2009 年 4 月墨西哥城外猪流感的爆发造成一百多人死亡。

7. 【答案】A

   【解析】画线单词 discharge 意思是"释放，散发"，与 put out 同义。pass off 意为"消失"；pull out 意为"拔出来，驶出"；send out 意为"派出"。故本题选 A。

   题干译文：森林起火燃烧时，会释放成百上千种化合物，包括一氧化碳。

8. 【答案】A

   【解析】画线单词 from scratch 的意思是"从头做起，从零做起"，与 from the beginning 同义。from now on 意为"从现在"；from time to time 意为"时不时，经常"；from the bottom 意为"从底部"。故本题选 A。

   题干译文：不幸的是，修建中的桥在地震中坍塌了，他们不得不从头开始。

9. 【答案】D

   【解析】画线单词 promise 的意思是"承诺，保证"，与 ensure 含义相同。administer 意为"管理"；nurture 意为"培育"；inspire 意为"鼓励"。故选 D。

   题干译文：双胞胎姐妹让英国科学家在白血病研究上有了突破，能使治疗方案效果更好，副作用更少。

10. 【答案】A

    【解析】画线单词 disruption 的意思是"破坏"，与 disturbance 含义相近。distraction "分散"；intersection "横断，交叉"；interpretation "解释"。故本题选 A。

    题十译文：激进的环境保护主义者谴责杀虫剂中的污染物和合成化学物质破坏了人体荷尔蒙。

2013 年真题

1. 【答案】C

   【解析】画线词 defect 的含义是"缺陷，缺点"。选项 A 为"赤字"，选项 B 为"误差"，选项 C 为"缺点，缺陷"，选项 D 为"差异，矛盾"。

   题干译文：圣诞节期间的购物者应该知道打折销售的产品可能是残次品。

2. 【答案】D

   【解析】画线词组 take on 的含义是"承担"。选项 A 为"轻视"，选项 B 为"逃避"，选项 C 为"要求"，选项 D 为"承担"。

   题干译文：这个培训项目的目的就是要提高孩子们的责任心以及乐于迎接挑战的勇气。

3. 【答案】B

   【解析】画线词 tax 在题干中的含义是"使……承担过重"。选项 A 为"改善"，选项 B 为"使烦恼，负担"，选项 C 为"检查"，选项 D 为"征税"。

   题干译文："9.11"事件后，奥运会使得东道国的安保服务承担更大的压力。

4. 【答案】C

   【解析】画线词的含义是"惊厥，痉挛，震动，动乱，哄堂大笑"。此题可根据题干信息得出答案。

   题干译文：小丑的表演很搞笑，观众无论大人还是小孩都在大笑。

5. 【答案】A

【解析】画线词的含义是"抵押贷款"，因而答案为 A。

题干译文：我们向中国银行申请抵押借款，并被通知年底还清。

6. 【答案】D

【解析】画线词的含义是"完全的，绝对的"。题干中 hypocrisy 的含义是"伪善"。

题干译文：提倡者高度重视体育精神，而反对者则贬低它，声称这完全就是伪善与自我欺骗。

7. 【答案】A

【解析】画线词的含义是"不安的，激动的，焦虑的"。选项 A 为"恼怒的，生气的"，选项 B 为"顺从的"；选项 C 为"盖戳的，铭刻的"；选项 D 为"探测"。

题干译文：每当响尾蛇躁动时，它就开始摇摆尾巴并发出很大的响声。

8. 【答案】B

【解析】画线词的含义是"洞察力"，选项 A 为"归纳，感应"；选项 B 为"感觉，洞察力"，选项 C 为"解释"；选项 D 为"渗透"。

题干译文：这个侦探对罪犯的伎俩有着不寻常的洞察力，清楚如何抓捕他们。

9. 【答案】A

【解析】画线词的含义是"演讲"（传递信息给听众）。

题干译文：我弟弟一遍遍地练习演讲，直到他的发言和时间都很完美为止。

10. 【答案】C

【解析】画线词的含义是"不合理地"。选项 A 为"不合时宜地，过早地"；选项 B 为"意外地"；选项 C 为"不合理地"；选项 D 为"异常地，不依惯例地"。

题干译文：近几周房价和股价开始从不合理的惊人高位回落。

2014 年真题

1. 【答案】D

【解析】画线词 indispensable 的含义是"必不可少的"。选项 A 为"不可抗拒的"，选项 B 为"珍视的"，选项 C 为"不可分割的"，选项 D 为"必备的"。

题干译文：所有诺贝尔文学奖获得者的成功都是长期积累的过程，坚持不懈的努力是不可或缺的。

2. 【答案】A

【解析】画线词 impart 的含义是"赋予"，选项 A 为"授予，放置"，选项 B 为"展示"，选项 C 为"强加，施加"，选项 D 为"放射，发出"。

题干译文：女王的到来使伦敦白金汉宫的接待酒会多了一份高雅。

3. 【答案】B

【解析】画线词 manifest 作为形容词的含义是"明显的，显然的"。选项 A 为"加强的"，选项 C 为"代表性的"，选项 D 为"阴险的，隐伏的"。

题干译文：医生清楚甲状腺功能不全在生长期儿童身上非常明显，表现为身心发展迟缓。

4. 【答案】C

【解析】画线词 accommodate oneself to 的含义是"适应"，A 选项与 to 连用，含义为"屈服，让步"，选项 B 的含义是"扩大"。

题干译文：眼睛能自动调节适应不同距离，这一机制被应用在自动照相机技术上，并带来一个革命性的技术飞跃。

5. 【答案】B

【解析】画线词 exacerbate 的含义是"使加剧，恶化"。选项 A 为"根除"，选项 C 为"征服，击败"，选项 D 为"避免，防止"。

题干译文：不同宗教信仰者之间的区别是常见的，然而正是宗教迫害的压力加剧了冲突，造成了联盟的分崩离析。

6. 【答案】B

【解析】画线词 obliterate 的含义是"抹去，擦去"。选项 A 为"复制"，选项 C 为"代替"，选项 D 为"编纂"，只有 B 表示"除去，消除"。

题干译文：毕加索特别贫穷的时候，他可能曾经尝试在帆布上抹掉原始创作重新作画。

7. 【答案】A

【解析】画线词 deplore 的含义是"谴责，哀叹"。选项 B 的含义是"鄙视，轻视"，选项 C 的含义是"推翻，拆除"；选项 D 的含义是"腐烂"。

题干译文：为了保护动物，环境保护者谴责核工厂修建项目。

8. 【答案】A

【解析】画线词 fidelity 的含义是"忠诚"，选项 B 为"道德"，选项 D 为"稳定"。

题干译文：尤其是政治人物，需要严格遵守道德忠贞的标准。

9. 【答案】C

【解析】画线词 negligent 的含义是"疏忽的，粗心大意的"。选项 A 为"暴怒的"，选项 B 为"热心的"，选项 D 为"残暴的"。

题干译文：病人抱怨医生疏忽大意，给他的检查不够全面。

10. 【答案】A

【解析】画线词 wrath 的含义是"发怒"，选项 B 的含义是"混乱"，选项 C 为"绝望"，选项 D 为"苦恼，痛苦"。

题干译文：她整个早晨都在心平气和地处理所有投诉。

2015 年真题

1. 【答案】A

【解析】画线词 prompt 的含义是"激起，促使"。选项 A 为"促使"，选项 B 为"延长"，选项 C 为"迷惑"，选项 D 为"承诺"。

题干译文：英国每年有 1000 多个病人因等不及器官捐赠而死亡，这促使科学家去考虑其他制造器官的方式。

2. 【答案】A

【解析】画线词 stigma 的含义是"耻辱，污名"。选项 A 为"耻辱"，选项 B 为"歧视"，选项 C 为"骚扰"，选项 D 为"隔离"。

题干译文：治疗方案的改进改变了艾滋病人的前景，但是对艾滋病仍有严重的歧视。

3. **【答案】C**

   【解析】画线词 lassitude 的含义是"无精打采"。选项 A 为"消耗",选项 B 为"脱水",选项 C 为"筋疲力尽",选项 D 为"残废"。

   题干译文:船只失事的幸存者在因为体力透支而导致无力坚持的时候最终获救。

4. **【答案】D**

   【解析】画线词 illegible 的含义是"难以辨认的,不清楚的"。选项 A 为"负面的",选项 B 为"令人疑惑的",选项 C 为"雄辩的",选项 D 为"不清楚的"。

   题干译文:科学家发明了立体扫描技术来阅读原本无法辨认的木雕石头,这是一种可以应用在其他领域的方式,比如医疗。

5. **【答案】C**

   【解析】画线词 scrutinize 的含义是"仔细研究"。选项 A 为"期望",选项 B 为"澄清",选项 C 为"检查",选项 D 为"证实,核对"。

   题干译文:顶尖的运动员会和教练仔细研究成功和失败,并从中吸取教训,但他们从不会远离自己长期的目标。

6. **【答案】D**

   【解析】画线词 imperative 的含义是"必需的,义务的"。选项 A 为 challenging "挑战的",选项 B 为"庄严的",选项 C 为"有敌意的",选项 D 为"苛刻的,苛求的"。

   题干译文:他毋庸置疑的语气显示了他的傲慢自大和刚愎自用。

7. **【答案】C**

   【解析】画线词 eclipse 的含义是"淹没重要性,使失色"。选项 A 为"擦掉",选项 B 为"激发",选项 C 为"使有阴影",选项 D 为"搁置"。

   题干译文:美国和欧盟关于经济合作的讨论可能因为近期日益增多的贸易摩擦而前途叵测。

8. **【答案】A**

   【解析】画线词 foster 的含义是"培育,培养"。选项 A 为"培育",选项 B 为"消除",选项 C 为"同化,吸收",选项 D 为"刺穿,戳穿"。

   题干译文:价格快速的增长促使大家相信,未来也会呈更大幅度的增长,高价促进需求,而非压制需求。

9. **【答案】C**

   【解析】画线词 unprecedented 的含义是"前所未有的"。选项 A 为"难以预料的",选项 B 为"非传统的",选项 C 为"无法媲美的",选项 D 是"无法预料的"。

   题干译文:摄像技术近期的一些发展允许动物在以前难以接近的地方,以前所未有的详细方式被研究。

10. **【答案】B**

    【解析】画线词 manipulating 的含义是"操纵,应付"。选项 A 为"估计",选项 B 为"处理",选项 C 为"改正,校正",选项 D 是"期望"。

    题干译文:一个经验丰富的谈判专家在处理棘手问题时应该很有技巧。

2016 年真题

1. 【答案】D

   【解析】画线词 scrutiny 彻底检查；A. sanction 准许，批准；B. restriction 限制；C. census 统计，调查；D. examination 检查。

   题干译文：无论怎样，注射死刑都要经过联邦政府审查。

2. 【答案】B

   【解析】画线词 potent 有效的；A. inexpensive 廉价的；B. powerful 强有力的；C. conventional 传统的；D. lethal 致命的。

   题干译文：不起眼的西红柿可能成为抗击前列腺癌的利器。

3. 【答案】D

   【解析】画线词组 at odds with 与……不一致；A. in tune with 与……一致；B. in favor of 赞成，支持，有利于；C. for the sake of 为了……利益；D. in disagreement with 与……不一致。

   题干译文：男性对于他们应该照料多少的看法与女性截然不同。

4. 【答案】A

   【解析】画线词 eminent 著名的；A. renowned 著名的；B. notorious 臭名昭著的；C. popular 受欢迎的；D. mysterious 神秘的。

   题干译文：黄山以其自然风光著名，值得一去。

5. 【答案】C

   【解析】画线词 diversity 多样性；A. severity 严重性；B. reliability 可靠性；C. variety 种类；D. specificity 特性。

   题干译文：肥胖是多种因素造成的持续性状态。

6. 【答案】A

   【解析】画线词 lapse 过失，小错，疏忽；A. error 错误；B. sin 罪恶；C. guilt 罪行；D. offense 冒犯。

   题干译文：通常他行为举止端正，这次无礼仅仅是一个过失。

7. 【答案】D

   【解析】画线词 jaundice 黄疸，偏见；A. grievance 委屈，冤情；B. 同情；C. 嫉妒；D. indignation 愤怒，愤慨。

   题干译文：你能感受到他评论中的偏见吗？

8. 【答案】B

   【解析】画线词组 to little avail 的意思是"没什么用，不奏效"。by no means 绝不；in vain 徒劳无功；of no account "没有考虑到"；at stake "处于危险中"。

   题干译文：1902 年，德国医生尝试使用甲状腺细胞米治疗甲状腺功能低下的孩子，但丝毫不奏效。

9. 【答案】C

   【解析】画线词 lavishly 的意思是"非常浪费地，奢华地"。fearlessly 无畏地；conspicuously 显著地，明显地；wastefully 浪费地；ferociously 厉害地，

激烈地。

题干译文：在很多人看来，他挥霍无度。

10. 【答案】A

【解析】画线词 progression 的意思是"进展"。要注意，"疾病的进展"言下之意是疾病恶化了。deterioration 恶化；accumulation 积累；expansion 扩展；promotion 提升。

题干译文：现在，没有医疗手段可以阻止风湿性二尖瓣狭窄的恶化。

2017 年真题

1. 【答案】B

【解析】如果你服用的药物让你昏昏欲睡，就向经理汇报。画线单词 drowsy 的意思是"打瞌睡的，想睡觉的"，与 sleepy 含义相近，故本题选 B。

2. 【答案】D

【解析】糖尿病是世界上最普遍和最具潜在危险的疾病之一。画线单词 prevalent 的意思是"流行的，常见的"。crucial "至关重要的"，virulent "有毒的"，colossal "庞大的"，widespread "普遍的"，本题正确答案为 D。

3. 【答案】C

【解析】同样，烟灰和烟雾中含有大量的致癌物质。a multitude of 的意思是"大量的，很多"，与 plenty of 含义相近。

4. 【答案】C

【解析】关于雌激素效应的许多问题仍有待阐明，各种调查正在通过持续的实验室研究和临床研究来寻求答案。画线单词 elucidate 的意思是"阐明，解释"。implicate "暗示"，imply "暗示，暗含"，illuminate "阐明，启示"，initiate "发起，开始"。正确答案为 C。

5. 【答案】D

【解析】网络聊天是面对面交友的暗淡无力的替代品。画线单词 substitute 的意思是"代替，替代"。accomplishment "成就"，refreshment "提神，恢复精神"，complement "补充"，replacement "代替"。正确答案为 D。

6. 【答案】A

【解析】患者在医院住院时间长了，往往会形成过度依赖，不再愿意自理。画线单词 overly 的意思是"过度地，极端地"。extremely "极端地"，exclusively "仅仅"，exactly "精确地"，explicitly "清楚地"。本题正确答案为 A。

7. 【答案】C

【解析】限制市中心的停车场的尝试进一步加剧了交通堵塞问题。画线单词 aggravate 的意思是"使恶化"。ameliorate "改善"，aggregate "合计"，deteriorate "恶化"，duplicate "复制"。正确答案为 C。

8. 【答案】C

【解析】据报道，细菌污染了美国国内 80% 的零售生鸡。画线单词 contaminate 的意思是"污染"。inflame"发炎"，inflict"痛苦"，infect"传染，感染"，infiltrate"浸润"。本题正确答案为C。

9. 【答案】A

【解析】研究人员最近发布了美国枪支暴力数据，并认为合法持枪的规定并不能阻止暴力犯罪。画线单词 inhibit 的意思是"抑制，遏制"。curb"控制"，induce"诱导"，lessen"减少"，impel"促使"。curb 与 inhibit 含义最相近，因此最佳答案为A。

10. 【答案】C

【解析】无论我们对固定印象如何不安，许多研究仍然显示中西教育差异明显。画线单词 stereotype 的意思是"刻板印象"。specification"尺寸，规格"，sensation"感觉，感情"，convention"传统，规约"，conservation"保护，保守"。根据题意，这里强调的是"长久以来形成的固定看法"，与 conventions 的含义最相近，因此最佳答案为C。

2018 年真题

1. 【答案】B

【解析】句意：真正称职的医生，能坐下来，感受他人的"秘密"，表现出对病人的个人兴趣和充分理解。competent"合格的，胜任的"，与 capable 含义相同。

2. 【答案】B

【解析】句意：医生通常认为治疗是由病人发起的。perceive"认为，认知"。conserve"保留"，theorize"理论化"，realize"意识到"，persist"坚持己见"。本题最佳答案为 realized。

3. 【答案】A

【解析】句意：大型社区聚餐或许能作为社会联系的润滑剂，缓解紧张关系。lubricate"润滑"。facilitate"帮助，促进"，intimidate"威吓"，terminate"终结"，mediate"调解"。本题 mediate 为混淆选项，调解往往指有矛盾时才调解，而 lubricate 在这里是明显的褒义，表达将社区关系向更好的方向发展的只有facilitate。

4. 【答案】D

【解析】句意：过氧化氢酶活性降低了谷胱甘肽，维生素 E 水平仅在具有活动性疾病的受试者中降低。exclusively"独一无二地"，与 solely 含义相同。simply也有"only"的含义，但没有排外性，更多地强调"少"的意义。

5. 【答案】B

【解析】句意：体外受精繁衍出的后代序列中经常出现眼部异常。offspring"后代,子孙"。fetus"胚胎"，descendant"后代，继承者"，seed"种子"，orphan"孤儿"。根据题意，正确答案为B。

6. 【答案】C

【解析】句意：儿童贫困应被视为儿童面临的唯一最大的公共健康威胁。menace"威胁"，与 threat 同义。breach "违背"，grief "痛苦"，abuse "滥用"。

7. 【答案】C

    【解析】句意：一个未来的理想是特意引发地震，以可控的方式释放地球构造应力。deliberately "故意地，有意地"，与 intentionally 含义相同。definitely "确定地"，desperately "绝望地"，identically "相同地"。

8. 【答案】D

    【解析】巨大的挑战仍然横亘在企业将二氧化碳转化成汽油的道路上。convert "转化，转变"，与 transform 的含义相同。apply "应用"，relate "联系"，relay "接力，中继"。

9. 【答案】D

    【解析】句意：最近有人担心这些药物会引起对认知方面意料之外的副作用，如记忆力减退、思维模糊和学习障碍。elicit "引起，诱发"，与 induce 的含义相同。ensue "随之而来"，encounter "遭遇，碰到"，impede "妨碍"。

10. 【答案】A

    【解析】句意：一叶障目，不见泰山，意思是人们对重要事情的看法被琐碎事物所蒙蔽。trivial "琐碎，细小的事情"。insignificant "不重要的"，insufficient "不充足的"，substantial "实质的，重要的"，unexpected "意料之外的"。根据题意，正确答案为 A。

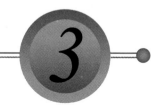

第三章 CHAPTER 3 完形填空

一、考试大纲的要求

根据考试大纲的要求，这部分考题主要侧重测试考生在篇章中理解、运用语言知识的综合能力。此部分的篇章约为 200 个词的短文，短文中有 10 处空白。要求考生在理解全文大意和上下文的基础上，从每题的四个备选选项中选出一个最佳答案，使得所填内容符合语法、句型结构以及上下文的逻辑关系。此部分共 10 道小题，每题 1 分，共计 10 分，考试时间约为 10 分钟。通过这一考试要求的表述，我们可以得出这样的结论：完形填空的特点在于它的综合性，考查考生的阅读能力、语法分析能力、词汇掌握熟练程度，因而具有相当的难度。

二、真题演练与解析

最新真题解析（2018 年真题）

Directions: *In this section there is a passage with ten numbered blanks. For each blank, there are four choices marked A, B, C and D listed on the right side. Choose the best answer and mark the letter of your choice on the **ANSWER SHEET**.*

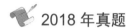 2018 年真题

The same benefits and drawbacks are found when using CT scanning to detect lung cancer — the three-dimensional imaging improves detection of disease but creates hundreds of images that increase a radiologist's workload, which, __51__, can result in missed positive scans.

Researchers at University of Chicago Pritizker School of Medicine presented

52 data on a CAD (computer-aided diagnosis) program they've designed that helps radiologist spot lung cancer 53 CT scanning. Their study was 54 by the NIH and the university.

In the study, CAD was applied to 32 low-dose CT scanning with a total of 50 lung nodules, 38 of which were biopsy-confirmed lung cancer that were not found during initial clinical exam. 55 the 38 missed cancers, 15 were the result of interpretation error (identifying an image but 56 it as non cancerous) and 23 57 observational error (not identifying the cancerous image).

CAD found 32 of the 38 previously missed cancers (84% sensitivity), with false-positive 58 of 1.6 per section.

Although CAD improved detection of lung cancer, it won't replace radiologists, said Sgmuel G. Armato, PhD, lead author of the study. "The computer is not perfect," Armato said. "It will miss some cancers and call some things cancer that 59 . The radiologists can identify normal anatomy that the computer may 60 something suspicious. It's a spell-checker of sorts, or a second opinion.

51. A. in common   B. in turn   C. in one   D. in all
52. A. preliminary   B. considerate   C. deliberate   D. ordinary
53. A. being used   B. to use   C. using   D. use
54. A. investigated   B. originated   C. founded   D. funded
55. A. From   B. Amid   C. Of   D. In
56. A. disseminating   B. degenerating   C. dismissing   D. deceiving
57. A. were mistaken for   B. were attributed to
    C. resulted in   D. gave way to
58. A. mortalities   B. incidences   C. images   D. rates
59. A. don't   B. won't   C. aren't   D. wasn't
60. A. stand for   B. search for   C. account for   D. mistake for

答案及解析

51. 【答案】B

【解析】本题考查上下文关系。第一段讲到用 CT 扫描的优劣势。优势为 3D 成像可以帮助筛查疾病，但同时因为成百上千张影像增加了放射科医生的工作量，这相应也会增加漏筛。in turn 是正确答案。

52. 【答案】A

【解析】本题考查句意。preliminary "初期的"，considerate "体贴的"，deliberate "特意的"，ordinary "普通的"。根据上下文的语义，初期数据是符合题意的搭配。

53. 【答案】C

【解析】本题考查非谓语动词。这里用现在分词的主动形式做方式状语，help sb. do sth. using…。这里非谓语动词的逻辑主语为 radiologist，是主动关系。

54. 【答案】D

【解析】本题考查动词。该项目受到了 NIH 的资助，而不是"调查""起源"或是"建立"。

55. 【答案】D

【解析】通过介词考查逻辑关系。本段第一句讲到，在该研究中，将 CAD 应用于 32 个低剂量 CT 扫描，总共 50 个肺结节，其中 38 个是经初步临床检查未发现的活检证实的肺癌。空格处紧跟其后，是在这 38 个漏掉的癌症病例中……，因此用 in 最合适。

56. 【答案】C

【解析】本题考查动词的含义。disseminating "传播"，degenerating "恶化，退化"，dismissing "打发"，deceiving "欺骗"。根据句意，本题选择 dismissing 最合适，意思是"……但却当成非癌来搁置了"。

57. 【答案】B

【解析】本题考查逻辑关系。38 个漏诊的案例中，15 个是阐释错误，23 个归因于观察失误。这里需要表示因果关系的词组，只有 B 和 C 符合题意，且前面是结果，observational error 是原因，只有 B 是正确的。

58. 【答案】D

【解析】本题考查名词辨析。本句的大意为 CAD 在 38 个以前错过的癌症中发现了 32 个（84% 的敏感性），假阳性率为每节 1.6 个。表示"概率"。

59. 【答案】C

【解析】本题考查句子结构。这里是个省略句，完整的表达应该是：It will miss some cancers and call some things cancer that are not cancers. 因此本题正确答案为 C。

60. 【答案】D

【解析】本题考查句意和词组。原句 The radiologists can identify normal anatomy that the computer may __60__ something suspicious 大意是，放射科医生能将电脑误诊的疑似病例通过正常的解剖手段识别出来。因此本题正确答案为 mistake for，形成前后的对照。

三、考查内容及相应的应试技巧

（一）考查内容

下面就完形填空所涉及的考查内容进行简单讲述。

1. 阅读能力是考查的难点和重点

完形填空是以篇章的形式设置考题，因而值得考生注意的是，此部分考查内容首要就是测试考生的阅读能力。具体地说，这种考查内容主要涉及考生对阅读文章整体脉络、文章上下文逻辑关系的把握。考生在阅读完形填空的篇章时，要注意每一个自然段落的主旨大意，不要仅仅局限于空白处所在的句子。每个段落的主旨大意联系起来就是文章内容的脉络。例如前面的真题演练，篇章的前后都紧密相连，从阅读第 1 段了解 Robert Spring 是个伪造者，如何成为伪造者；第 2 段主要讲述伪造者的伪造手段；这两段的信息对第 3 段考题的解题大有帮助。另外，考生在阅读篇章段落时，对于衔接词应充分注意，例如：so that, however 等。这些衔接词体现了文章上下文的逻辑关系，对于掌握文章脉络有着重要的意义。以上面真题为例，10 道题中，用到文章上下文解题的题目就有 8 个。

2. 词汇、语法是考查的基础

对于词汇的考查，形式和内容类似于词汇部分的 Section A，考查内容涉及形近词的辨认能力、对同义词或近义词的识别能力、对短语或词组的熟悉程度、对短语或词组搭配的掌握，例如上面真题中的第 1 和第 5 题。

完形填空考查内容不仅涉及以上要点，而且还涉及语法的应用，主要包括以下一些内容：动词题（时态、语态、非谓语动词）、从句、特殊句型、虚拟语气、倒装等。因而考生要对这些语法项目的内容有所了解，并能灵活运用。

（二）应试技巧

1. 完形填空的解题步骤

第一，通读完形篇章，把握文章脉络

考生不要在不了解篇章大意的情况下，匆忙解题，这会有可能出现由于文章大意掌握不准确，或偏差，连续出现解题错误的情况。所以，考生首先应该将文章快速通读一遍，了解大意，确定每个段落的主旨内容。

第二，进行选择，分析判断

如果是根据上下文解题，就要抓住解题信息。当在句内无法解题时，可以参看上下文多一点的信息，或者暂时跳过该题，不要在一道题上耽误过多时间，因为有时候前面题的答案就在后面的篇章里出现。例如上面真题中的第 5 题，答案就在第 3 段的第 2 行里。进行选择后，还要根据上下文反复推敲，随时调整选项。

第三，再次通读全文，检查结果

做完所有题目后，还要通读一遍全文，从语义、逻辑结构、语法、搭配等方面考虑得出的答案是否合理。

2. 解题策略以及应注意的问题

第一，充分利用篇章知识

通过分析上面的真题，可以很清楚地发现上下文信息对于解题帮助很大。出题人在设置题目的时候，也是要考虑到篇章中是否存在解题信息。基于这两点，考生要把文章发展的脉络、线索作为解题的主要手段，切忌只看到题目出现的某一句上。通常没有出现考题的内容对解题很有帮助，不要忽略。

第二，注重表示逻辑关系的衔接词

文章的各种逻辑关系，如列举、结果、让步、对比、目的、条件、转折等，需要通过

各种衔接词加以体现和表达。没有这些逻辑词，文章就显得语义模糊不清，不能形成篇章。因而考生要重视这些逻辑词，它们可帮助考生理解文章发展的脉络。

第三，**注意答案就在文中**

在有些情况下，某一题的答案就隐藏在篇章中，因而考生在理解上下文的时候，要做个敏感的有心人，随时根据自己的发现调整选项的选择。

四、完形填空专项练习及最新真题解析

历年真题精析

 2017 年真题

It was the kind of research that gave insight into how flu strains could mutate so quickly. The same branch of research concluded in 2005 that the 1918 flu started in birds before passing

to humans. Parsing (分析) this animal-human __51__ could provide clues to __52__ the next potential superflu, which already has a name: H5N1, also known as avian flu or bird flu.

This potential killer also has a number: 59%. According to WHO, nearly three-fifths of the people who __53__ H5N1 since 2003 died from the virus, which was first reported __54__ humans in Hong Kong in 1997 before a more serious __55__ occurred in Southeast Asia between 2003 and 2004. Some researchers argue that those mortality numbers are exaggerated because WHO only __56__ cases in which victims are sick enough to go to the hospitals for treatment.

__57__, compare that to the worldwide mortality rate of the 1918 pandemic; it may have killed roughly 50 million people, but that was only 10% of the number of people infected, according to a 2006 estimate.

H5N1's saving grace — and the only reason we're not running around masked up in public right now — is that the strain doesn't jump from birds to humans, or from humans to humans, easily. There have been just over 600 cases (and 359 deaths) since 2003. But __58__ its lethality, and the chance it could turn into something far more transmissible, one might expect H5N1 research to be exploding, with labs __59__ the virus's molecular components to understand how it spreads between animals and __60__ to humans, and hoping to discover a vaccine that could head off a pandemic.

51. A. rejection   B. interface   C. complement   D. contamination

52. A. be stopped   B. stopping

     C. being stopped   D. having stopped

53. A. mutated   B. effected   C. infected   D. contracted
54. A. in   B. on   C. with   D. from
55. A. trigger   B. launch   C. outbreak   D. outcome
56. A. counts   B. amounts to   C. accounts for   D. accumulates
57. A. Thereafter   B. Thereby   C. Furthermore   D. Still
58. A. given   B. regarding   C. in spite of   D. speaking of
59. A. parses   B. parsed   C. parsing   D. to parse
60. A. potently   B. absolutely
     C. potentially   D. epidemiologically

答案及解析

51. 【答案】B

【解析】本题考查上下文语义和名词含义。rejection "排异"，interface "结合，交界"，complement "补充物"，contamination "接触，传染"。空白处前一句话讲到这种流感在鸟类中出现了很多起，才开始向人类传播。因此 parsing（分析）鸟类和人类的交叉感染是符合上下文语义走向的。

52. 【答案】B

【解析】本题考查固定搭配。a clue to doing sth 的结构中，to 为介词，后面常常跟名词或者动名词形式，意思是"做某事的线索"。

53. 【答案】D

【解析】本题考查动词词义辨析。mutate "变异"，effect "引起"，infect "使感染"。infect 用于疾病感染人，而 contract 用于人感染疾病，文中是人感染疾病，故答案为 contract。

54. 【答案】A

【解析】本题考查介词。"在某个方面"介词常常用 in。on 表示"以……为主题"。

55. 【答案】C

【解析】本题考查语义。疾病"爆发"的表达方式为 outbreak。trigger "诱因"，launch "发起"，outcome "结果"。根据语义，C 为正确选项。

56. 【答案】A

【解析】本题考查语义和动词含义。account for "解释，说明"。count "把……算入"，amount to "达到"，accumulate "积累"。句意：有些研究者认为这些死亡数据有些夸大，因为 WHO 只会将严重到需要去医院就诊的病例算在内。count 是最贴切的选项。

57. 【答案】D

【解析】本题考查逻辑关系。still 有让步的含义，意思是"尽管如此"。thereby 表示因果关系，furthermore 表示递进关系，thereafter 表示"之后"。该题上一句讲到有些研究者认为这些死亡数据有些夸大，因为 WHO 只会将严重到需要去医院就诊的病例算在内。空格后则强调该数字仍然是惊人的。因此这里选择有让步含义的副词 still。

58. 【答案】A

【解析】本题考查逻辑关系。这里需要原因和条件，只有 given 能有此功能，意思是"鉴于，因为"，这里是连词。speaking of 的意思是"谈到，谈起"。

59. 【答案】C

【解析】本题考查 with 引导的介宾短语充当状语。with sth doing sth 结构，在本句中意思是"同时，实验室要探究病毒的分子构成"。

60. 【答案】C

【解析】本题考查句子含义和副词。这里表示可能对人类的传染，只有 potentially 表示"可能地，潜在地"。

2016 年真题

Humans are the only species known to have consciousness, awareness that we have brains and bodies __51__ adaptability, that we can affect the course our lives take, that we can make choices __52__ that vastly affect the quality of our lives—biologically, intellectually, environmentally, and spiritually. As humans, we have the ability to mold our __53__ beings to become what or who we wish to become. While some of us may, __54__, have genetic and biological imperatives that may require medication or training to overcome, or at least to modulate, the vast majority of us do, in fact, hold our emotional __55__ in our bank.

All that __56__, until the last decade, scientists believed that the human brain and its connections were formed during gestation and infancy and remained __57__ unchanged through childhood. They believed that humans had a given number of neurons in a specific brain structure, and __58__ the number might vary among people, once you were done with childhood development, you were set in this __59__. Your connections were already made, and the learning and growing period of your brain was over. In the last decade, however, researchers have found __60__ evidence that this is not so, and that something called neuroplasticity continues throughout our lives.

51. A. careful about   B. capable of   C. accessible to   D. susceptible to
52. A. in the event   B. in an attempt   C. at the moment   D. along the way
53. A. exclusive   B. very   C. just   D. exact
54. A. indeed   B. however   C. moreover   D. therefore
55. A. demonstration   B. dimension   C. destiny   D. determination
56. A. has been said   B. being said   C. was said   D. is said
57. A. more or less   B. pretty much   C. as ever   D. if any
58. A. while   B. despite   C. nevertheless   D. since
59. A. case   B. mold   C. sense   D. condition
60. A. different   B. similar   C. insufficient   D. significant

✝ 答案及解析

51. 【答案】B
    【解析】文章第一句的大意是：人类是唯一有意识的物种：我们的大脑和肢体能够适应选择的生活轨迹……careful about "仔细的，小心的"，capable of "能够"，accessible to "可接近的"，susceptible to "易于，敏感的"。根据题目含义，本题最佳答案为B。

52. 【答案】D
    【解析】根据选项可知，本题考查句意和词组。"…that we can make choices __52__ that vastly affect the quality of our lives…"的大意是"这种意识能让我们一直做出对自己生活产生重大影响的决策"。in the event "在某个事件上"，in an attempt "尝试"，at the moment "当下"，along the way "一路上，沿途"。根据题意，D为最佳选项。

53. 【答案】B
    【解析】本题考查句意和形容词含义。该句的大意为"作为人类，我们都有将自己_____的存在变成自己希望变成的样子"。exclusive "专用的，独家的"，very "特有的，正好的"，just "正直的，公正的"，exact "精确的"。根据题干意思判断，very 是最佳答案。

54. 【答案】A
    【解析】本题考查逻辑关系。indeed "实际上"，however "然而"表示转折，moreover "并且"表示递进，therefore "因此"表示因果。该句句首 while 表示让步"虽然"，根据语法规则，however 在这里就不能再添加。该句大意是"尽管一些人_____有需要药物或者训练才能克服的生理冲动，但绝大多数人可以将情绪_____"，第一个空格处填入 indeed 表示强调某种事实，承认这种现象的存在，是最符合语义走向的。

55. 【答案】C
    【解析】根据该句的大意为"……大多数人能将情绪控制好"。demonstration "展示"，dimension "体积，范围"，destiny "命运"，determination "决定，意志"。根据题意，选项C（dimension）是最佳答案。

56. 【答案】B
    【解析】本题考查非谓语动词和习惯用法。该句的主谓结构为 scientists believe，因此 all that 后的谓语动词应该相应变成非谓语结构。纵观四个选项，只有B符合要求。all that being said 是独立主格结构，充当状语，意思是"综上所述"。

57. 【答案】B
    【解析】more or less "或多或少"，pretty much "十分，非常"，as ever "和以往一样"，if any "即使有的话也……"。该句的下文说到，科学家们认为一旦人脑成形，神经元便会保持稳定。由此信息便可知空格中应该为 pretty much unchanged，意思是"保持高度稳定"。

58. 【答案】A
    【解析】本题考查逻辑关系。while 放在句首，表示让步，放在句中表示对比；despite

"尽管"，表示让步，后面连接的是 that 从句；nevertheless "然而"，表示转折，放在句中时往往用标点隔开；since "因为，既然"，表示因果。"They believed that humans had a given number of neurons in a specific brain structure..."讲到，科学家们相信在人类某个大脑结构中存在一定数量的神经元。and 后的句子中含有两个信息的缺失，需要我们找到语义线索来确定逻辑关系。vary "变化"，done with childhood development "童年发展完成"，be set "定型"，由以上三个重点线索可知，这里的逻辑关系应该为"虽然……变化，但是一旦完成童年发展，你就会……成形"。因此这里应该选择表示"尽管"的连词。因引导句子，故 while 是正确答案。

59. 【答案】B

【解析】该句的意思是"一旦儿童发展阶段完成，大脑便会成形"。in the mold 是正确答案。in this case "这种情况"，in this sense "在这个意义上"，in this mold "以这种形式"，in this condition "在这种条件下"。

60. 【答案】D

【解析】本题考查语义走向和形容词。different "不同的"，similar "相似的"，insufficient "不充足的"，significant "重要的，有意义的"。文章的最后两句话大意是：你的神经元连接已经成型，大脑的学习和生长阶段已然结束。但是，在最近十年里，研究者们却发现了_____的证据，证明情况并非如此，神经重构贯穿人类的一生。这里找到的证据应为"重要的，关键的"。此处并非谈论证据的"相似"或"不同"，而是强调证据对论点的支持力度。因此本题正确答案为 significant。

2015 年真题

A mother who is suffering from cancer can pass on the disease to her unborn child in extremely rare cases, ___51___ a new case report published in PNAS this week.

According to researchers in Japan and at the Institute for Cancer Research in Sutton, UK, a Japanese mother had been diagnosed with leukemia a few weeks after giving birth, ___52___ tumors were discovered in her daughter's cheek and lung when she was 11 months old. Genetic analysis showed that the baby's cancer cells had the same mutation as the cancer cells of the mother. But the cancer cells contained no DNA whatsoever from the father, ___53___ would be expected if she had inherited the cancer from conception. That suggests the cancer cells made it into the unborn child's body across the placental barrier.

The *Guardian* claimed this to be the first ___54___ case of cells crossing the placental barrier. But this is not the case — microchimerism, ___55___ cells are exchanged between a mother and her unborn child, is thought to be quite common, with some cells thought to pass from fetus to mother in about 50 to 75 percent of cases and to go the other way about half ___56___.

As the BBC pointed out, the greater ___57___ in cancer transmission from mother to fetus had been how cancer cells that have slipped through the placental barrier could survive in the fetus without being killed by its immune system. The answer, in this case at least, lies in a second mutation of the cancer cells, which led to the __58__ of the specific features that would have allowed the fetal immune system to detect the cells as foreign. As a result, no attack against the invaders was launched.

__59__, according to the researchers there is little reason for concern of "cancer danger". Only 17 probable cases have been reported worldwide and the combined __60__ of cancer cells both passing the placental barrier and having the right mutation to evade the baby's immune system is extremely low.

51. A. suggests B. suggesting C. having suggested D. suggested
52. A. since B. although C. whereas D. when
53. A. what B. whom C. who D. as
54. A. predicted B. notorious C. proven D. detailed
55. A. where B. when C. if D. whatever
56. A. as many B. as much C. as well D. as often
57. A. threat B. puzzle C. obstacle D. dilemma
58. A. detection B. deletion C. amplification D. addition
59. A. Therefore B. Furthermore C. Nevertheless D. Conclusively
60. A. likelihood B. function C. influence D. flexibility

答案及解析

51. 【答案】A

【解析】本题考查动词时态。文章第一句为主题句：本周发布的一份新案例研究表明，患癌母亲在极为罕见的情况下，才会将疾病传染给未出生的婴儿。因为本题有非常明确的时间状语 this week，同时医学权威发布的结果应当为有一定代表性的结论，故选用动词的一般现在时。因此本题正确答案为 A。这与第二段中的 This suggests... 形成呼应。

52. 【答案】C

【解析】本题考查逻辑关系引导词。本句大意是：一位母亲在分娩的几周后被诊断为白血病，而女儿在 11 个月大的时候，在其脸颊和肺部都发现了肿瘤。根据题意，两个分句之间有对比和转折的逻辑关系，因此本题正确答案为 C。

53. 【答案】D

【解析】本题考查从句引导词。本题的主句结构完整，意思是该女婴癌细胞中未发现父亲的 DNA，这就让大家认为她是在受孕过程中染上疾病的。这里需要一个引导词，能指代主句内容，同时还能引导从句，只有 as/which 才有此功能。因此本题正确答案为 D。

54. 【答案】C

【解析】本题考查句意和形容词。本句大意是：《卫报》称这是第一个得以证实的细胞穿透胎盘屏障的案例。上文用一个日本病人的案例对此进行了证明，因此本题正确答案为 C。

55. **【答案】A**
　　【解析】 本题考查逻辑关系和从句引导词。本句大意是：这不是微嵌合状态的病例，在该状态下，细胞在母体和胎儿之间发生交换，非常常见。50% 到 75% 的情况下，一些细胞从胚胎游向母体，50% 的情况下则是反向行之。此处从句表示该种情况发生的状态，用 where 最合适。因此本题正确答案为 A。

56. **【答案】D**
　　【解析】 本题考查副词。这里表示细胞从母亲到胎儿和胎儿到母亲两种方式的概率，能表示"概率，频率"的，只有 often。因此本题正确答案为 D。

57. **【答案】B**
　　【解析】 本题考查句意和名词。这里的大意为：这些越过胎盘障碍的癌细胞如何不会被免疫系统杀死，这是个令人费解的事情。因此本题正确答案为 B。

58. **【答案】B**
　　【解析】 本题考查句意与名词。对上面提出的 puzzle，答案是癌细胞进行了第二次变异，使检测异质细胞的免疫系统丧失功能。这里只能选择能表示"消失，磨灭"含义的词，才能符合文意。因此 deletion 是正确答案。

59. **【答案】C**
　　【解析】 本题考查逻辑关系。这里上文讲的是母体向胎儿传染癌症的情况，空格后则在舒缓对 cancer danger 的紧张情绪，这是明显的转折关系。因此本题正确答案为 C。

60. **【答案】A**
　　【解析】 本题考查句意和名词。这里进一步解释为何不用担心 cancer danger，因为全世界范围内只有 17 个可能性案例，能突破胎盘障碍的癌细胞同时能避免胎儿免疫系统筛查的免疫，两种方式结合起来的可能性实在很低。因此本题选 likelihood。

仿真模拟练习

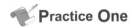 **Practice One**

If we accept that we cannot prevent science and technology from changing our world, we can at least try to __1__ that the changes they make are in the right directions. In a democratic society, this means that the public needs to have a basic understanding of science, __2__ it can make informed decisions and not __3__ them in the hands of experts. At the moment, the public has a rather ambivalent attitude __4__ science. It has come to expect the steady increase in the standard of __5__ that new developments in science and technology have brought to continue, but it also distrusts science because it doesn't understand it. This distrust is evident in the cartoon __6__ of the mad scientist working in his laboratory to produce a Frankenstein. It is also an important __7__ behind support for the Green parties.

What can be done to __8__ this interest and give the public the scientific background it needs to make informed decisions on subjects like acid rain, the greenhouse effect, nuclear weapons, and genetic engineering? Clearly, the basis must lie in what is taught in schools. But in schools science is often __9__ in a dry and uninteresting manner. Children learn it by rote to pass examinations, and they don't see its __10__ to the world around them. Moreover, science is often taught in terms of equations. Although equations are a concise and accurate way of describing mathematical ideas, they frighten most people.

1.　A. assess　　　　B. discern　　　　C. ensure　　　　D. anticipate
2.　A. because　　　B. so that　　　　C. despite that　　D. though
3.　A. clutch　　　　B. leave　　　　　C. fabricate　　　D. nurture
4.　A. about　　　　B. with　　　　　C. upon　　　　　D. toward
5.　A. living　　　　B. life　　　　　C. survival　　　　D. lives
6.　A. literature　　B. person　　　　C. art　　　　　　D. figure
7.　A. role　　　　　B. concept　　　　C. element　　　　D. index
8.　A. constrain　　B. harness　　　　C. foster　　　　　D. extinguish
9.　A. presented　　B. conducted　　　C. portrayed　　　D. utilized
10.　A. meaning　　B. contribution　　C. application　　D. relevance

短文概要

对科学基本的了解和认知。

答案及解析

1.　【答案】C
　　【解析】本题考查句意和动词辨析。题干大意为：我们至少要努力确保科技带来的变化方向是正确的。A 项 assess "评定，估价"；B 项 discern "识别；领悟"；C 项 ensure "确保，保证"；D 项 anticipate "预期，抢先"。

2.　【答案】B
　　【解析】本题考查逻辑关系。题干大意为：在民主社会，这就意味着公众需要对科学有一个基本的了解，以便它做出的明智决策能为公众所知情。A 项 because "因为"；B 项 so that "以便，所以"；C 项 despite that "尽管，不管"；D 项 though "虽然，尽管"。

3.　【答案】B
　　【解析】本题考查动词词组。题干大意为：……而不是在专家的掌握之中。leave... in the hands of "把……掌控在某人手中"。

4.　【答案】D
　　【解析】本题考查介词。题干大意为：目前，公众对于科学的态度相当矛盾。attitude toward 是固定搭配，表示"对……的态度"。

5. 【答案】A。
   【解析】本题考查固定搭配。题干大意为：一方面公众期望科技新发展继续稳定提高生活水平……根据句意可知本处是指"生活水平"的提高，其正确表达法是 the standard of living。故选 A。

6. 【答案】D
   【解析】本题考查名词词义。题干大意为：这种不信任在卡通人物疯狂科学家身上体现得尤为明显，他创造了一个科学怪人。

7. 【答案】C
   【解析】本题考查名词词义，题干大意为：它也是支持绿党背后的一个重要元素。A 项 role "角色"；B 项 concept "观念"；C 项 element "元素"；D 项 index "指标"。

8. 【答案】B
   【解析】本题考查动词词义。题干大意为：怎样利用这个兴趣给公众补充科学背景知识。A 项 constrain "束缚"；B 项 harness "治理；利用；驾驭"；C 项 foster "培养，养育"；D 项 extinguish "熄灭，扑灭"。

9. 【答案】A
   【解析】本题考查动词词义。题干大意为：在学校，科学常常以枯燥乏味的形式出现。A 项 present "介绍，呈现"；B 项 conduct "管理，引导"；C 项 portray "描绘，扮演"；D 项 utilize "利用"。

10. 【答案】D
    【解析】本题考查名词词义。题干大意为：孩子们为了通过考试只会死记硬背，他们看不到科学与世界的相关性。A 项 meaning "意义，含义"；B 项 contribution "贡献"；C 项 application "申请"；D 项 relevance "相关性"。

Practice Two

The problem of caring for the weak and sick members of society has existed from the very earliest times. But the idea is a new one in the history of man.

The Greek, for instance, had ___1___ public institutions for the sick. Some of their doctors maintained surgeries where they could carry on their work, but they were very small, and only one patient could be treated ___2___. The Romans, in times of war, established infirmaries, ___3___ were used to treat sick and injured soldiers. Later on, infirmaries were founded in the larger cities and were ___4___ out of public funds.

___5___, the Roman influence was responsible for the establishment of hospitals. As Christianity grew, the care of the sick became the duty of the Church. During the Middle Ages monasteries and convents provided most of the hospitals monks and nuns were the nurses.

The custom of making pilgrimages to religious shrines also helped advance the ___6___ of hospitals. These pilgrimages were often long, and the travelers had to stop overnight at small inns along the road. These inns were called hospitalia, or guest houses, from the Latin word "hospes", meaning "a guest". The inns connected with the monasteries ___7___ themselves to caring for travelers who were ill or lame or weary. In this way the name "hospital" became connected with __8__ for the afflicted.

Since living conditions during the Middle Ages were not very comfortable or hygienic, the hospitals of those days were __9__ clean or orderly. In fact, many a hospital would put two or more patients in the same bed!

During the seventeenth century, there was a general improvement in living conditions. People began to feel that it was the duty of the state to care for its ailing citizens. But it wasn't __10__ the eighteenth century that public hospitals became general in the larger towns of England. Soon, the idea of public hospitals began to spread and they appeared all over Europe.

1. A. a few   B. no   C. many   D. few
2. A. at a time   B. at no time   C. once and again   D. once for all
3. A. they   B. that   C. in which   D. which
4. A. supplied   B. recruited   C. built   D. supported
5. A. In the same way   B. In a big way
   C. In a way   D. In the way
6. A. history   B. idea   C. condition   D. equipment
7. A. devoting   B. that devoted   C. devoted   D. for devoting
8. A. housing   B. hospitality   C. casing   D. friendship
9. A. far from being   B. far to being
   C. so far as to be   D. so much from being
10. A. in   B. by   C. up to   D. until

短文概要

医院发展的历史。

答案及解析

1. 【答案】B

   【解析】本题考查句意。根据后文可知，Greek 是没有公共医疗机构的，于是有些医生自行建立了一些小的手术室，故 B 项正确。

2. 【答案】A

   【解析】本题考查句意和词组。此处句意为：手术室非常小，一次只能为一个病人做手术。故 at a time "一次"是正确答案。at no time "任何时候都不"，once and again "再次"，没有 once for all 这个词组。

3. 【答案】D

   【解析】本题考查定语从句。根据所填词前面的逗号可知，此处为非限制性定语从句，因此 which 是正确的，指代上文的 infirmaries。

4. 【答案】D

   【解析】本题考查句意和动词。此处指这些医务室是由公共资金支持赞助的，因此

support 是正确答案。supply "供应"，recruit "招聘"，build "建立"。

5. 【答案】C

【解析】本题考查词组。in a way "在某种程度上"，in the same way "同样地"，in the way "挡道"，in a big way "彻底地，大规模地"。

6. 【答案】B

【解析】本题考查句意和搭配。根据下文可知朝圣的风俗使许多 inns 出现，从而演变成为 hospital，故此处应是帮助提出了 "医院" 的概念。同时四个选项中，只有 idea 可与 advance "提出" 搭配，故本题正确答案为 B。

7. 【答案】C

【解析】本题考查句意和动词。devote oneself to 表示 "投身于……"。

8. 【答案】C

【解析】本题考查句意和名词。casing "包装，保护性的外套"。housing "提供住宅"，hospitality "好客，盛情"，friendship "友谊"。

9. 【答案】A

【解析】本题考查词组。句意：因为中世纪生活条件既不舒适也不卫生，所以那时的医院既不干净也无秩序。far from "没有"，so far as "就……而论，在……的范围内"。

10. 【答案】D

【解析】本题考查固定搭配。句意：直到 18 世纪，在英国一些较大的城镇，公立医院才变得普遍起来。not until "直到……才"。

Practice Three

Women appear to be more vulnerable than men ___1___ many ___2___ consequences of alcohol use. A recent *NIAAA Alcohol Alert* reports that women achieve higher concentrations of alcohol in the blood and become more ___3___ than men after drinking equivalent amounts of alcohol. They are more ___4___ than men to alcohol-related organ damage and to trauma resulting ___5___ traffic crashes and interpersonal violence. This *Alcohol Alert* examines gender differences in alcohol's effects and considers some factors that may place women at risk for alcohol-related problems.

Women's drinking is most common between ages 26 and 34 and among women who are ___6___ or separated. Binge drinking (i.e., consumption of five or more drinks per occasion on 5 or more days in the past month) is most common among women ages 18 to 25. Among racial groups, women's drinking is more prevalent among whites, although black women are more likely to drink heavily.

Household surveys indicate that alcohol use is more ___7___ among men than women in the United States. In one survey, 34 percent of women reported ___8___ at least 12 standard drinks during the previous year compared with 56 percent of men. Among drinkers surveyed, 10 percent of women and 22 percent of men consumed two or more drinks per day on average. Men are also more likely than women to become alcohol __9__ . Men have greater rates of alcohol-use disorders than women. A new study of emotional and alcohol- __10__ responses to stress has found that when men become upset, they are more likely than women to want alcohol.

1. A. for　　　　B. in　　　　　C. to　　　　　D. at
2. A. positive　　B. adverse　　　C. side　　　　D. significant
3. A. sober　　　B. drunk　　　　C. robust　　　D. impaired
4. A. susceptible　B. adaptable　　C. accustomed　D. related
5. A. in　　　　　B. from　　　　C. of　　　　　D. as
6. A. unmarried　B. housebound　C. divorced　　D. hospitable
7. A. prevalent　　B. unpopular　　C. ordinary　　D. preferable
8. A. digested　　B. digesting　　C. consumed　　D. consuming
9. A. dependent　B. independent　C. predominant　D. disorders
10. A. sensitive　　B. insensitive　　C. craving　　D. crazy

短文概要

本文论述男女饮酒后的影响差异。

🕊 答案及解析

1. 【答案】C
【解析】此题解题的关键在于"动词＋介词搭配"。be vulnerable to sth. 表示"更易受……影响"。故答案为 C。

2. 【答案】B
【解析】此题解题的关键在于上下文信息。A 项 positive "积极的"；B 项 adverse "相反的，不利的"；C 项 side "旁边的"，side effect "副作用"；D 项 significant "重要的"。根据下文内容提到喝酒的不利结果，本段逻辑关系为总分，例证关系。此句含义：女性看上去要比男性更容易受饮酒不利结果的影响。因而答案为 B。

3. 【答案】D
【解析】A 项 sober "清醒的"；B 项 drunk "喝醉的"；C 项 robust "强有力的"；D 项 impaired "削弱的"。仅参考此句不能解题，下文提到女性容易患上器官损伤等疾病，因而此处与上下文逻辑关系最吻合的就是 D 项。此句含义：据报告称，与男性相比，饮用同等量酒后，女性血液中的酒精浓度更高，身体更加衰弱。

4. 【答案】A
【解析】解题关键在于固定搭配。A 项 be susceptible to sth. "对……敏感"，与 be vulnerable to 同义；B 项 be adaptable to "使适应"；C 项 be accustomed to "习惯于"；D 项 be related to "和……有关"。根据介词 to 后面的名词可知，此处含义为"患病"，因而 A 项为答案。

5. 【答案】B
【解析】此题考点为"动词＋介词搭配"。result in 含义为"导致……发生"，例如：Carelessness resulted in the accident. 粗心导致这个事故的发生。result from 意为"由于"，表示原因，例如：The accident resulted from his carelessness. 事故的发生是因为他的粗心。此处表示原因，因而为 from，选 B。

6. 【答案】C

   【解析】此题解题的关键在于和空白处并列的 separated，因而空白处应该为 separated 的近义词，故答案为 C。

7. 【答案】A

   【解析】根据空白处下一句的数据可以判断此题空白处的词义，故答案为 prevalent，意为"普遍的，流行的"。D 项 preferable 表示"更适合，更可取"，与介词 to 连用，例如：Anything is preferable to the tense atmosphere at home. 什么都比家里气氛紧张要好。

8. 【答案】D

   【解析】根据句意此处含义应该为"饮酒"，故 A、B 可以排除。digest 的含义为"消化，吸收"。根据语法知识，report 为谓语动词，故 consume 应该是表示主动的非谓语动词，答案即为 D。此句含义：在一项调查中，与 56% 的男士相比，有 34% 的女士报告说在去年至少饮用了 12 标准杯的酒。

9. 【答案】A

   【解析】根据下文的含义，男士在遇到情感问题或压力的时候，要比女性更想饮酒。所以此空白处的含义应该为"对酒精的依赖"，答案为 A。B 项 independent "独立的"；C 项 predominant "处于主导地位的"；D 项 disorders 为名词，指的是"紊乱，失调"。

10. 【答案】C

    【解析】根据句意可以得出答案，句意参考第 9 题。A 项 sensitive "敏感的"；B 项 insensitive "不敏感的"；C 项 craving "渴望的"；D 项 crazy "疯狂的"。

Practice Four

Elderly people respond best to a calm and __1__ environment. This is not always easy to provide as their behaviour can sometimes be __2__. If they get excited or upset they may become more confused and more difficult to look after. Although sometimes it can be extremely difficult, it is best to be patient and not get upset yourself. You should always encourage old people to do as much as possible for themselves but be ready to __3__ a helping hand when necessary.

__4__ memory makes it difficult for the person to recall all the basic kinds of information we take for granted. The obvious way to help in this situation is to supply the information that is missing and help them __5__ what is going on. You must use every opportunity to provide information but remember to keep it simple and __6__.

"Good morning, Mum. This is Fiona, your daughter. It is eight o'clock, so if you get up now, we can have breakfast downstairs."

When the elderly person makes confused statements, such as, about going out to his or her old employment or visiting a dead relative, correct him or her in a __7__ matter-of-fact fashion: "You don't work in the office any more. You are retired now. Will you come and help me with the dishes?"

We rely heavily on the information provided by signposts, clocks, calendars and newspapers. These assist us to organise and direct our behavior. __8__ old people need these aids __9__ to __10__ their poor memory. Encourage them to use reminder boards or diaries for important coming events and label the contents of different cupboards and drawers. Many other aids such as information cards, old photos, scrap books, addresses or shopping lists could help in individual case.

1. A. excited   B. hasty   C. unhurried   D. nervous
2. A. ridiculous   B. childlike   C. unacceptable   D. irritating
3. A. carry   B. offer   C. lend   D. provide
4. A. Implicit   B. Failing   C. Sensory   D. Semantic
5. A. make sense of   B. make sense
    C. see sense   D. knock some sense into
6. A. complicated   B. implicit   C. straightforward D. ambiguous
7. A. calm   B. impatient   C. fussy   D. furious
8. A. Excited   B. Irritated   C. Disappointed   D. Confused
9. A. all the time   B. at times   C. in no time   D. at a time
10. A. remind of   B. compensate for C. prevent from   D. derive from

短文概要

本文讨论如何照料老人，尤其是该如何帮助记忆力不好的老年人。

答案及解析

1. 【答案】C
    【解析】A 项 excited "兴奋的"；B 项 hasty "匆忙的"；C 项 unhurried "不慌不忙的，从容的"；D 项 nervous "紧张的"。此题解题关键在于 calm，空白处应该为 calm 的近义词，故答案为 C。

2. 【答案】D
    【解析】此题解题的关键在于后面具体的表述。我们可以得知如果老年人很激动或者紧张不安，他们就会变得很困惑，也很难照料。因而空白处所在句子的含义为：因为他们的行为有时候很恼人，所以这并不容易。A 项 ridiculous "荒谬可笑的"；B 项 childlike "幼稚的"；C 项 unacceptable "不可接受的"；D 项 irritating "恼人的"。

3. 【答案】C
    【解析】此题考点为固定搭配 be ready to lend a helping hand，表示 "乐于助人"。

4. 　【答案】B

　　【解析】A 项 implicit "暗示的"；B 项 failing "失败的"；C 项 sensory "感官的"，sensory memory 表示 "感官记忆"；D 项 semantic "语义的"，semantic memory 表示 "语义记忆"。此句含义：对于一个记忆力下降的人来说，要想回想起我们认为理所当然的基本信息是很困难的。根据句意，B 项正确。

5. 　【答案】A

　　【解析】A 项 make sense of "理解，弄懂"，例如：I can't make sense of the novel. 我读不懂这本小说。B 项 make sense 有两种含义。①有道理，有意义，例如：Your explanation doesn't make sense. 你的解释不通。②明智的，例如：It makes sense to buy the most up-to-date version. 买最新版本是明智的。C 项 see sense 搭配不存在。D 项 knock some sense into sb. "强使某人理智行事"。此句含义：在这种状况下最直接的办法就是提供已经消失的信息并且帮助他们明白正在发生的事情。

6. 　【答案】C

　　【解析】A 项 complicated "复杂的"；B 项 implicit "暗示的"；C 项 straightforward "直截了当的"；D 项 ambiguous "模棱两可的"。根据此句中的 simple 可以推断空白处为 simple 的近义词，故 C 项为答案。此句含义：你一定要利用每一个机会提供信息，但是记得让信息简单且直白。

7. 　【答案】A

　　【解析】根据后面引语里面的话，可以推断：更正的方式应该是温和且实事求是的。A 项 calm "冷静的"，为答案；B 项 impatient "不耐心的"；C 项 fussy "急躁的"；D 项 furious "发怒的"。此句含义：当老年人出现困惑的时候（因为记忆不好了），要用温和、实事求是的方式纠正他们。

8. 　【答案】D

　　【解析】四个备选单词的含义比较简单，关键看语境含义。"我们通常很依赖路标、时钟、日历和报纸提供给我们的信息。这些帮助我们安排、指导我们的行为。"根据这句话的含义我们知道这些都是提醒的作用。那么对于老人来说，尤其是对于记忆力不好的老人来说他们尤其需要这些帮助。根据推断，答案为 confused，表示 "困惑的"。

9. 　【答案】A

　　【解析】A 项 all the time "总是，一贯"；B 项 at times "有时，间或"；C 项 in no time "立即"；D 项 at a time "每次，一次"。

10. 　【答案】B

　　【解析】remind sb. of "使某人想起"，例如：The picture reminds me of France. 这张图片让我想起了法国。B 项 compensate for "弥补"；C 项 prevent from "防止"；D 项 derive from "从……获得"。此句含义：使用这些提示可以帮助老年人弥补他们很差的记忆。

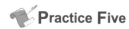 **Practice Five**

Many theories concerning the causes of juvenile delinquency (crimes committed by young people) focus either on the individual or on society as the major contributing influence. Theories ___1___ on the individual suggest that children engage in criminal behavior because they were not sufficiently penalized for previous misdeeds or that they have learned criminal behavior through ___2___ with others. Theories focusing on the role of society suggest that children commit crimes in ___3___ to their failure to rise above their socioeconomic status or as a rejection of middle-class values.

Most theories of juvenile delinquency have focused on children from disadvantaged families, ___4___ the fact that children from wealthy homes also commit crimes. The latter may commit crimes for lack of adequate parental control. All theories, however, are tentative and are ___5___ to criticism.

Changes in the social structure may indirectly ___6___ juvenile crime rates. For example, changes in the economy that lead to fewer job opportunities for youth and rising unemployment ___7___ make gainful employment increasingly difficult to obtain. The resulting discontent may in ___8___ lead more youths into criminal behavior.

Families have also experienced changes these years. More families consist of one parent households or two working parents. Consequently, children are likely to have less supervision at home than was common in the traditional family ___9___. This lack of parental supervision is thought to be an influence on juvenile crime rates. Other identifiable causes of offensive acts include frustration or failure in school, the increased availability of drugs and alcohol, and the growing ___10___ of child abuse and child neglect. All these conditions tend to increase the probability of a child committing a criminal act, although a direct causal relationship has not yet been established.

1. A. acting   B. relying   C. centering   D. commenting
2. A. interactions   B. assimilation   C. cooperation   D. consultation
3. A. return   B. reply   C. reference   D. response
4. A. considering   B. ignoring   C. highlighting   D. discarding
5. A. immune   B. resistant   C. sensitive   D. subject
6. A. affect   B. reduce   C. chock   D. reflect
7. A. in general   B. on average   C. by contrast   D. at length
8. A. case   B. short   C. turn   D. essence
9. A. system   B. structure   C. concept   D. heritage
10. A. incidence   B. awareness   C. exposure   D. popularity

短文概要

本文介绍与青少年犯罪相关的几个理论。

答案及解析

1. **【答案】C**

   【解析】文中第一句的含义：许多有关青少年犯罪的理论把个人或社会作为主要成因。此处空白需要一个非谓语动词来修饰 theories，表示"侧重于"，因而选项 C centering 为正确答案，同时 center on 为 focus on 的近义改写。A 项 act on "充当"；B 项 rely on "依靠，依赖"；D 项 comment on "评论"。此句含义：侧重于个体的理论认为儿童参与犯罪是因为他们没能从上一次犯罪中受到充分的惩罚，或者他们从和别人的交往中学会了犯罪。

2. **【答案】A**

   【解析】此句中 through 表示学会犯罪的途径或手段。A 项 interactions "交往"；B 项 assimilation "同化"；C 项 cooperation "合作"；D 项 consultation "咨询，请教"。只有选项 A 在逻辑关系和句意上能与 learn criminal behavior 吻合，故答案为 A。

3. **【答案】D**

   【解析】A 项 in return 与介词 for 连用，而不与介词 to 搭配（原文中介词为 to），表示"对……的回报"，例如：Can I buy you lunch in return for your help? 我能请你吃个饭吗？以表示感谢你的帮忙。B 项 in reply to 表示"回答，回复"，例如：I wrote to you in reply to your letter. 给你写信，以回复你的来信。C 项 in/with reference to 表示"关于"，例如：In / With reference to the plan, I have to say something. 就这个计划，我有话要说。D 项 in response to 表示"对……的回应"，体现一种因果关系。例如：The shop improved its service in response to customers' demands. 应顾客要求，这个商店改进了服务。此句含义：侧重社会角色的理论认为，青少年犯罪是对其社会经济地位提升的失败或者被中产阶级价值观所抛弃的一种回应。

4. **【答案】B**

   【解析】A 项 considering "认为"；B 项 ignoring "忽视"；C 项 highlighting "强调，突出"；D 项 discarding "抛弃"。此题要依据上下文信息。下文提到：The latter may commit crimes for lack of adequate parental control. the latter 这里指的是 children from wealthy homes（有钱人家的孩子犯罪是因为缺乏父母足够的管教）。此句含义：大多数青少年犯罪的理论侧重于那些来自不富裕家庭的孩子，而忽略了富家子弟也同样犯罪。所以答案应该为 B。

5. **【答案】D**

   【解析】A 项 be immune to "不受……的影响"，例如：He was immune to all persuasion. 他对所有的劝说都无动于衷。B 项 be resistant to "对……有抵抗力"，例如：These plants are resistant to cold weather. 这些植物抗寒。C 项 be sensitive to "对……敏感"。D 项 be subject to "易受……的影响"。根据上文的信息可以了解，这些青少年犯罪的理论都存在缺陷，因而容易备受批评。所以答案为 D。

6. 【答案】**A**

【解析】A 项 affect "影响"；B 项 reduce "减少"；C 项 chock "用楔子塞住"；D 项 reflect "反映"。从本段首句就可以判断该段落要讲述社会对青少年犯罪的影响，因而选项 A 为正确答案。此句含义：社会结构的变化可能间接地影响青少年犯罪率。

7. 【答案】**A**

【解析】A 项 in general "大体上，一般来说"；B 项 on average "平均"；C 项 by contrast "与……成对比"；D 项 at length "详尽地"。此句含义：例如，总的来说，经济上的变化导致年轻人的就业机会越来越少，失业率越来越高，找到一份有收入的工作越来越难。四个备选词组中只有 A 符合此句语境。

8. 【答案】**C**

【解析】A 项 in case "以免，以防"；B 项 in short "简而言之"；C 项 in turn 的含义为：①依次，轮流，例如：The children called out their names in turn. 孩子们依次报姓名。②相应地，例如：Increased production will, in turn, lead to increased profits. 增加生产会继而增加利润。D 项 in essence "本质上"，例如：The two arguments are in essence the same. 这两个论点大致相同。C 符合句子的逻辑关系。此句含义：这种不满可能导致更多的年轻人犯罪。

9. 【答案】**B**

【解析】根据此句话的含义可以判断这个段落讲述的是家庭对青少年犯罪的影响。此句含义：家庭这些年来也发生了变化。更多的家庭是单亲家庭或者父母双方都是外出上班族。结果孩子很可能比传统家庭疏于管教。这说明家庭结构发生了变化，所以选择 B。A 项 system "制度"；C 项 concept "理念"；D 项 heritage "传统"。

10. 【答案】**A**

【解析】A 项 incidence "影响范围，发生率"；B 项 awareness "意识"；C 项 exposure "暴露"，常与介词 to 连用，例如：Much exposure to the strong sunlight will lead to skin damage. 在强太阳光下晒太久会导致皮肤损伤。D 项 popularity "流行"。此句含义：缺少父母管教会影响青少年犯罪率。其他可以确定的犯罪原因有：在学校受到挫折和失败，越来越容易得到毒品和酒，虐待和忽视孩子的现象日益增多。故答案为 A。

Practice Six

It is natural for young people to __1__ their parents at times and to blame them for most of the misunderstandings between them. They have always complained, more or less justly, that their parents are out of touch with modern ways; that they are possessive and __2__ that they do not trust their children to deal with crises; that they talk too much about certain problems and that they have no sense of humour, at least in parent-child relationships.

I think it is true that parents often ___3___ their teenage children and also forget how they themselves felt when young. Young people often ___4___ their parents with their choices in clothes and hairstyles, in entertainers and music. This is not their motive. They feel cut off from the adult world into which they have not yet been accepted. So they create a culture and society of their own. Then, if it turns out that their music or entertainers or vocabulary or clothes or hairstyles irritate their parents, this gives them additional ___5___ . They feel they are ___6___ , at least in a small way, and that they are leaders in style and taste.

Sometimes you are ___7___ , and proud because you do not want your parents to approve of what you do. If they did approve, it looks as if you are ___8___ your own age group. But in that case, you are assuming that you are the underdog: you can't win but at least you can keep your honour. This is a passive way of looking at things. It is natural enough after long years of childhood, when you were completely under your parents' control. But it ignores the fact that you are now beginning to be responsible for yourself.

If you plan to control your life, co-operation can be part of that plan. You can charm others, especially parents, into doing things the way you want. You can ___9___ others with your sense of responsibility and initiative, so that they will give you the ___10___ to do what you want to do.

1. A. comment on   B. be critical of   C. be indifferent to   D. be content with
2. A. wordy   B. righteous   C. bounteous   D. dominant
3. A. underestimate B. blame   C. overrate   D. criticize
4. A. are satisfied B. are content   C. irritate   D. inspire
5. A. puzzle   B. enjoyment   C. trouble   D. criticism
6. A. superior   B. inferior   C. satisfied   D. proud
7. A. confident   B. resistant   C. selfish   D. indifferent
8. A. comforting   B. deceiving   C. pleasing   D. betraying
9. A. impress   B. charm   C. cheer   D. fascinate
10. A. specification B. authority   C. priority   D. instruction

短文概要

本文谈论父母对孩子生活的过多干涉可导致父母和孩子关系的紧张。

答案及解析

1. 【答案】B

【解析】A 项 comment on "对……加以评论"；B 项 be critical of "不满，批评"，例如：Parents are always highly critical of the school. 家长总是对学校不满，提出批评。C 项 be indifferent to "对……冷漠"；D 项 be content with "对……感到满意"。根据上下文我们可以知道：年轻人总是对他们的父母不满，对父母对他们因为误解而进行的批评颇有微词。所以答案应改为 B。

2. 【答案】D

【解析】A 项 wordy "唠叨的，话多的"；B 项 righteous "正直的"；C 项 bounteous "宽宏大量的"；D 项 dominant "处于支配地位的"。此题根据前面的单词 possessive（占有的），可以推断 D 为答案，此句含义：年轻人经常抱怨他们的父母与时尚脱节、占有欲强、总是想支配人等。

3. 【答案】A

【解析】这篇短文主要谈论父母对孩子的生活干涉过多导致孩子与父母之间互相不理解，甚至针锋相对的状况。本题这句话的含义是父母经常低估了他们。A 项 underestimate "低估"；B 项 blame "批评"；C 项 overrate "对……估计过高"；D 项 criticize "批评"。

4. 【答案】C

【解析】根据上下文信息可以得知，父母和孩子在各方面存在代沟，无法互相理解，因而这句意思也一样，孩子们和父母在衣服的选择、发型、娱乐明星和音乐方面有代沟。四个备选项表示"双方观点不一致"的就只有 C 项 irritate with "对……恼怒"。并且在下面的原文信息当中答案复现：Then, if it turns out that their music or entertainers or vocabulary or clothes or hairstyles irritate their parents…

5. 【答案】B

【解析】此句含义：如果因为上述方面与父母看法不同而惹恼了父母，对于孩子来说就会是一种额外的快乐。符合句意的只有 B。下一句信息证实了这个答案。

6. 【答案】A

【解析】此句含义：至少在一定程度上他们感到高人一等，他们是时尚和品位方面的潮流人士。联系第 5 题，可以得出正确答案。A 项 superior "高人一等的"；B 项 inferior "自卑的"；C 项 satisfied "满足的"；D 项 proud "自豪的"。

7. 【答案】B

【解析】根据原因状语从句的内容：因为你不想让你父母同意你所做的，所以结果就是有时你很反叛，很自负。与语境符合的备选单词就是 resistant。

8. 【答案】D

【解析】此句含义：如果他们同意了，这就好像你脱离了你的年龄群。与这个语句含义推断相近的选项为 D 项 betray "背叛"。

9. 【答案】A

【解析】此句含义：你可以给别人留下很负责任、很主动的印象。此题考点为固定搭配，impress sb. with "给……留下印象"。

10. 【答案】B

【解析】此句含义：如果你给别人上述印象，别人就会让你去做自己想做的事情。A 项 specification "规格"；B 项 authority "权利，职权"；C 项 priority "优先权"；D 项 instruction "指导"。

Practice Seven

Fear is often a(n) __1__ emotion. When you become frightened, many physical changes occur within your body. Your heartbeat and __2__ quicken; your pupils expand to admit more light; large quantities of energy-producing adrenaline（肾上激素）are poured into your bloodstream. __3__ a fire or accident, fear can __4__ life-saving flight. Similarly, when a danger is psychological rather than physical, fear can force you to take self-protective measures. It is only when fear is disproportional to the danger __5__ that it becomes a problem.

Some people are simply more vulnerable __6__ fear than others. A visit to the newborn nursery of any large hospital will demonstrate that, from the moment of their births, a few fortunate infants respond calmly to sudden fear-producing situations such as a loudly slammed door. Yet a neighbour in the next bed may cry out with profound fright. From birth, he or she is more __7__ learn fearful responses because he or she has inherited a tendency to be more __8__.

Further, psychologists know that our early experiences and relationships strongly __9__ and determine our later fears. A young man named Bill, for example, grew up with a father who regarded each adversity as a __10__ obstacle to be overcome with imagination and courage. Using his father as a model, Bill came to welcome adventure and to trust his own ability to solve problem.

1. A. useful   B. unbeneficial   C. strong   D. mixed
2. A. steps   B. pace   C. responses   D. breath
3. A. Suffering from   B. Confronted with
   C. In relation to   D. In the face of
4. A. avoid   B. hinder   C. delay   D. fuel
5. A. at hand   B. in hand   C. to hand   D. by hand
6. A. in   B. to   C. at   D. on
7. A. tend to   B. attendant upon   C. prone to   D. subjected to
8. A. sensory   B. sensible   C. sensational   D. sensitive
9. A. affect   B. hinder   C. avoid   D. shape
10. A. temporary   B. permanent   C. unconquered   D. formidable

短文概要

本文讨论恐惧的好处以及早期经历对人以后恐惧心理的影响。

答案及解析

1. 【答案】A

【解析】解此题需要参看下面的信息来确定哪个形容词适合在这里形容恐惧。当你害怕的时候，出现许多身体变化。后面的内容就要具体看出现哪些变化，而且要看出这些变化是积极的还是消极的。因而这道题需要解决所有其他题目之后再决定。此句属于主题句。整个段落都在讲述恐惧的好处，故答案为 A。

2. 【答案】C

【解析】根据具体的身体变化可以推断空白处的答案。"你的心跳加快，瞳孔放大以接受更多的光，大量用来产生能量的肾上腺激素进入血流。"如果仅仅看本句，可以排除 A 和 B。这时需要继续往下看相关信息。"当遇到火灾或事故的时候，恐惧有助于逃命。"看到这里就可以判断此题 C 项 response 反应加快要比 breath 呼吸加快更恰当。

3. 【答案】B

【解析】在做出正确选项前，可以推断此处的含义为"遇到火灾或事故"。可以排除 C项 in relation to "和……有关"。A 项 suffer from "遭受"，D 项 in the face of "面对"；二者虽然含义与此句吻合，但是这两个词组的主语通常为人，因而在这里不合语法。故答案为 B。

4. 【答案】D

【解析】此题解题的关键在于 similarly，意为"同样"，即用后面的已知信息推知前面的含义。"同样，当危险是心理上的而不是身体上的，恐惧可以迫使你启用自我保护的措施。"因而可以推断前面的未知信息是有助于或者促进逃命的含义。答案为 fuel，原意为"提供燃料"。

5. 【答案】A

【解析】此题考点为形近词组辨析。A 项 at hand 意为"在手边，在附近，即将到来"；B 项 in hand "在手头，在进行中"；C 项 to hand "在手边，随时可以得到"，例如：I'm afraid I don't have the latest figures to hand. 恐怕我手头没有最新的数据。D 项 by hand "手工的，专人送递的"。此句为强调句，含义为：只有当恐惧与即将到来的危险不成比例的时候，它才成为一个问题。

6. 【答案】B

【解析】此题为固定搭配，be vulnerable to "易受……影响"，此句含义：一些人比其他人更容易受恐惧的影响。

7. 【答案】C

【解析】本段举例新生儿。A 项 tend to "倾向于"，意思吻合但不合语法，这个词组为动词短语，不与 be 动词连用。B 项 be attendant upon "随之而来的"，例如：We had all the usual problems attendant upon starting a new business. 我们遇到了创业时通常会出现的所有问题。C 项 be prone to "易于遭受，有做……的倾向"。D 项 be subjected to "使服从"。此句含义：从出生开始，他或她就更容易开始学习恐惧的反应，因为他或她与生俱来有一种对事物更敏感的趋势。故答案为 C。

8. 【答案】D

【解析】此题考点为形近词辨析。A 项 sensory "感官的"；B 项 sensible "明智的"；C 项 sensational "轰动性的，极好的"；D 项 sensitive "敏感的"。句意参看第 7 题。

9. 【答案】D

   【解析】此题解题关键在于后面的例子，由例子的含义可以推断出主题句的大意。D 项 shape 表示"形成"，与 determine 近义，故 D 为答案。

10. 【答案】A

   【解析】事例告诉我们这个叫 Bill 的年轻人由他父亲抚养长大，他的父亲把每一个挫折视为暂时的困难，并且相信智慧和勇气可以战胜困难。根据这句话的含义，他父亲坚定地认为困难不是不可战胜的。A 项 temporary "暂时的"；B 项 permanent "永久的"；C 项 unconquered "不可战胜的"；D 项 formidable "令人可怕的"。只有 A 符合他父亲对困难的态度。

Practice Eight

Statuses are marvelous human __1__ that enable us to get along with one another and to determine where we "fit" in society. As we __2__ our everyday lives, we mentally attempt to place people __3__ their statuses. For example, we must judge whether the person in the library is a reader or a librarian, whether the telephone caller is a friend or a salesman, whether the unfamiliar person on our property is a thief or a meter reader, and so on.

The statuses we __4__ often vary with the people we encounter, and change throughout life. Most of us can, at very high speed, assume the statuses that various situations require. Much of social interaction consists of __5__ and selecting among appropriate statuses and allowing other people to assume their statuses in relation to us. This means that we fit our actions to those of other people based on a __6__ mental process of __7__ and interpretation. Although some of us find the task more difficult than others, most of us perform it rather __8__.

A status has been compared to ready-made clothes. Within certain limits, the buyer can choose style and fabric. But an American is not free to choose the costume（服装）of a Chinese peasant or that of a Hindu prince. We must choose from among the clothing presented by our society. Furthermore, our choice is limited to a size that will fit, as well as by our pocketbook（钱包）. Having made a choice within these limits we can have certain __9__ made, but __10__ minor adjustments, we tend to be limited to what the stores have on their racks. Statuses too come ready-made, and the range of choice among them is limited.

1. A. discoveries   B. inventions   C. creations   D. innovation
2. A. go about   B. go by   C. go down   D. go through
3. A. in relation to   B. in line with   C. in the light of   D. on account of
4. A. resume   B. assume   C. consume   D. distinguish
5. A. recognizing   B. realizing   C. identifying   D. interpreting
6. A. instant   B. temporary   C. permanent   D. constant
7. A. trials   B. praise   C. appraisal   D. consideration

8.　A. effortlessly　　B. unendurably　　C. knottily　　D. smoothly
9.　A. alternations　　B. alterations　　C. alternatives　　D. decisions
10.　A. far from　　B. in terms of　　C. apart from　　D. in view of

短文概要

本文就人类的身份进行讨论。

答案及解析

1.　【答案】B
　　【解析】A 项 discovery "发现"，常表示 "原来存在，后来被发现的事物"；B 项 invention "发明"；C 项 creation "创造"；D 项 innovation 作为不可数名词，含义为 "创新，改革"，作为可数名词含义为 "新思想，新方法"。此句含义：身份地位是人类的发明创造，它使我们能够彼此相处，并且决定了我们在社会中适合的位置。故 B 为答案。

2.　【答案】A
　　【解析】此题为形近词组辨析。A 项 go about "着手做某事"，例如：How can I go about a part-time job? 我怎样才能找到一份兼职呢？B 项 go by 有两个含义。①（时间）逝去，过去，例如：Things will get easier as time goes by. 随着时间的推移，事情会越来越简单。②遵循（某事物），例如：That is the rule you have to go by. 这个规则你必须遵守。C 项 go down "下沉，下跌"，例如：The price of oil is going down. 油价正在下跌。D 项 go through 有三个含义。①仔细察看，例如：I used to start the day by going through e-mails. 过去我常常是从查看邮件开始我新的一天。②经历，遭受，例如：He went through a tough period during the war. 战争期间他经历了很困难的时期。③用完，耗尽，例如：The child went through the whole loaf of bread after school. 放学后这个孩子吃光了整条面包。此句含义：当我们开始一天的生活时，我们会试图从情感上根据地位将人们划分归类。故答案为 A。

3.　【答案】C
　　【解析】A 项 in relation to "和……有关"；B 项 in line with "符合"；C 项 in the light of "根据，依照"；D 项 on account of "由于，因为"，例如：She retired earlier on account of poor health. 她因为身体不好提早退休了。原句含义参见第 2 题。

4.　【答案】B
　　【解析】A 项 resume "恢复"；B 项 assume "假定"；C 项 consume "消费"；D 项 distinguish "分辨"。根据原文大意：我们假定的身份地位因我们遇到的人而有所不同，并且在一生中都会发生变化。

5.　【答案】C
　　【解析】A 项 recognize "认出某人"；B 项 realize "认识到……"；C 项 identify "鉴别，确定"；D 项 interpret "解释，说明"。此句含义：社会交往包含在适

合的身份地位中确定、选择并且允许其他的人认定他们和我们有关的身份地位。C 项符合句意。

6. 【答案】**D**

【解析】此题较难。A 项 instant "立即的，快速的"；B 项 temporary "临时的"；C 项 permanent "永久的"；D 项 constant "持续的"。此句含义：这就意味着我们要根据时刻进行的解释和评价使我们的行为符合其他人的行为。这一过程不是一朝一夕，应该是持久的。这也符合本段第 1 句话告诉我们的：变化调整要伴随一生。（The statuses we assume often vary with the people we encounter, and change throughout life.）

7. 【答案】**C**

【解析】A 项 trial "试验"；B 项 praise "表扬"；C 项 appraisal "评价，评估"；D 项 consideration "考虑"。只有 C 符合本句含义。原文含义参看第 6 题。

8. 【答案】**A**

【解析】此题解题关键在于 although 这个连词，这就告诉我们空白处应该为 difficult 的反义词。A 项 effortlessly "不费力气地"；B 项 unendurably "无法忍受地，不能持久地"；C 项 knottily "棘手地，困难多地"；D 项 smoothly "平稳地"。

9. 【答案】**B**

【解析】此段落用一个比喻做进一步的阐述。A 项 alternation "交替，轮流"；B 项 alteration "改变"；C 项 alternative "选择"；D 项 decision "决定"。此题关键在于 but 后面的 minor adjustments（微调）。因而答案为 B。

10. 【答案】**C**

【解析】A 项 far from "远离，远非"；B 项 in terms of "根据，按照"；C 项 apart from "除⋯⋯之外"；D 项 in view of "考虑到，由于"。此句含义：除了做一点微调，我们总是局限于货架上现有的货品。只有 C 项符合此句的逻辑关系。

Practice Nine

Most children with healthy appetites are ready to eat almost anything that is offered them and a child rarely dislikes food __1__ it is badly cooked. The __2__ a meal is cooked and served is most important and an __3__ served meal will often improve a child's appetite. Never ask a child whether he likes or dislikes a food and never __4__ likes and dislikes in front of him or allow anybody else to do so. If the father says he hates fat meat or the mother __5__ vegetables in the child's hearing he is __6__ to copy this procedure. Take it for granted that he likes everything and he probably will. Nothing healthful should be __7__ from the meal because of a __8__ dislike. At meal time it is a good idea to give a child a small __9__ and let him come back for a second helping rather than give him as much as he is likely to eat all at once. Do not talk too much to the child during meal time, but let him get on with his food; and do not allow him to leave the table immediately after a meal or he will soon learn to swallow his food so he can hurry back to his toys. Under ___10___ circumstances must a child be coaxed or forced to eat.

1. A. if　　　　　B. until　　　　　C. that　　　　　D. unless
2. A. procedure　B. process　　　C. way　　　　　D. method
3. A. adequately　B. attractively　C. urgently　　　D. eagerly
4. A. remark　　　B. tell　　　　　C. discuss　　　D. argue
5. A. opposes　　B. denies　　　　C. refuses　　　D. offends
6. A. willing　　　B. possible　　　C. obliged　　　D. likely
7. A. omitted　　B. allowed　　　C. served　　　D. prevented
8. A. supposed　B. proved　　　C. considered　　D. related
9. A. part　　　　B. portion　　　C. section　　　D. quotient
10. A. some　　　B. any　　　　　C. such　　　　　D. no

短文概要

本文讲述如何促进孩子食欲以及一些教育方面的禁忌。

答案及解析

1. 【答案】D
   【解析】解此题的关键在于此句的含义及逻辑关系。"许多胃口好的孩子总是能够把食物几乎都吃掉。他们几乎不会讨厌食物，除非食物做得太难吃了。"根据句意和逻辑关系，只有 unless 这个含有否定含义的连词最合适。

2. 【答案】C
   【解析】A 项 procedure "程序，手续"；B 项 process "过程"；C 项 way "方式"；D 项 method "方法"。此句含义为：烹饪方式和色泽很关键，菜色很好的食物会促进孩子的食欲。根据这个含义，此题空白处应该为 C，意为"做菜和上菜的方式"。

3. 【答案】B
   【解析】A 项 adequately "充足地"；B 项 attractively "诱人地，吸引人地"；C 项 urgently "迫切地"；D 项 eagerly "热心地"。根据第 2 题的大概含义，应该是菜色好的饭菜会促进孩子的食欲，所以 attractively 符合句意。

4. 【答案】C
   【解析】A 项 remark "评论"，与介词 on 或者 upon 连用，例如：remark on the subject 对于题目的评论。D 项 argue "争论"，与介词 for 或者 against 连用。此句含义：永远不要问孩子是否喜欢还是不喜欢某种食物，也不要在孩子面前讨论喜欢吃的和不喜欢吃的，也不要别人这样做。只有 C 项既符合句意又符合语法。

5. 【答案】C
   【解析】A 项 oppose "反对，对抗"，例如：oppose war and violence 反对战争、暴

力；B 项 deny "否认"；D 项 offend "冒犯，违反"。此题空白处单词应该是 hate 的近义词，本句大概含义为：如果孩子听到父亲说他不喜欢吃肥肉或者母亲不吃蔬菜，他也可能会这样。C 项 refuse 为答案。

6. 【答案】D

【解析】此题表示孩子也有可能像父母那样。表示可能性的说法只有 D 项 be likely to do sth.。A 项 be willing to do "自愿做某事"；B 项 possible，句型为 it is possible for sb. to do sth.；C 项 be obliged to do sth. "不得不，必须做"，例如：I felt obliged to leave after such an unpleasant quarrel. 发生了这样不愉快的争吵之后，我觉得有必要离开。

7. 【答案】A

【解析】此题解题的关键在于主语 nothing healthful。根据对文章主旨含义的掌握可以判断，有营养的食物绝对不应该因为认为不喜欢就不去吃，主语为否定词，因而 A 为正确答案。

8. 【答案】A

【解析】参照此句的大意：有营养的食物不应该因为认为不喜欢就不去吃。只有 A 符合句意。

9. 【答案】B

【解析】此句大意：就餐时，给孩子一小份比较好，让他能再要一次（食物），而不是一次就给他可能吃完的量。根据句中的 as much as he is likely to eat all 以及 come back for a second helping 可以推断前面为一小份。A 项 part "部分，部件"；B 项 portion "（食物）一份"；C 项 section "部门"；D 项 quotient "份额"。故 B 为答案。

10. 【答案】D

【解析】此句话为倒装句。根据全文对于孩子吃饭的观念，可以判断这里的含义大概为：不要哄骗或者强迫孩子吃饭。因而空白处应该为否定词，under no circumstance 这里的含义就是 "在任何情况下都不要……"。

Practice Ten

In __1__ children, every parent watches eagerly the child's __2__ of each new skill — the first spoken words, the first independent steps, or the beginning of reading and writing. It is often __3__ to hurry the child beyond his natural learning rate, but this can set up dangerous feelings of failure and states of worry in the child. This might happen at any stage. A baby might be forced to use a toilet too early; a young child might be encouraged to learn to read before he knows the meaning of the words he reads. On the other hand, though, if a child is left alone too much, or without any learning opportunities, he loses his natural __4__ for life and his desire to find out new things for himself.

Parents vary greatly in their degree of strictness towards their children. Some may be especially strict in money matters. Others sever over time of coming home at night or punctuality for meals. __5__, the controls imposed represent the needs of the parents and the values of the community as much as the child's own happiness.

As regards the development of moral standards in the growing child, __6__ is very important in __7__ teaching. To forbid a thing one day and excuse it the next is no foundation for morality. Also, parents should realize that "example is better than __8__". If they are not sincere and do not practise what they preach（说教）, their children may grow __9__, and emotionally insecure when they grow old enough to think for themselves, and realize they have been to some extent fooled.

A sudden awareness of a marked difference between their parents' __10__ and their morals can be a dangerous disappointment.

1. A. bringing about　B. bringing up　　C. bringing down　D. bringing in
2. A. acquisition　　B. attainment　　C. achievement　　D. performance
3. A. forcing　　　B. persuading　　C. allowing　　　D. tempting
4. A. potential　　B. talent　　　C. enthusiasm　　D. capability
5. A. First of all　B. In detail　　C. Above all　　D. In general
6. A. patience　　B. consistency　C. consideration　D. strictness
7. A. maternal　　B. paternal　　C. parental　　　D. school
8. A. blame　　　B. precept　　　C. action　　　　D. revile
9. A. timid　　　B. naughty　　　C. confused　　　D. disappointed
10. A. principles　B. principals　　C. morale　　　D. instructions

短文概要

本文论述父母应该如何教育孩子，以及在教育过程中父母的一些错误行为。

答案及解析

1. 【答案】B
【解析】A 项 bring about "引起，导致"，例如：What brought about the change in his attitude? 什么使得他改变了态度？B 项 bring up"抚养，提出（讨论等），呕吐"；C 项 bring down "减少，打败"；D 项 bring in "提出（新法案等）"。这句话是指在抚养孩子过程中，因而答案为 B。

2. 【答案】A
【解析】A 项 acquisition "（知识、技能等）获得，得到"；B 项 attainment "成就，造诣，达到，获得（success in achieving sth.）"；C 项 achievement "成就"；D 项 performance "表演，表现"。此句含义：父母们总是很热切地观察自己的孩子学会每一个新技能。所以答案为 A。

3. 【答案】D

【解析】此句解题的关键在于上下文的逻辑关系。根据第 2 题可以知道在抚养孩子的过程中，父母们都急切地观察孩子学会每一个新技能。此题所在句子继续告诉我们：这也就使得家长急切地希望孩子能超越自然学习的频率而超前学习，但是这就导致孩子心理上危险的失败感和担忧。与上下文父母急切的心情和做法一致的选项只有 tempt to do sth.，表示"诱使，对做什么事情动了心"。

4. 【答案】C

【解析】前文提到由于父母急切的心情，使得孩子会超前学习的情况。on the other hand 表示"另一方面"。"如果一个孩子不被关注，或者没有学习机会，他就失去了自己学习新知识的愿望。"此空白处应该为 desire 的近义词。A 项 potential "潜能"；B 项 talent "才能，天赋"；C 项 enthusiasm "热情"；D 项 capability "能力"。只有 C 项表示一种愿望和想法，因而为正确答案。

5. 【答案】D

【解析】A 与 C 选项为近义词组，表示"首先，首要的是"；B 项 in detail "详尽地"；D 项 in general 表示总结性，意思是"概括地说，总的来说"。此句话是基于上述父母对孩子的限制和严格管教做出的总结性论述，因而 D 为答案。

6. 【答案】B

【解析】as regards "关于，至于"。此句含义为：就儿童成长过程中道德标准的形成而言，某事是至关重要的。此题解题的关键在于下面的具体论述。下一句话提到：不要一天禁止一件事，而第二天就原谅了，毫无道德基础。这也就说明：在教育孩子的时候，要前后保持一致。四个备选单词中只有 B 项 consistency 表示"一致性，连贯性"，为正确选项。

7. 【答案】C

【解析】通篇在讲述父母应该如何教育孩子。A 项 maternal "母亲的"；B 项 paternal "父亲的"；C 项 parental "父母的"。文章没有提到学校教育该如何进行，因而 D 项与文章无关。

8. 【答案】B

【解析】此题解题的关键也在于下一句话。这句话大意为：榜样比某某更好。下一句提到如果父母不真诚，并不按照他们说教的去做，他们的孩子……。从这句话可以判断题目真正的含义为"身教胜于言教"。B 项 precept 为"规则"，与"言教"近义，是正确选项。D 项 revile 为"辱骂，斥责"。

9. 【答案】C

【解析】前句中提到父母要注意"身教胜于言教"。如果父母不这样去做，说一套做一套，孩子就会……。从字里行间可以推断孩子可能会不知所措，很困惑。A 项 timid "胆小的，怯懦的"；B 项 naughty "淘气的"；C 项 confused "困惑不解的"；D 项 disappointed "失望的"。故答案为 C。

10. 【答案】A

【解析】此题解题的关键在于后面的单词 morals（道德标准），空白处需要一个与之近义的单词。principle 含义为"原则"；principal 为名词时，含义为"校长"，为形容词时，含义为"主要的"；morale 含义为"士气"；instruction 含义为"指示，指导"。A 项与 morals 近义。

Practice Eleven

With 950 million people, India ranks second to China among the most populous countries. But since China __1__ a family planning program in 1971, India has been __2__ the gap. Indians have reduced their birth rate but not nearly as much as the Chinese have. If current growth rates continue, India's population will __3__ China's around the year 2028 at about 1.7 billion. Should that happen, it won't be the __4__ of the enlightened women of Kerala, a state in southern India. __5__ India as a whole adds almost 20 million people a year, Kerala's population is virtually stable. The reason is no mystery: nearly two-thirds of Kerala women practice birth control, compared with about 40% in the entire nation.

The difference __6__ the emphasis put on health programs, including birth control, by the state authorities, which in 1957 became India's first elected Communist government. And an educational tradition and matrilineal（母系的）customs in parts of Kerala help girls and boys get equally good schooling. While one in three Indian women is __7__, 90% of those in Kerala can read and write.

Higher literacy rates __8__ family planning. "Unlike our Parents, we know that we can do more for our children if we have fewer of them," says Laila Cherian, 33, who lives in the Village of Kudamaloor. She has limited herself to three children — one below the national __9__ of four. That kind of restraint will keep Kerala from putting added __10__ on world food supplies.

1. A. discovered   B. circulated   C. launched   D. transmitted
2. A. closing   B. widening   C. getting   D. bridging
3. A. shake   B. pass   C. rocket   D. impress
4. A. force   B. fight   C. false   D. fault
5. A. As   B. When   C. While   D. Since
6. A. lies in   B. shows off   C. results in   D. departs from
7. A. cultural   B. literate   C. native   D. responsible
8. A. foster   B. hamper   C. reform   D. advocate
9. A. statistics   B. average   C. tendency   D. category
10. A. increase   B. challenge   C. pressure   D. complaint

短文概要

本文讲述了印度人口增长的状况，以及通过印度的一个城市人口控制的成功说明计划生育的实施与受教育程度的关系。

答案及解析

1. 【答案】C

   【解析】文章首句提到世界上人口最众多国家中，印度人口9.5亿，仅次于中国。rank second to 含义为"排名在……之后"。family planning "计划生育"。A 项 discover "发现"；B 项 circulate "使流通，使运行"；C 项 launch "（计划等）发动，发起"；D 项 transmit "传输，传播"。

2. 【答案】A

   【解析】由于中国在 1971 年实行了计划生育，因而印度缩小了差距。（由于实行计划生育，中国人口数下降或增长缓慢，而印度人口发展趋势不减，所以两国之间的差距在缩小。）正确答案为 A，相当于 narrow；B 项 widen 含义为"扩大"；D 项 bridge 作为动词，表示"弥补差距"或"消除隔阂"。

3. 【答案】B

   【解析】此句话上下文的含义为：印度的出生率已经下降，但下降速率不及中国。如果现有的增长继续，到了 2028 年印度人口将会超过中国，达到 17 亿。根据上下文含义推测，只有 B 符合句意，表示"超过"。C 项 rocket "飞速上升"；D 项 impress "给……留下印象"。

4. 【答案】D

   【解析】此句为省略 if 的虚拟条件句。"如果这一切真的发生，这不是位于印度南部的 Kerala 这个地区开明女性的错误。"此空白处需要一个名词表示"错误"，因而选项 D 为正确答案。

5. 【答案】C

   【解析】此句含义：印度每年整体人口增长大约为 2000 万，Kerala 地区人口增长很稳定。此句话的逻辑关系为对比，因而选项 C 为正确选项。as a whole "总体上"，stable "稳定的"。

6. 【答案】A

   【解析】此句含义：这一差异在于对医疗项目的重视，包括对计划生育的重视。lie in 表示"（问题、差异）在于……"，例如：The key to teaching lies in patience. 教学的关键在于耐心。B 项 show off "卖弄，炫耀"；C 项 result in "导致"；D 项 depart from "离开"。

7. 【答案】B

   【解析】while 表示对比，此句含义：三分之一的印度妇女能够……，在 Kerala 地区的 90% 妇女可以读写。数量上的对比，因而空白处应该是 read and write 的近义词。B 项 literate 的含义为"有文化的，能读写的"，为正确选项。并且，在下面一句话也再次出现正确答案，literacy 为 literate 的名词，意为"读写能力，识字"。

8. 【答案】A

   【解析】解此题的关键在于后面的具体论述。根据对具体论述的理解可知，Kerala 地区人口增长平稳的原因就在于这个地区的妇女文化水平较高。因而此题的大概含义就是高文化水平推动了计划生育。A 项 foster "培养，鼓励"；B 项

hamper "妨碍，牵制"；C 项 reform "改革"；D 项 advocate "鼓吹"。与句意最接近的选项为 A。

9. 【答案】B

【解析】举例说明这个地区人口平稳的原因。Laila 这个妇女由于有文化，因而认识到如果孩子少一些的话她可以为孩子做更多的事情。因而她只有 3 个孩子，这要比印度平均数低。所以答案为 average。

10. 【答案】C

【解析】此句含义：这样的抑制（人口控制）使得该地区远离日益严重的全球粮食供应压力。故答案为 C。

Practice Twelve

Reading involves looking at graphic symbols and formulating mentally the sounds and ideas they represent. Concepts of reading have changed ___1___ over the centuries. During the 1950's and 1960's especially, increased attention has been devoted to defining and describing the reading process. Although specialists agree that reading involves a complex organization of higher mental functions, they disagree on the exact nature of the process. Some experts, who regard language primarily as a code using symbols to represent sounds, view reading as simply the decoding of symbols into the sounds they stand ___2___ .

These authorities ___3___ that meaning, being concerned with thinking, must be taught independently of the decoding process. Others maintain that reading is ___4___ related to thinking, and that a child who pronounces sounds without ___5___ their meaning is not truly reading. The reader, according to some, is not just a person with a theoretical ability to read but one who actually reads.

Many adults, although they have the ability to read, have never read a book in its entirety. By some expert they would not be ___6___ as readers. Clearly, the philosophy, objectives, methods and materials of reading will depend on the definition one use. By the most ___7___ and satisfactory definition, reading is the ability to ___8___ the sound-symbols code of the language, to interpret meaning for various ___9___ , at various rates, and at various levels of difficulty, and to do so widely and enthusiastically. ___10___ reading is the interpretation of ideas through the use of symbols representing sounds and ideas.

1. A. substantively B. substantially C. substitutively D. subjectively
2. A. by B. to C. off D. for
3. A. content B. contend C. contempt D. contact
4. A. inexplicably B. inexpressibly C. inextricably D. inexpediently
5. A. interpreting B. saying C. explaining D. reading
6. A. regarded B. granted C. classified D. graded
7. A. inclusive B. inclinable C. conclusive D. complicated
8. A. break up B. elaborate C. define D. unlock

9.   A. purposes   B. degrees   C. stages   D. steps

10. A. By the way   B. In short

      C. So far   D. On the other hand

短文概要

本文讨论阅读的含义。

✝ 答案及解析

1. 【答案】B

【解析】文章首句提出此短文的话题：阅读包括看图解符号以及明确地叙述它们所呈现的声音和观点。A 项 substantively "实质上"；B 项 substantially "非常，大量"；C 项 substitutively "替代地"；D 项 subjectively "主观地"。此空白处需要一个程度副词修饰动词 change，因而 B 为正确选项。

2. 【答案】D

【解析】A 项 stand by "袖手旁观"，例如：How could you stand by and do nothing for the poor girl? 你怎么能袖手旁观，不为这个可怜的小女孩做点儿什么呢？B 和 C 选项的词组不存在。stand for "代表"，例如：WTO stands for World Trade Organization. WTO 代表世界贸易组织。此句含义：一些专家把语言看作是用符号做代表声音的编码，这些人把阅读简单地看成是把符号解码成它们所代表的声音。

3. 【答案】B

【解析】A 项 content "内容，满意"；B 项 contend "主张"；C 项 contempt "轻蔑"；D 项 contact "接触，联系"。此处的含义为：这些权威们认为……因而 B 项为正确选项。并且下面一句话中，others 与 these authorities 相对应，而 maintain（主张）则与 contend 对应，为答案复现。

4. 【答案】A

【解析】A 项 inexplicably "费解地，无法解释地"；B 项 inexpressibly "不能表达地"；C 项 inextricably "无法分开地"；D 项 inexpediently "不适宜地"。此句含义：另一些专家认为，阅读和思维有着一种无法解释的关系。

5. 【答案】A

【解析】此句含义：（那些专家）还认为一个孩子只发音但没有明白含义，就没有真正地阅读。interpret 的含义为 "用语言解释、说明"。

6. 【答案】C

【解析】此段落首句告诉我们：尽管许多成年人有能力阅读，但他们从没完整地阅读。A 项 be regarded as "被看作是……"。B 项 granted，固定搭配通常为 take sth. for granted "认为……理所应当"；C 项 be classified as "被划分、被界定为……"。D 项 be graded as "划分等级"。此句的含义为：根据某类专家的观点，他们不能界定为阅读者。下一句中的 definition 也给出了此题解题的关键词。

7. 【答案】**C**

【解析】解此题的关键在于 satisfactory，意为"令人满意的"，空白处应该为 satisfactory 的近义词。此句含义为：根据最确实的、最满意的定义，阅读……。A 项 inclusive "包含的，包括的"；B 项 inclinable "倾向于……"；C 项 conclusive "最后的，确实的"；D 项 complicated "复杂的"。

8. 【答案】**D**

【解析】此句为阅读的定义：阅读就是为了解释说明各种目的的含义，解开语言声音符号密码的能力。A 项 break up "破裂，中断"；B 项 elaborate "精心制作，详尽阐述"；C 项 define "下定义"；D 项 unlock "解开"。故 D 项符合句意。

9. 【答案】**A**

【解析】此句含义参看第 8 题，为了各种目的。正确选项为 A。

10. 【答案】**B**

【解析】根据此句话可以推断出这句话为总结性的语句。A 项 by the way "顺便说一下"；B 项 in short "简而言之"；C 项 so far "迄今为止"；D 项 on the other hand "另一方面"。只有 B 项为总结性的短语。

Practice Thirteen

Culture shock might be called a(n) __1__ disease of people who have been suddenly transplanted abroad. Like most ailments, it has its own symptoms cure.

Culture shock is precipitated by the anxiety that results from losing all our familiar signs and __2__ of social intercourse. Those signs or cues include the thousand and one ways in which we __3__ ourselves to the situation of daily life: when to shake hands and what to say when we meet people, when and how to give tips, how to __4__ purchases, when to accept and when to refuse invitations, when to take statements seriously and when not. These cues, which may be words, gestures, facial expressions, customs, or norms, are __5__ by all of us in the course of growing up and are as much a part of our culture as the language we speak or the beliefs we accept. All of us depend on our peace of mind and our efficiency on hundreds of these cues, most of which we do not carry on the level of conscious awareness.

Now when an individual enters a strange culture, all or most of these familiar cues are __6__ . He or she is like a fish out of water. No matter how broad-minded or full of goodwill you may be, a series of props have been knocked from under you, followed by feeling of frustration and __7__ . People react to the frustration in much the same way. First they __8__ the environment which causes the discomfort. "The ways of the __9__ country are bad because they make us feel bad." When foreigners in a strange land get together to __10__ about the host country and its people, you can be sure they are suffering from culture shock.

1. A. acute 　　　　 B. chronic 　　　　 C. infectious 　　　　 D. occupational
2. A. symbols 　　　 B. signals 　　　　 C. indications 　　　　 D. clues

3.   A. familiarize   B. orient   C. convert   D. contribute

4.   A. do   B. accomplish   C. complete   D. make

5.   A. required   B. inquired   C. acquired   D. acknowledged

6.   A. adjusted   B. modified   C. rejected   D. removed

7.   A. nervousness   B. anxiety   C. excitement   D. grief

8.   A. remove   B. refuse   C. reject   D. leave

9.   A. guest   B. target   C. host   D. master

10. A. grouse   B. be appraised   C. comment   D. be unsatisfied

短文概要

本文简述文化冲击的成因以及表现。

✝ 答案及解析

1. 【答案】D

   【解析】空白处需要一个形容词修饰 disease（疾病）。A 项 acute disease "急性病"；B 项 chronic disease "慢性病"；C 项 infectious disease "传染性疾病"；D 项 occupational "职业病"。正确选项由后面的定语从句界定：文化冲突可以称作是一种职业病，突然移居国外的人常患此病。根据句意，正确选项为 D。

2. 【答案】A

   【解析】解此题的关键在于前面的单词 signs，空白处应该为这个单词的近义词。symbol "符号，标志"；signal "信号"；indication "指示"；clue "线索"。此句含义：文化冲突是由于在社会交往中，我们所有熟悉的标志和符号的消失引起的。

3. 【答案】B

   【解析】此题解题的关键在于后面的介词搭配 to。A 项 familiarize oneself / sb. with sth. "使熟悉，了解"，例如：I need time to familiarize yourself with our office procedures. 我需要时间熟悉办公程序。B 项 orient sb. to / towards to sth. "使适应，确定方向"，例如：New students should orient themselves to everything in the new school soon. 新生应该尽快适应新学校的一切。C 项 convert sth. (from sth.) into sth. "使转变"，例如：The hotel is going to be converted into a nursing home. 这家旅馆将要变成一所养老院。D 项 contribute to "为……做贡献"。此句含义：那些符号包括一千零一种使我们适应日常生活各种状况的方式。根据句意，正确选项为 B。

4. 【答案】D

   【解析】此题考点为固定搭配，含义为 "买东西"，只有 D 项 make 可以与 purchases 搭配。

5. 【答案】C

   【解析】此题考点为形近词辨析。require "要求"；inquire "询问"；acquire "获得"；

acknowledge "承认"。此句含义：这些暗示，也许是文字、手势、面部表情、习俗或者规则，都是在成长的过程中获得的。C 项 acquire 吻合句意。in the course of "在……过程中"。

6. 【答案】D

　　【解析】此题解题需要了解本句和下一句的含义。"当一个人进入到一个陌生的文化中，所有或者大多数熟悉的暗示都不见了。他或她就像是离开水的鱼。" A 项 adjust "调整"；B 项 modify "更改"；C 项 reject "拒绝，抛弃"；D 项 remove "移动，消除"。D 项符合句意。

7. 【答案】B

　　【解析】此题解题的关键在于 frustration（沮丧），空白处应该为这个词的近义词。原文大意是：无论心胸多么宽阔，多么善意，你都可能遇到一系列的问题，随之而来的就是沮丧和不安。

8. 【答案】C

　　【解析】根据原文大意，首先人们会排斥让他们感到不适的环境。因而空白处的含义为"拒绝接受，排斥"。只有 C 项符合此意。

9. 【答案】C

　　【解析】此题为答案复现，在最后一句话中出现了答案 host。这里 host country 的含义为"东道国"。

10. 【答案】A

　　【解析】此题解题的关键在于"动词 + 介词搭配"，grouse about "埋怨，发牢骚"；appraise "评价，评估"；comment 与介词 on 或者 upon 连用，含义为"表达意见"；unsatisfied 为形容词，固定搭配为 be unsatisfied with，意为"对……不满意"。

Practice Fourteen

One aspect of American culture is a great belief in independence and __1__. Children are encouraged to be independent. Many children are given __2__ Americans call a "weekly allowance" and are __3__ to have part-time jobs at young age: for boys, newspaper routes, and for girls, baby-sitting. Parents often encourage their children to open bank accounts, and some high school and college students have their own credit cards.

Although American families stress independence, America is also a youth-oriented nation, and a great deal of public attention is paid to children. In many American families, husband and wife will __4__ up their own plans to go to a vacation __5__ in order to please their children by choosing amusement parks like Disney World and Disneyland. The toy industry in America is large and __6__ rapidly. Americans buy expensive toys for their children. For an American family, Christmas, Easter, and a child's birthday are __7__ events. All of these holidays __8__ on the children. Many American couples form friendships based upon their children's friendships. For instance, two couples often become friends because their children are friends. Television shows on Saturday morning are __9__ to children, and a lot of advertising is aimed __10__ children.

1. A. self-respect   B. self-defence   C. self-discipline   D. self-reliance
2. A. what   B. which   C. that   D. when
3. A. forced   B. inspired   C. considered   D. forbidden
4. A. keep   B. turn   C. give   D. put
5. A. spot   B. district   C. zone   D. park
6. A. enlarging   B. increasing   C. growing   D. enhancing
7. A. major   B. critical   C. familiar   D. domestic
8. A. depend   B. fall   C. concentrate   D. center
9. A. turned   B. devoted   C. adapted   D. adjusted
10. A. to   B. for   C. at   D. on

短文概要

本文讲述美国文化中的独立特性以及父母对孩子的重视。

答案及解析

1. 【答案】D
    【解析】此题解题的关键在于 independence 的近义词。self-respect "自尊"；self-defence "自我防卫"；self-discipline "自律"；self-reliance "依靠自己"。

2. 【答案】A
    【解析】此题考点为语法知识中的名词从句。从句中缺少宾语因而正确选项为 A。weekly allowance 指的是 "零花钱"。

3. 【答案】B
    【解析】根据上文含义，美国父母希望自己的孩子独立。因而这里应该是父母鼓励孩子在小时候就做兼职。与 "鼓励" 近义的选项为 inspire，意为 "激励，鼓励"。

4. 【答案】C
    【解析】此段首句告诉我们美国家庭重视独立，但是美国同时也是一个关注孩子的国家。因而此句话应该是父母为了取悦孩子放弃自己的度假计划，答案为 give up，意为 "放弃"。keep up "跟上，保持"；turn up "出现"；put up "表现，推荐，提升"。

5. 【答案】A
    【解析】此题为固定搭配，vacation spot "旅游胜地"。

6. 【答案】C
    【解析】此句含义：由于美国家庭十分重视孩子，因而美国的玩具业也很庞大，发展迅速。只有 C 项表示 "发展"。enlarge "扩大"；enhance "提高，增强"。

7. 【答案】A
    【解析】此句含义：对于美国家庭来说，圣诞节、复活节和孩子的生日都是重大活动。

critical "关键的"；domestic "国内的"。

8. 【答案】D

   【解析】depend on "依靠，依赖"；concentrate on "集中于"；center on "以……为中心"。

9. 【答案】B

   【解析】此句含义：电视节目和大量广告都以孩子为目标。turn to "转向"；be devoted to "致力于"；adapt to "使适合于"；adjust to "调整以适合于"。

10. 【答案】C

   【解析】aim at 表示 "以……为目标"，是固定搭配。

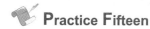 ## Practice Fifteen

In the last fifty years, modern medical research has made a number of important __1__ in heart surgery. For example, in 1954, Henry Swan, an American, established cryosurgery — surgery in which the tissue to be cut up is frozen — as a standard procedure. In that landmark operation, Swan __2__ the patient's body temperature and slowed down the patient's circulation. This __3__ the surgeon to perform the operation in a dry area. This technique was successful ever since.

Another major advance was the development of open heart surgery. C. Walter Lillehie first accomplished this in 1954. Although open heart surgery is still a __4__ operation, recently surgeons perform it __5__ greater and greater success. A discovery that __6__ to the success of heart surgery was the use in 1963 of an artificial heart to circulate blood during the operation. This gave the patient greater safety and the doctor, Michael De Baker, more working time. Perhaps the most famous and most promising action in heart surgery was made in 1967 by Christian Barnard, a South African. He attempted to __7__ healthy human heart into a person who had a __8__ heart. Although the patient only lived for a short while after the operation, Barnard continued his transplants in other patients __9__ he hoped to perfect the transplanting operation. We all hope that this important advance in heart surgery can be __10__ in the future.

1. A. moves   B. changes   C. advances   D. programs
2. A. maintained   B. leveled   C. measured   D. lowered
3. A. encouraged   B. acquired   C. required   D. urged
4. A. fatal   B. dangerous   C. rare   D. pilot
5. A. with   B. by   C. for   D. in
6. A. contributed   B. attributed   C. distributed   D. committed
7. A. transmit   B. employ   C. transform   D. transplant
8. A. faulty   B. defective   C. weak   D. fragile
9. A. although   B. even if   C. because   D. when
10. A. fostered   B. perfected   C. promised   D. forwarded

短文概要

本文介绍在心脏手术方面的进展。

答案及解析

1. 【答案】C

【解析】根据下文可知：近50年来，现代医学研究在心脏手术方面取得了许多重要的进步。advance 为"进步"的含义。

2. 【答案】D

【解析】根据前文可知，cryosurgery 是一种在手术中被切开的细胞组织，是冷冻的。因而此题部分的含义就是病人的体温要降下来，使病人的血液循环缓慢。所以 lower 正确。

3. 【答案】C

【解析】此句含义为：这就要求外科医生要在比较干燥的环境下进行手术。require "要求做……"。

4. 【答案】B

【解析】本句前文提到另一个开心脏手术的进步。根据此句话中的 although 所提示的逻辑关系，再加上后面的 success，因而可以判断这样的手术风险大。A 项 fatal "致命的，致死的"；B 项 dangerous "危险的"。

5. 【答案】A

【解析】此题为介词搭配。with success 相当于 successfully。

6. 【答案】A

【解析】此题考点为固定搭配，contribute to 含义为"贡献于"，此句含义为：促成心脏手术的发现是 1963 年在手术中使用人造心脏形成血液循环。

7. 【答案】D

【解析】根据上下文可以推断，这个医生试图将一个健康人的心脏移植到有心脏病的病人身上。符合这一含义的只有 D 项 transplant "移植（器官）"。并且在下文出现答案选项，属于答案复现。

8. 【答案】B

【解析】根据第 7 题得知空白处应该为有心脏病缺陷的病人。A 项 faulty "有错误的"；B 项 defective "有缺陷的，有毛病的"；C 项 weak "虚弱的"；D 项 fragile "易碎的，脆弱的"。故答案为 B。

9. 【答案】C

【解析】此题测试考生对原文语句逻辑关系的理解。"尽管那个进行心脏移植手术的病人术后只存活了一小会儿，但这个医生继续在其他病人身上进行移植，因为他希望能完善移植手术。"空白处应该为因果关系，故 C 为正确答案。

10. 【答案】B

【解析】第 9 题提到这个医生的不懈努力，因而在这句话中"我们也希望心脏手术这一重大进步能在今后更加完善"。B 符合句意。

Practice Sixteen

American and Chinese cultures are __1__ in some ways. An American hostess, __2__ for her culinary（烹饪）skill, is likely to say, "Oh, I'm so glad you liked it. I cooked it especially for you." Not so a Chinese hostess, who will instead __3__ for giving you nothing even slightly __4__ and for not showing you enough honor __5__ providing proper dishes.

The same rules hold true __6__ children. American parents speak proudly of their children's achievements, telling how Johnny made the school team or Jane made the honor roll. Not so Chinese parents, whose children, even if at the top of their class in school, are always so "naughty", never studying, never listening to their elders, and so forth.

The Chinese take pride in "modesty"; Americans __7__ "straightforwardness". This modesty has left many a Chinese hungry at an American table, for Chinese __8__ __9__ three refusals before one accepts an offer, and American hosts take a "no" to mean "no", whether it's the first, second, or third time.

Recently, a member of a delegation sent to China by a large American corporation complained to me about how the Chinese had asked them three times if they would be willing to change some proposal, and each time the Americans had said "no" clearly and __10__. My friend was angry that the Chinese had not taken his word the first time. I recognized the problem immediately and wondered why the Americans had not studied up on cultural difference before coming to China. It would have saved everyone a lot of perplexity and needless frustration in their negotiations.

1. A. similar   B. familiar   C. opposite   D. adverse
2. A. complimented   B. compiled   C. complemented   D. commented
3. A. praise   B. apologize   C. be disappointed D. be satisfied
4. A. eligible   B. illegible   C. suitable   D. edible
5. A. for   B. on   C. by   D. in
6. A. regard for   B. with regard to C. regardless of   D. regard as
7. A. in   B. of   C. for   D. on
8. A. frankness   B. cautions   C. uprightness   D. politeness
9. A. calls on   B. calls for   C. calls up   D. calls in
10. A. ambiguously   B. roughly   C. definitely   D. arbitrarily

短文概要

本文介绍中美两国餐桌文化的差异。

答案及解析

1. 【答案】C

【解析】根据下文美国文化和中国文化的对比，可以得知文章首句的含义为"两国文化在某种程度上完全相反"。这样可以排除 A 项 similar 和 B 项 familiar。D 项 adverse "敌对的，对立的"。

2. 【答案】A

【解析】根据后面美国女主人的回答，可以知道此空白处的含义为"称赞"。compliment "称赞"；compile "编纂"；complement "补充"；comment "评价"。故答案为 A。

3. 【答案】B

【解析】此句话一开头就知道中国女主人不是这样的。根据对中国文化的背景知识再加上对此句句意的理解，此题应该为 B。此句含义为：中国女主人会因没有为客人准备什么而道歉。

4. 【答案】D

【解析】此句含义上接第 3 题，指的是没什么可吃的。A 项 eligible "符合条件的"；B 项 illegible "字迹模糊的，难以辨认的"；C 项 suitable "适合的"；D 项 edible "可以食用的"。

5. 【答案】C

【解析】此句含义为：通过……方式表达对客人的尊敬。因而使用介词 by。

6. 【答案】B

【解析】此题考点为形近词词组辨析。A 项 regard for 表示"对……的尊敬"，例如：He had a high regard for the professor. 他非常敬重这位教授。B 项 with regard to "关于，至于"。C 项 regardless of "不管，不论"；D 项 regard...as "把……看作是……"。符合句意的只有 B。

7. 【答案】A

【解析】此题解题的关键在于前面的词组 take pride in "为……感到自豪"。分号连接两个并列成分，因而此空白处相当于省略了 take pride，介词应该为 in。

8. 【答案】D

【解析】此题与前面中国人对自己的 modesty（谦虚）感到自豪有关，因而此处应该为 politeness，意思是：中国人这种谦虚使得中国人在饭桌上会挨饿，因为他们的礼貌客气使他们在接受一次食物之前要拒绝三次。A 项 frankness"坦率"；B 项 caution "谨小慎微"；C 项 uprightness "正直"；D 项 politeness "礼貌客气"，可知 D 与文中语境相吻合。

9. 【答案】B

【解析】此题为形近词组辨析。call on "号召，呼吁"；call for "需要"；call up "使想起"；call in "召集"。句意参看第 8 题。

10. 【答案】C

【解析】此空白处需要一个与 clearly 意思相近的副词。A 项 ambiguously "模棱两可地"；B 项 roughly "大概地"；C 项 definitely "明确地，一定"；D 项 arbitrarily "武断地"。

Practice Seventeen

Planning is a very important activity in our lives yet really sophisticated. It can give pleasure, even excitement, __1__ cause quite severe headaches. The more significant the task __2__ is, the more careful the planning requires. Getting to school or to work on time is a task requiring little or no planning, and it is almost a __3__. A month's touring holiday abroad, or better __4__, getting married, it would be a different matter altogether. If the holiday involves a church wedding, with fifty guests, a reception, a honeymoon in Venice, and __5__ to a new home, this requires even more planning to make sure that it is successful. Planning is our way of trying to ensure success and __6__ avoiding costly failures we cannot afford. It is equally essential and fundamental to mankind as a whole, to individual nations, to families and single people; the __7__ may vary, but the degree of importance does not. In essence, a nation planning its resources and needs does not differ from the familiar weekly shopping or monthly household budget. __8__ are designed to ensure an adequate supply of essentials, at a rate of spending within the limits of __9__, and if properly carried out, will __10__ shortages, wastage and over-expenditure.

1. A. on the end   B. or   C. least   D. more or less
2. A. arrangement   B. aside   C. ahead   D. above
3. A. assignment   B. burden   C. endeavor   D. routine
4. A. more   B. otherwise   C. still   D. moreover
5. A. attending   B. gripping   C. returning   D. staying
6. A. of   B. for   C. with   D. between
7. A. scale   B. scope   C. extent   D. range
8. A. Some   B. All   C. Both   D. Many
9. A. production   B. wage   C. income   D. property
10. A. avoid   B. keep   C. solve   D. cause

短文概要

规划的定义和重要性。

答案及解析

1. 【答案】B
   【解析】本题考查句子结构。or 表示选择。这里前后两个单词 excitement 和 headache 的意思是相反的，表示选择的话只能用 or。on the end 没有这种搭配，least "最小的，最少的"，more or less "或多或少"，放在文中语义不对。

2. 【答案】C
   【解析】本题考查句意和形容词。ahead "在前面，前面的"。该句的意思是：要使将来的任务有意义，就需要用更多的心思来做规划。

3. 【答案】D
   【解析】本题考查句意和形容词。routine "日常工作，日常的事情"。该句的意思是：去上学或者工作不需要做什么规划，这几乎是我们每天都做的事情。assignment "分配，安排"，burden "负担"，endeavor "努力"。

4. 【答案】C
   【解析】本题考查逻辑关系。该句的意思是"如果你幸运的话，你就会在国外度过一个月的假期，或者更好的，你结婚了"。more "更加"，只能放在被修辞词的前面。otherwise "否则"，moreover "甚至，并且"。

5. 【答案】C
   【解析】本题考查句意和动词。return "返回"，后面用 to 加上地方，表示"回到某地"，这里指"回到家"。attend "出席"，grip "紧握"，stay "停留"。

6. 【答案】A
   【解析】本题考查并列结构。and 前后的成分要一致，前面用的 of 词组，and 后也应用 of，做 our way of 的并列成分。

7. 【答案】A
   【解析】本题考查句意和名词辨析。scale "规模"，scope "范围，眼界"，extent "程度，长度"，range "幅度"。这里的意思是：尽管规模不同，但是重要性的程度却是一样的。

8. 【答案】C
   【解析】本题考查不定代词。both "两者都"，这里指代国家预算和家庭预算。

9. 【答案】C
   【解析】本题考查名词辨析。income "收入"，这里指的一个家庭所有的收入来源，范围比其他三个词广。意思是：以收入限制范围内的速度花钱。production "生产"，wage "工资"，property "财产"（包括不动产）。一个家庭的花销一般是根据收入情况来决定的。

10. 【答案】A
    【解析】本题考查句意和动词。avoid "避免"。该句的意思是：如果计划实施顺利，将会避免资金不足、浪费，以及过度消费的情况。

Practice Eighteen

Visual impairment carries with __1__ ability to travel through one's physical and social environment until adequate orientation and mobility skills have been established. Because observational skills are more limited, self-control within the immediate surroundings is limited. The visually impaired person is less able to anticipate __2__ situations or obstacles to avoid.

Orientation refers to the __3__ map one has of one's surroundings and to the relationship between self and that environment. It is best generated by moving through the environment and __4__ together relationships, object by object, in an organized approach. With __5__ visual feedback to reinforce this map, a visually impaired person must rely on memory for key landmarks and other clues, which enable visually impaired persons to __6__ their position in Space.

Mobility is the ability to travel safely and efficiently from one point to another within one's physical and social environment. Good orientation skills are necessary to good mobility skills. Once visually impaired students learn to travel safely as pedestrians（行人）they also need to learn to use public transportation to become as __7__ as possible.

To meet the __8__ demands of the visually impaired person, there is a sequence of instruction that begins during the preschool years and may continue after high school. Many visually impaired children lack adequate concepts regarding time and space or objects and events in their environment. During the early years much attention is focused on the development of some fundamental __9__, such as inside or outside, in front of or behind, fast or slow, which are essential to safe, __10__ travel through familiar and unfamiliar settings.

1. A. complex   B. vital   C. restricted   D. remarkable
2. A. varying   B. difficult   C. hazardous   D. distressful
3. A. mental   B. visual   C. graphic   D. demographic
4. A. putting   B. getting   C. reinforcing   D. piecing
5. A. few   B. little   C. much   D. inadequate
6. A. testify   B. affirm   C. identify   D. certify
7. A. flexible   B. independent   C. frequent   D. skillful
8. A. expanding   B. extending   C. continual   D. desperate
9. A. behaviors   B. concepts   C. awareness   D. memory
10. A. comfortable   B. effective   C. efficient   D. efficacious

短文概要

本文介绍了视觉障碍的两个关键因素——定位和移动，以及如何帮助视觉障碍的人群。

答案及解析

1. 【答案】C
    【解析】此题考点为上下文。第 1 句话是视觉障碍的定义，故应该是能力不足或有限，选项 C 正确。
2. 【答案】C
    【解析】此题考点为上下文。此题解题关键可以参考 or 所连接的并列名词 obstacle。这句话的含义是：因为有视觉障碍的人的观察技能比较有限，所以他们在所处环境中的自控能力有限，因此不能预先估计危险状况或者应该避免的障碍。
3. 【答案】A
    【解析】此题考点是上下文。本段讲述定位，并且第 1 句话即为定义。根据本段的细节信息可知视觉障碍的人无法形成视觉图像，故只能依靠移动过程中对于所触及的物体或者地标进行记忆，形成大脑中的图像以保证确定自己的方位。故选项 A 最符合本段含义。graphic 的含义是"图表的"；demographic 的含义是"人口统计学的"。

4. 【答案】D

   【解析】此题考点为上下文。在移动中，把物体之间的关系按照有序的方式结合起来，这样形成最好的心理地图。piece 作为动词其含义是"把碎片结合起来"，故为正确答案。

5. 【答案】B

   【解析】此题考点为上下文。视觉障碍的人应该是没有视觉反馈的，因而选项 B 符合句意。本句含义为：作为视觉障碍的人，他们不能对物体产生视觉反馈以加强心理地图，因而他们要靠记忆重要地标或线索来确定他们的方位。

6. 【答案】B

   【解析】此题考点为上下文，且需要形近词辨析。A 项 testify "证明，作证"；B 项 affirm "确定，断定"；C 项 identify "识别，鉴定"；D 项 certify "保证"。此处含义应该是"通过记忆中的主要地标或者线索确定自己在空间中的位置"，故选项 B 符合句意。

7. 【答案】B

   【解析】此题考点为上下文。这个段落介绍移动能力的定义以及对于视觉障碍的人来说移动能力的重要性。段落最后提到"视觉障碍的人既要学会安全行走又要学会使用公共交通，这样做的目的应该是使得他们能够在社会上独立"，故选项 B 符合语义。句意：一旦视觉障碍的学生学会如何作为行人在路上安全行走，他们也需要学会使用公共交通，以便能够尽可能地独立。

8. 【答案】A

   【解析】此题考点为固定搭配。A 项 expanding "扩展的，扩充的"；B 项 extending "伸展的"；C 项 continual "不断的"；D 项 desperate "绝望的，不顾一切的"。根据句意可知应该是满足视觉障碍人更多的需求，所以选项 A 符合句意。

9. 【答案】B

   【解析】此题考点为原词再现。上一句提到：许多视觉障碍的孩子缺乏对时间、空间、物体或者环境中事件的概念。所以下一句提到在他们早期培训中，重点要集中在他们一些基本概念的建立上。根据这一逻辑关系，选项 B 为答案。

10. 【答案】C

    【解析】此题考点为上下文。B 项"有效的"，尤指能看得到效果和成效的；D 项 efficacious 的含义是"灵验的，有效的"。最后一句提到这些基本的概念是他们在熟悉或不熟悉环境中安全行走的基础。除了"安全的"以外，符合句意的形容词只有 C。

Practice Nineteen

Man is the only animal that laughs. Why is this true? What makes us respond as we do to pleasurable experiences? What is the history of this "happy ___1___ ", as someone once termed it, and just what is its function?

We are not short of theories to explain the mystery; for centuries, biologists, philosophers, psychologists, and medical men have sought a definitive explanation of laughter. One writer ___2___ that its function is to ___3___ others or to prove to be better than them by insulting them. Another took the opposite view: that we laugh in order not to cry. A psychologist offered the explanation that laughter functions as a(n) ___4___ for painful experiences, and that it serves to defend a person against what the psychologist termed "the many minor pains to which man is ___5___ ". In the 17th century a writer set forth the theory that we laugh when we compare ourselves with others and find ourselves superior; ___6___ , we laugh at the weakness of others.

Virtually every theory has been concerned with either the structure or the function of laughter, whereas relatively few have been devoted to the question of its ___7___ . I propose to offer a theory which, so far as I am aware, has not previously been set forth: that only those animals capable of ___8___ are capable of laughter; and that therefore man, being the only animal that speaks, is the only animal that laughs.

Those of us who have observed chimpanzees closely feel quite confident that the chimpanzee occasionally exhibits behavior that looks very much like a primitive human laughter. This behavior, however, has been observed only in a human context; ___9___ it occurs under natural conditions is dubious; but ___10___ that under any conditions an ape is capable of such behavior is of more than passing interest—for does it not indicate that early man had the basics of laughter?

1. A. conviction   B. condition   C. convulsion   D. contraction
2. A. theorized   B. projected   C. asserted   D. hypothesized
3. A. evaluate   B. stimulate   C. imitate   D. intimidate
4. A. remedy   B. medication   C. anesthetics   D. placebo
5. A. accustomed   B. exposed   C. addicted   D. attached
6. A. instead   B. however   C. in effect   D. for instance
7. A. mechanism   B. rationale   C. source   D. origin
8. A. speech   B. judging   C. thoughts   D. communication
9. A. no matter if   B. whenever   C. however   D. whether or not
10. A. a fact   B. the very fact   C. an interesting fact   D. the exact fact

短文概要

人类是唯一能笑的物种，文中对其做出了理论解释。

答案及解析

1. 【答案】C
    【解析】考查形近词辨析。本段首句主要是说的 laugh，可知空格处也讲的是快乐的笑的历史作用。C. convulsion（大笑，痉挛）与"laugh"义同，为正确答案。A. conviction（确信，信心），B. condition（状态）和 D. contraction（收缩）为干扰项，与"laugh"的意思不符，置入空格后不能体现"笑"的面部特征。故选 C。

2. 【答案】A

【解析】考查对上下文的理解。本段句首指出，解释这一神秘现象的理论并不少见；几百年来，生物学家、哲学家、心理学家和医护工作者一直在为"笑"寻求一个明确的解释。因此可以推测，后面的句子应该是对各种"笑"的理论的客观介绍。空格所在的句子是对其中一种理论的介绍。A. theorized（创建理论）表明短文在介绍一种理论，与本段句首的 theories 相对应，是正确答案。由本段首句definitive一词可以推测，各方对自己理论的合理性都相当有把握，因而B. projected（预测）和 D. hypothesized（假设）不合题意。C. asserted（断言）有主观色彩，与作者客观描述各种理论的语气不符。故选 A。

3. 【答案】D

【解析】D。考查对上下文的理解和形近词辨析。本题空格所在的 that 从句意思是："笑的作用是_____他人或通过羞辱他人证明自己比他人优秀"。从句中 or 表并列，前后表达的意思应该大致相近，因而，一旦"自己比他人优秀"，最有可能的表现就是威胁他人，故 D. intimidate（恐吓，威胁）为正确答案。A. evaluate（评价）和 B. stimulate（刺激）不合题意，C. imitate（模仿）为干扰项，亦不属于"笑"的作用。故选 D。

4. 【答案】A

【解析】A。考查近义词辨析。本题空格所在的句子中有两个 that 从句，且由 and 连接，因而两个从句意思相近。第二个 that 从句提到笑帮助人抵御心理学家所谓的许多微小伤痛。因而本题空格部分应表达类似的意思。A. remedy（治疗，补救）符合语义，在文中表达抽象意义上的疗伤，为正确答案。B. medication（药物，药剂）多指具体的药物疗伤，C. anesthetics（麻醉剂）和 D. placebo（安慰剂）不能体现"笑"的积极防御作用，三者皆不合题意。

5. 【答案】B

【解析】B。考查对上下文的理解。上题已分析了空格所在句子的部分意思。此题需要一个限定 many minor pains 的词，many minor pains 做 is_____to 短语中 to 的宾语。空格所在的句子提到了"笑"对许多微小伤痛的抵御。A. accustomed 意为"习惯的"。如若人们习惯了小伤痛，便不易察觉到小伤痛造成的伤害，亦不会积极抵御。因而 A. accustomed 不正确，与题意不符。另外，人们一般也不会对小伤痛上瘾或喜爱小伤痛，这与常理相违背，故 be addicted to 与 be attached to 不合适；B. exposed 为正确答案。be exposed to 意为"遭受"，符合题意。故选 B。

6. 【答案】C

【解析】C。考查对上下文的理解和衔接词的选择。空格前面的部分提到，"17 世纪的一种理论便是：当我们和他人相比，发现自己优越时，我们会笑"。空格后面的部分意思为"我们嘲笑他人的软弱"。后者提到对别人软弱的嘲讽，隐含了自己的优越，和前者表达的意思一致。因而，C. in effect（事实上）是正确答案；A. instead（相反）和 B. however（然而）表示转折关系，不合逻辑。空格后面部分不是例子，故 D. for instance（例如）不合题意。故选 C。

7. 【答案】D

【解析】D。考查对上下文的理解。本题空格所在的句子意思是："几乎每一种理论都讲到笑的构造和作用，而研究笑的_____问题的研究却相对较少。"因此，空格部分应填的词汇应该与构造和作用无关。A. mechanism（构造，机制）与 structure 意思相近，故不符合题意。短文第 2 段在提到笑的作用的时候，解释了人们为什么笑，故 B. rationale（理由，逻辑依据）不合逻辑。C. source 和 D. origin 均指来源。前者多指起因或资料来源，后者多表起源。文章开始就提到"笑"的历史，后面部分又提到黑猩猩的笑，可知作者是研究笑的起源的。故选 D。

8. 【答案】A

【解析】A。考查对上下文的理解。本题空格所在的分句意思是："只有会_____的动物才会笑。"因此，空格部分应关乎笑的唯一条件。空格所在的分句后面又提到："因此，人作为唯一能说话的动物，是唯一会笑的动物"。此句揭示了笑的条件：能说话。根据前后两句话的因果关系，可以推断 A. speech（说话，言语）是正确答案。B. judging（判断），C. thoughts（思想）和 D. communication（交流）不合逻辑。故选 A。

9. 【答案】D

【解析】D。考查语法结构。本题空格所在的分句中，is 是谓语动词，故空格部分要求一个引导词，引导句子 it occurs under natural conditions，从而使整个从句 it occurs under natural conditions 做 is 的主语。四个选项中，只有 D. whether or not（是否）可以引导主语从句，符合条件。其余三个选项 A. no matter if（无论是否），B. whenever（无论何时）和 C. however（无论多么）通常用来引导让步状语从句，故选 D。

10. 【答案】B

【解析】考查语法结构。本题空格所在的从句是同位语从句，而同位语从句前的先行词（此题中先行词为 fact）多用定冠词修饰，故首先排除 C. an interesting fact。另外，在同位语从句中，如若强调先行词，则要在先行词前加形容词 very，故排除 D. the exact fact。A. the fact 和 B. the very fact 皆符合语法和语义，区别仅在于后者表示强调。从文中可以看出作者十分注重这一事实，将此事实作为探究笑的起源的依据，故选 B。

Practice Twenty

Without exposure to the cultural, intellectual, and moral traditions that are our heritage, we are excluded from a common world that __1__ generations. On the one hand, such exclusion tends to __2__ us to recreate everything, a needless and largely impossible task; on the other hand, it tends to make us __3__, to suggest that we are indeed the creators of the world and of all good ideas— __4__ in fact we are only a fragment of the history of man. __5__ entirely to ourselves, we could make only the slimmest contributions to wisdom.

While the humanities overlap the fine and liberal arts, they are also related of necessity to the science and to technology. Some of the __6__ of the humanities raise questions about what ends are worthy to be __7__, what ideals deserve __8__. But since it is futile to know what is worth doing without having any idea of how to get things done, effective study in the humanities requires respect for and attainment of factual knowledge and technological skill. __9__, it is pointless to know how to get things done without having any idea what is worth doing, so that informed study in applied science demands __10__ in the humanities.

1. A. crosses   B. passes down   C. survives   D. exists
2. A. warn   B. facilitate   C. compel   D. encourage
3. A. arrogant   B. exhausted   C. productive   D. reliable
4. A. since   B. when   C. whereas   D. which
5. A. Provided   B. Left   C. Reserved   D. Kept
6. A. arenas   B. communities   C. subjects   D. disciplines
7. A. followed   B. investigated   C. served   D. abandoned
8. A. identification   B. maintenance   C. reverence   D. endeavor
9. A. Similarly   B. Contrarily   C. Virtually   D. Literally
10. A. concentration   B. presupposition   C. revelation   D. reflection

短文概要

人文学科与应用科学的关系。

答案及解析

1. 【答案】B
   【解析】B。本题考查文意和动词。cross "交叉，横断"，pass down "传承"。survive "生存"，exist "存在"。B符合文意。
2. 【答案】C
   【解析】本题考查文意和动词。warn "警告，提醒"，facilitate "促进，帮助"，compel "强迫，迫使"，encourage "鼓励，怂恿"。C项符合文意。
3. 【答案】A
   【解析】A。本题考查文意和形容词。arrogant "自大的，傲慢的"，exhausted "疲惫的，耗尽的"，productive "能生产的，有生产力的"，reliable "可靠的，可信赖的"。

根据句意，正确答案为 A。

4. 【答案】C

【解析】C。本题考查上下文逻辑关系。空格前后的句子是转折关系。since 表示因果，when 表示时间，whereas 表示转折和对比，which 则表示"哪一个"。故本题正确答案为 C。

5. 【答案】D

【解析】D。本题考查动词的固定搭配。provide for sb. "为……提供"，leave to sb. "留给……，交托……"，reserve "预防，储备"，keep to oneself "不交际，独居"。根据句意，正确答案为 D。

6. 【答案】C

【解析】C。本题考查文意和名词。arenas "竞技场"，communities "社区，团体"，subjects "学科，科目"，disciplines "纪律"。空格前提到 to the science and to technology，这些都属于 subjects。故本题正确答案为 C。

7. 【答案】A

【解析】A。本题考查上下文语义和动词的惯用法。follow "听从，跟随"，investigate "研究，调查"，serve "服务"，abandon "放弃"。根据句意，正确答案为 A。

8. 【答案】B

【解析】B。本题考查文意和名词。identification "鉴定，识别"，maintenance "维护，维修"，reverence "敬畏，尊敬"，endeavor "努力，尽力"。根据文意，正确答案为 B。

9. 【答案】A

【解析】A。空格上句提到的 futile 意思是"无用的，无效的"。空格所在的句子中 pointless "无意义的"，前后语义走向是一致的。similarly "同样地，类似地"，contrarily "相反地，反之"，virtually "事实上，几乎"，literally "逐字地，照字面意义地"。根据题意，正确答案为 A。

10. 【答案】D

【解析】D。本题考查句意和名词。concentration "浓度，集中"，presupposition "假定，预想"，revelation "启示，揭露"，reflection "反射，沉思"。根据题意，正确答案为 D。

Practice Twenty-One

Despite the common belief that high stress can trigger a stroke, a new study finds no evidence that distressing life events __1__ the risk of a particularly deadly type of stroke.

It's common for people to attribute a __2__ medical problem like stroke to stress, noted senior researcher Dr. Craig S. Anderson, of the George Institute of International Health and the University of Sydney in Australia. In the case of subarachnoid hemorrhage（蛛网膜下出血）, he said it is possible for a sudden rise in blood pressure to cause a rupture in an aneurysm — a weakened area in an artery wall. And subarachnoid hemorrhage does sometimes follow a sudden exertion, during exercise or sex, for example.

However, whether life's __3__ experiences are associated with a higher risk of the strokes has been __4__. For their study, Anderson and his colleagues interviewed 388 subarachnoid-hemorrhage __5__ about stressful life events they had experienced in the one-month-and-one-year __6__ the stroke. Overall, the study found, most forms of stressful life events showed no relationship with the risk of subarachnoid hemorrhage.

When it came to events __7__ in the month before the subarachnoid hemorrhage, two types of stressors — financial or legal problems and the catch-all category of "other significant event" — were associated with an increased risk. Ten percent of survivors reported a financial or legal problem over that month, versus 4 percent of the control group.

However, the researchers report, when they __8__ factors like high blood pressure, smoking and drinking, the links between those two __9__ and subarachnoid hemorrhage were only "__10__" significant.

1. A. lower   B. induce   C. eliminate   D. raise
2. A. chronic   B. fatal   C. sudden   D. sticky
3. A. distressing   B. disturbing   C. distasteful   D. disruptive
4. A. definite   B. infinite   C. ambiguous   D. uncertain
5. A. victims   B. survivors   C. sufferers   D. casualties
6. A. exceeding   B. preceding   C. conceding   D. proceeding
7. A. experiencing   B. to be experienced
    C. experienced   D. having experienced
8. A. accounted for B. sought for   C. cleared up   D. showed up
9. A. stressors   B. factors   C. risks   D. components
10. A. greatly   B. marginally   C. less   D. increasingly

短文概要

本文指出高压力或者痛苦的经历对中风的影响不大。

答案及解析

1. 【答案】D
    【解析】此题考点是上下文。根据第 1 段这句话的逻辑关系，可以做出正确判断。本句含义是：尽管普遍认为高压力可以引发中风，但一项新的研究发现，没有证据能够证明痛苦的生活事件会提高致命型中风的危险。

2. 【答案】C
    【解析】此题为原词再现。在本文第 2 段，可以根据线索找到本题答案。句意：人们通常把像中风这种突然性的疾病归因于压力。

3. 【答案】A

   【解析】此题考点为上下文。A 项 distressing "令人苦恼、痛苦的"；B 项 disturbing "令人不安的"；C 项 distasteful "令人反感的"；D 项 disruptive "捣乱的，破坏性的"。根据本段提到的具体信息 stressful life experiences 可知，这里应该是指令人痛苦的含义。

4. 【答案】D

   【解析】此题考点为上下文。根据本句第 1 个词 however 可以得知两者的相关性还不确定。A 项 definite "确定的"；B 项 infinite "无限的"；C 项 ambiguous "模棱两可的"。故选项 D 为答案。

5. 【答案】B

   【解析】此题考点为词语辨析。根据句意得知这位专家和同事访问了 388 名曾经患过蛛网膜下出血的患者，以调查他们发病前所经历的压力生活事件是否和他们的中风有关。这说明他们曾经有过这样的情况,但活下来了,故选项 B 最接近含义。victim 指的是"受害者"。D 项 casualty 的含义是"伤亡者"。

6. 【答案】B

   【解析】此题考点是形近词辨析。A 项 exceeding "超过的"；B 项 preceding "之前的"；C 项 conceding "让步，承认"；D 项 proceeding "进行中的"。句意参考第 5 题。

7. 【答案】C

   【解析】此题考点是语法结构。空白处需要一个形容 events 的定语，表示"经历过的事件"，应该是被动结构，并且是已经发生过的，故选项 C 过去分词 experienced 是正确答案。

8. 【答案】A

   【解析】此题考点是词组含义。A 项 account for "解释，占……比例，查明"；B 项 seek for "寻求"；C 项 clear up "天气放晴，痊愈，清理，解决"；D 项 show up "出现，使人难堪"。这句话的含义：然而，研究者们报告说当他们查明例如高血压、吸烟、喝酒这些因素时……故选项 A 为正确答案。

9. 【答案】A

   【解析】此题考点为原词再现。根据 those two，可以在倒数第 2 段的第 1 句话找到所指代的内容: two types of stressors。故选项 A 正确，指的是"经济和法律问题"。

10. 【答案】B

   【解析】此题考点为上下文。本文主旨是要通过实验揭示生活中的痛苦事件与中风发作关系不大，故选项 B 正确，含义是"微小的"。

Practice Twenty-Two

Vitamins are organic compounds necessary in small amounts in the diet for the normal growth and maintenance of life of animals, including man.

They do not provide energy, __1__ do they construct or build any part of the body. They are needed for __2__ foods into energy and body maintenance. There are thirteen or more of them, and if __3__ is missing a deficiency disease becomes __4__.

Vitamins are similar because they are made of the same elements—usually carbon, hydrogen, oxygen, and __5__ nitrogen. They are different __6__ their elements are arranged differently, and each vitamin __7__ one or more specific functions in the body.

__8__ enough vitamins is essential to life, although the body has no nutritional use for __9__ vitamins. Many people, __10__, believe in being on the "safe side" and thus take extra vitamins. However, a well-balanced diet will usually meet all the body's vitamin needs.

1. A. either   B. so   C. nor   D. never
2. A. shifting   B. transferring   C. altering   D. transforming
3. A. any   B. some   C. anything   D. something
4. A. serious   B. apparent   C. severe   D. fatal
5. A. mostly   B. partially   C. sometimes   D. rarely
6. A. in that   B. so that   C. such that   D. except that
7. A. undertakes   B. holds   C. plays   D. performs
8. A. Supplying   B. Getting   C. Providing   D. Furnishing
9. A. exceptional   B. exceeding   C. excess   D. external
10. A. nevertheless   B. therefore   C. moreover   D. meanwhile

短文概要

维生素的重要性。

答案及解析

1. 【答案】C

【解析】选项必须既能引导倒装句，又能与前面的否定相呼应。either 表示"也"，可以用在否定句中，但一般放在句尾；so 可以引导倒装句，但它用在肯定句中，表示"也"；nor 也可以引导倒装句，并可用在否定句中，构成 not...nor...（既不……也不……）固定结构；never 也可以引导倒装句，表示否定，但它必须放在句首。故选 C。

2. 【答案】D

【解析】由文意可知，空格填入的分词需和 into 搭配，并符合文意。transform 常与 into 搭配，强调的是"事物大的变革或质的改变"。在此从 food（食物）到 energy（能量）的转变是一种质的改变，因此 D 符合句意。shift 不与 into 搭配；transfer 多用于位置的改变，也不与 into 搭配；alter 强调部分或少量的变动，程度较轻。以上三个词都不能表示事物质的改变，故选 D。

3. 【答案】A

【解析】空格所在句子是一个由 and 连接的并列句，前一个分句 There are thirteen or more of them 中的 them 指的是 vitamins，后一个分句是一个由 if 引导的条件状语从句，意为"如果……缺乏，（会出现）维生素缺乏症。"由于 if 引导的从句中谓语动词 is 是单数，因而只能由一个表示单数意义的不定代词作为被选项。首先排除 some，它一般用于肯定句，做主语时谓语动词用复数；其次 anything 与 something 泛指任何事或某些事，放入句中不符合句意；any 放入后相当于 any of them，即"任何维生素"。注意 any 一般用于否定或疑问句中，做主语时，谓语动词常用单数，故选 A。

4.　【答案】B

　　【解析】根据上下文，这里需要填入一个准确描述疾病症状的词。serious、severe 和 fatal 这几个词都表示程度严重，甚至危及生命。但上下文没有暗示缺乏一种维生素会导致严重的后果，因此这三个词都不可作为被选项。apparent 只是简单地描述了疾病的症状，为正确选项，故选 B。

5.　【答案】C

　　【解析】本句破折号后举例说明维生素的组成成分：碳、氢、氧和＿＿＿氮，and 表明各成分之间为并列关系，选项应与 usually 相呼应。usually 是频率副词，选项也应是频率副词。mostly 和 partially 不是频率副词，而是强调事物部分与整体的关系，rarely 是频率副词，但它含否定含义，若用于句中，之前的连词 and 应改为表示转折关系的 but。故选 C。

6.　【答案】A

　　【解析】上句提到维生素相似的原因，这句开始提到维生素也是有区别的，由于两个句子是平行的结构，本句的后半句也会解释为什么不同。因此空格处应填入表示因果关系并连接原因状语从句的短语。except that 不表示因果，so that 和 such that 后面接结果。只有 in that 后面接原因，并且空格前面的 different 与介词 in 连用，表示"在哪一方面不同"。故选 A。

7.　【答案】D

　　【解析】本题考查动词与 function 的搭配。四个选项中能与 function 搭配的只有 perform，即 perform a function（具有……的功能，发挥……的作用），其他选项的常用搭配有：undertake a mission/task/project "承担使命 / 任务 / 工程"；hold a share "持有股份"；play a role/part "扮演……角色"。故选 D。

8.　【答案】B

　　【解析】本题空格所在句子是让步状语从句的复合句，空格部分和 enough vitamins 构成动名词的复合结构做主句的主语。空格处填入的动名词的逻辑主语也就是后面 although 引导的让步状语从句中的主语，即：the body。动名词所表示的动作必须是 the body 发出来的，又能接 enough vitamins 做宾语。选项中，Supplying，Providing 和 Furnishing 均表示"提供，供应"，动作的发出者不是"身体"。句子表达的含义是身体需要获取维生素的营养，而不是"提供"，因此只有 Getting（获取，获得）符合。故选 B。

9.　【答案】C

　　【解析】本题空格所在部分是 although 引导的让步状语从句。have use for 是固定短语，意为"需要"，主要用于否定和疑问句中，因此根据所在从句的含义，判断出人体对什么维生素没有营养上的需要。首先排除 external 和 exceptional，因为不存在"外部的维生素"或"例外的维生素"；exceeding 用来指被修饰的成分超出了一般的限度，它不能直接修饰"维生素"；只有 excess 指"超过正常或所需数额的数量"，强调"摄入过多的维生素"符合逻辑。故选 C。

10. 【答案】A

　　【解析】由题意可知，空格处应填入一个逻辑连接词，上文提到，过量服用维生素对身体没有营养价值，接着作者指出很多人的心态：为"安全"考虑，而服用额外的维生素。从语意上看，两句之间存在转折关系，选择项应该是一个表示转折关系的词，因此 nevertheless 符合题意，故选 A。

Practice Twenty-Three

Video game players may get an unexpected benefit from blowing away bad guys — better vision. Playing "action" video games improves a visual ability __51__ tasks like reading and driving at night, a new study says.

The ability, called contrast sensitivity function, allows people to discern even subtle changes __52__ gray against a uniformly colored backdrop. It's also one of the first visual aptitudes to fade with age.

That's __53__ a regular regimen of action video game training can provide long-lasting visual power, according to work led by Daphne Bavelier of the University of Rochester.

Previous research shows that gaming improves other visual skills, such as the ability to track several objects at the same time and __54__ attention to a series of fast-moving events, Bavelier said.

"A lot of different aspects of the visual system are being enhanced, __55__ one," she said. The new work suggests that playing video games could someday become part of vision-correction treatments, which currently rely mainly on surgery or corrective lenses.

"__56__ you've had eye surgery or got corrective lenses, exposing yourself to these games should help the optical system to recover faster and better. You need to retrain the brain to make use of the better, crisper information that's coming in __57__ a result of your improved eyesight," Bavelier said.

Expert action gamers in the study played first-person shooters in *Unreal Tournament 2004* and *Call of Duty 2*. A group of experienced nonaction gamers played *The Sims 2*, a "life simulation" video game. The players of nonaction video games didn't see the same vision __58__, the study says.

Bavelier and others are now trying to figure out exactly why action games __59__ seem to sharpen visual skill. It may be that locating enemies and aiming accurately is a strenuous, strength-building workout for the eyes, she said.

Another possible __60__ is that the unpredictable, fast-changing environment of the typical action game requires players to constantly monitor entire landscapes and analyze optical data quickly. Finally, Bavelier said, the games' rich payoff may also play a role.

"It's pleasing to be successful in your mission," she said. "When you combine rewards with these other 'factors', then you get much more learning."

51. A. ascribe to   B. key for   C. inclined to   D. crucial for
52. A. in light of   B. in shades of   C. in terms of   D. in guidance of
53. A. why   B. how   C. what   D. as
54. A. drawing   B. having   C. paying   D. giving
55. A. not just   B. no only   C. no just   D. not almost
56. A. Unless   B. Although   C. Once   D. Since
57. A. for   B. as   C. in   D. from
58. A. shortcomings   B. benefits   C. drawbacks   D. advantages
59. A. in fact   B. in effect   C. in particular   D. in vain
60. A. result   B. reason   C. fact   D. guess

答案及解析

51. 【答案】D
   【解析】本题考查形容词充当后置定语。原文的主题句为首段第一句：游戏玩家可能会因为打跑坏蛋得到意料之外的好处——视力变得更好。空格前说到玩动作游戏需要一种视觉能力，这种能力对阅读或者夜间驾驶是非常重要的。key 也表示"重要的，关键的"，但常跟的介词搭配为 to。因此本题正确答案为 D（至关重要的）。

52. 【答案】B
   【解析】本题考查介词词组。第一句在解释这是一种什么能力（对比敏感度——contrast sensitivity function），以及这种能力的功能是什么。既然与 contrast 相关，那么往往会牵涉对比底色和对比内容，因此本题选用 in shades of，in shades of grey 指模糊不清的中间色。

53. 【答案】A
   【解析】本题考查逻辑关系词。空格处需要填入一个表示逻辑关系的表语从句引导词。That 指代上一段的内容，空格后从句的意思是"定期的动作游戏的训练能提供长期的视觉能力"，这是上一段"对比敏感度也是第一种会随着年龄衰退的能力（aptitude）"的结果。因此 why 能体现因果关系，是正确答案。

54. 【答案】C
   【解析】本题考查固定搭配。pay attention to 的意思是"关注，注意"，本题正确答案为 C。

55. 【答案】A
   【解析】本题考查语义。该句的意思是：视觉系统的很多方面都得到提高，而不只是一方面。not just 的意思是"不是只有，不仅仅"，是正确答案。not almost 的意思是"几乎不是"，与上文语义不符合。

56. 【答案】C
   【解析】本题考查逻辑关系。unless 意为"除非"；although 意为"尽管"，表示转折；once 意为"一旦"，表示条件；since 意为"因为"，表示因果。原文的意思是"如果你做了眼睛手术或者戴了纠正视力的镜片，多接触这样的游戏就可以让光学系统更快、更好地恢复。"很明显，主从句是条件关系，故本题答案为 C。

57. 【答案】B

【解析】本题考查固定搭配。as a result of 的意思是"结果是，作为……的结果"。因此正确答案为 B。

58. 【答案】B

【解析】本题考查上下文呼应。原句的意思是：非动作游戏玩家并没有同样的视力 ____。本题可以追溯到全文的中心句，即第一句：动作游戏可以带来意料之外的收益。反之，非动作游戏的玩家则没有同样的"收益"，即 benefits。故本题答案为 B。

59. 【答案】C

【解析】本题考查固定搭配和上下文语义。该句的意思是：Bavelier 和其他人正在研究为什么偏偏是动作游戏能让我们的视觉更敏锐（sharpen）。能表示"偏偏，尤其"含义的只有 in particular。in fact 的意思是"事实上"，in effect 意为"事实上"，in vain 意为"徒劳无功的"。故本题选 C。

60. 【答案】B

【解析】本题考查名词和上下文语义。该句中的 another 证明上文还提到一个。到上文的最后一句可以得知"或许（maybe）定位敌人和精确瞄准是强化视觉能力的高强度锻炼"，可知这是对 why 的第一个回答，即 reason，由此可推断 another 后的也应该是原因，即 reason。

Practice Twenty-Four

Dear Dr. Benjamin,

Congratulations on your nomination as United States Surgeon General. Based on your extraordinary career and your commitment to __51__ health disparities among underserved populations, no doubt your tenure will be marked by great progress toward the goal of improved health for all Americans.

Each United States Surgeon General has the unique opportunity to create his or her own lasting legacy. Dr. Koop focused on smoking prevention. Dr. Satcher, one of __52__ mentors, released the first comprehensive report on mental health. We encourage you to build your own legacy __53__ concept of prevention through healthy lifestyles — a legacy that is both sustainable and cost-effective. This also is an important issue for Members of Congress, many of whom believe that __54__ prevention and wellness initiatives will bring down costs and help people lead healthier lives. The American College of Sports Medicine (ACSM) would be honored to partner with you on such an initiative.

ACSM, the largest sports medicine and exercise science organization in the world, __55__ ready to work with you to increase healthy behaviors — especially physical activity — throughout the life span. During this crucial period of health system reform, we've been advocating for strategies that support preventive medicine not just through diagnostic testing, __56__ promoting healthy, active behaviors that all Americans can achieve at little or no cost.

In fact, ACSM already has a working agreement with the Surgeon General's office, focused on a series of healthy lifestyle public service announcements, for our Exercise Is Medicine™ program, a program that __57__ calls on doctors to encourage their patients to incorporate physical activity and exercise into their daily routine. As you are __58__ aware, physical activity can prevent and treat a host of chronic conditions — such as heart disease, type II diabetes, and obesity — that currently plague our country. Your example as __59__ whose family has suffered from preventable disease and who demonstrates healthy lifestyles can be powerful indeed.

Anytime either before or after your appointment is confirmed, we would __60__ the opportunity to meet with you and your staff to discuss how we, along with other leading health organizations, can enhance the prevention paradigm through physical activity.

Again, Dr. Benjamin, I extend our deepest congratulations and best wishes.

Sincerely,

James Pivarnik, Ph.D., ACSM

President, American College of Sports Medicine

51. A. handling   B. eliminating   C. achieving   D. addressing
52. A. his own   B. our own   C. your own   D. her own
53. A. around   B. above   C. at   D. across
54. A. promoted   B. promoting
     C. having been promoting   D. having been promoted
55. A. put   B. got   C. sits   D. stands
56. A. but for   B. but that   C. but by   D. but also
57. A. arguably   B. excessively   C. specifically   D. exceptionally
58. A. well   B. better   C. the very   D. the most
59. A. those   B. one   C. this   D. it
60. A. greet   B. welcome   C. deserve   D. celebrate

短文概要

本文借恭贺 Benjamin 被提名为美国卫生局局长的名义，介绍 ACSM。

答案及解析

51. 【答案】D

【解析】本题考查上下文语义和词汇。该句的意思是"基于您出色的职业成就和致力于解决医疗服务的不平等"。此处 address 表示"解决……的问题"，符合上下文含义，是正确答案。address 还有"地址，致辞"的含义。

52.【答案】C

【解析】本题考查代词。空格后的句子讲到"我们鼓励你建立你自己的遗产",因此空格处可推测是"你自己的导师"。故本题选 C。

53.【答案】A

【解析】本题考查介词。此处表示"基于……上;围绕……的观点",around 是最合适的介词,故选 A。

54.【答案】B

【解析】本题考查语法。空格前后的意思是"提倡防治和健康意识能降低成本,并帮助人们过上更健康的生活"。此处 believe 后的从句需要主语,而主语又表示一种动作或行动,因此直接使用 promote 的动名词形式即可。故本题选 B。

55.【答案】D

【解析】本题考查固定搭配。stand ready to 的含义是"准备好",是正确答案。

56.【答案】C

【解析】本题考查并列结构的固定搭配。not just...but 表示"不仅仅是,而是",同时 but by 与 not just through 是并列关系。故本题选 C。

57.【答案】C

【解析】本题考查词汇和上下文语义。空格前后的意思是"(那是)一个特意呼吁医生鼓励病人将体力活动和锻炼与日常生活结合起来的项目"。arguably "按理";excessively "额外地";specifically "特别地,具体地";exceptionally "排外地,特别地"。故本题选 C。

58.【答案】A

【解析】此题考查固定搭配。be well aware 意思是"很清楚地认识到"。此处 well 为程度副词,修饰 aware。故本题答案为 A。

59.【答案】B

【解析】本题考查代词做先行词。定语从句中 whose family has suffered... 的先行词只能用单数代词,同时要指代人,因此只有 one 符合要求。故本题正确答案为 B。

60.【答案】B

【解析】本题测试上下文含义。greet "打招呼";welcome "欢迎";deserve "值得";celebrate "庆祝"。此处表示欢迎或期待见面的机会,故本题正确答案为 B。

📝 Practice Twenty-Five

Whenever people go and live in another country they have new experiences and new feelings. They experience culture shock. Many people have a(n) __51__ about culture shock. They think that it's just a feeling of sadness and homesickness when a person is in a new country. But this isn't really true. Culture shock is a completely natural __52__, and everybody goes __53__ it in a new culture.

There are four stages, or steps, in culture shock. When people first arrive in a new country, they're usually excited and __54__. Everything is interesting. They notice that a lot of things are __55__ their own culture and this surprises them and makes them happy. This is Stage One.

In Stage Two people notice how different the new culture is from their own culture. They become confused. It seems difficult to do even very simple things. They feel __56__. They spend a lot of time __57__ or with other people from their own country. They think: "My problems are all because I'm living in this country."

Then in Stage Three they begin to understand the new culture better. They begin to like some new customs. They __58__ some people in the new country. They're __59__ comfortable and relaxed.

In Stage Four they feel very comfortable. They have good friends in the new culture. They understand the new customs. Some customs are similar to their culture and some are different but that's OK. They can __60__ it.

51. A. account   B. reflection   C. verification   D. misconception
52. A. transition   B. exchange   C. immigration   D. selection
53. A. for   B. through   C. after   D. about
54. A. frightened   B. confused   C. uneasy   D. happy
55. A. representative of   B. different from
    C. peculiar to   D. similar to
56. A. intoxicated   B. depressed   C. amazed   D. thrilled
57. A. lonely   B. alone   C. lone   D. only
58. A. make friends with   B. make transactions with
    C. hold hostility to   D. shut the door to
59. A. hardly   B. more   C. very   D. less
60. A. live with   B. do without
    C. hold up with   D. make a success of

短文概要

本文介绍文化冲击的四个阶段。

答案及解析

51. 【答案】D
【解析】此题考点为上下文信息推断，尤其是转折关系。本句话告诉我们，人们认为文化冲击指的是一个人在陌生国度里伤心和想家的情绪。紧接着转折结构否认了该观点。本段最后一句话揭示文化冲击是一个很自然的过渡，处于陌生文化中的每个人都会经历。通过转折结构前后对比，可以得知转折前的观点是误解，因而选项 D 正确。

52. 【答案】A
【解析】此题考点为上下文信息推断，详见第 51 题。

53. 【答案】B
【解析】此题考点为固定搭配。go through 的含义是"经历"。go for 指"争取，拥护，

外出（进行活动）"；go after 的含义是"追赶，力争"；go about 的含义是
"着手做，从事"。

54. 【答案】D

【解析】此题考点为上下文信息推断。根据并列结构，空白处需要选择与 excited 近义
的词汇，因而答案为 D。

55. 【答案】D

【解析】此题考点为上下文信息推断。根据第二段可知，在文化冲击第一阶段，身处陌
生国度的人们很快乐。根据第三段的首句可知，在第二阶段人们发觉陌生文化
和本国文化的差异。据此我们可以推断在文化冲击第一阶段，身边有很多与
本国文化很相似的事情使得人们很惊奇并且很快乐。所以选项 D 正确。A 项
representative of 的含义是"代表……的"；C 项 peculiar to 的含义是"特有的"。

56. 【答案】B

【解析】此题考点为上下文信息推断。根据第三段的首句可知，在文化冲击的第二阶段，
人们注意到文化差异，并由此感到困惑不解，甚至做一些很简单的事情都很困
难，因而感到沮丧，所以答案为 B。A 项 intoxicated 的含义是"醉酒的，兴奋的"；
D 项 thrilled 的含义是"激动的，毛骨悚然的"。

57. 【答案】B

【解析】此题考点为形近词辨析。根据上下文信息可得知，感到沮丧的人们会和来自本
国的人在一起或者独处。A 项 lonely 指的是"孤独感"；B 项 alone 的含义是"独
处的"，既是形容词又是副词；C 项 lone 的含义是"孤单的"，通常用作形容词。
句子结构空白处需要一个副词，表示"独处"，因而答案为 B。

58. 【答案】A

【解析】此题考点为上下文信息推断。第四段提到在文化冲击的第四阶段人们开始
更好地了解新文化，开始喜欢新的风俗，也开始和新国家的人交朋友。因
而答案为 A。B 项 make transactions with 的含义是"做交易"；C 项 hold
hostility to 的含义是"对……有敌意"；D 项 shut the door to 的含义是"把
……拒之门外"。

59. 【答案】B

【解析】此题考点为上下文信息推断。根据第 58 题解析可知，人们开始熟悉并喜欢新
的国家和新的文化，由此人们的情感也应该从沮丧开始向好的方面转化，因而
选项 B 更为贴切，即人们更舒适、放松。

60. 【答案】A

【解析】此题考点为上下文信息推断。最后一段提到文化冲击的第四个阶段人们已经熟
悉新文化的一切，文化习俗相似或是存在差异都没影响了，因而人们便开始接
受了。A 项 live with 的含义为"接受"；B 项 do without 的含义是"没有……
也行"；C 项 hold up with 的含义是"向……看齐"；D 项 make a success
of 的含义是"取得成功"。因而答案为 A。

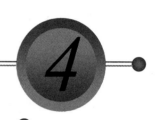

第四章 CHAPTER 4 阅读理解

一、考试大纲的要求

该测试部分由 6 篇阅读短文组成，每篇短文约有 300 个单词，每篇文章后有 5 个问题，要求考生根据对文章的理解，在每个问题后的四个备选选项中选出正确答案。此部分是测试考生通过阅读英文书刊获取信息的能力（包括阅读速度和理解程度）。要求考生在阅读完一篇短文后，能理解其主题思想、主要内容和主要细节；能根据所读材料的内容进行推理判断，理解某些单词和短语在具体语境中的意义，理解句与句之间的内在逻辑关系；能领会作者的观点和思想感情，判断其对事物的态度。测试材料主要涉及医学科普、自然科普和人文等各种题材和体裁的文章。此部分共 30 题，每题 1 分，共计 30 分。考试时间约为 65 分钟。

二、真题演练与解析

首先，请各位考生严格按照考试的时间要求，在 65 分钟内实际演练下面的真题。一方面，可正确且快速定位自己目前的水平，以便制订相应的复习策略；另一方面，可对医学博士英语统考的阅读部分测试有一个精准的把握，从而在复习过程中有的放矢，提高效率。

Reading Comprehension (30%)

Directions: *In this part there are six passages, each of which is followed by five questions. For each question there are four possible answers marked A, B, C and D. Choose the best answer and mark the letter of your choice on the **ANSWER SHEET**.*

Passage One

In a society where all aspects of our lives are dictated by scientific advances in technology, science is the essence of our existence. Without the vast advances made by chemists, physicists, biologists, geologists, and other diligent scientists, our standards of living would decline, our flourishing, wealthy nation might come to an economic depression, and our people would suffer from diseases that could not be cured. As a society we ignorantly take advantage of the amenities provided by science, yet our lives would be altered interminably without them.

Health care, one of the aspects of our society that separates us from our archaic ancestors, is founded exclusively on scientific discoveries and advances. Without the vaccines created by doctors, diseases such as polio, measles, hepatitis, and the flu would pose a threat to our citizens, for although some of these diseases may not be deadly, their side effects can be a vast detriment to an individual affected with the disease.

Yet another aspect of science, discoveries of the world beyond us, has increased our knowledge and contributed to our culture. Such discoveries were once viewed as an impossible task, but the technology brought to life by NASA employees has accomplished this aspiration, and numerous others. In addition, science has developed perhaps the most awe-inspiring, vital invention in the history of the world, the computer. Without the presence of this machine, our world could exist, but the conveniences brought into life by the computer are unparalleled.

Despite the greatness of present-day innovators and scientists and their revelations, it is requisite to examine the amenities of science that our culture so blatantly disregards. For instance, the light bulb, electricity, the telephone, running water, and the automobile are present-day staples of our society; however, they were not present until scientists discovered them.

Because of the contributions of scientists, our world is ever metamorphosing, and this metamorphosis economically and personally comprises our society, whether our society is cognizant of this or not.

61. In the first paragraph the author implies that we _____.
    A. would not survive without science
    B. take the amenities of science for granted
    C. could have raised the standards of living with science
    D. would be free of disease because of scientific advances

62. The author uses health care and vaccines to illustrate _____.
    A. how science has been developed
    B. what science means to society
    C. what the nature of science is
    D. how disease affects society

63. Nothing, according to the author, can match the invention of the computer in terms of _____.
    A. power   B. novelty   C. benefits   D. complexity

64. The author seems to be unhappy about _____.
    A. people's ignorance of their culture
    B. people's ignoring the amenities of science
    C. people's making no contributions to society
    D. people's misunderstanding of scientific advances

65. The author's tone in the passage is _____.
    A. critical   B. cognizant   C. appreciative   D. paradoxical

Passage Two

Biotechnology is expected to bring important advances in medical diagnosis and therapy, in solving food problems, in energy saving, in environmentally compatible industrial and agricultural production, and in specially targeted environmental protection projects. Genetically altered microorganisms can break down a wide range of pollutants by being used, for example, in bio-filters and wastewater-treatment facilities, and in the clean-up of polluted sites. Genetically modified organisms can also alleviate environmental burdens by reducing the need for pesticides, fertilizers, and medications.

Sustainability, as a strategic aim, involves optimizing the interactions between nature, society, and the economy, in accordance with ecological criteria. Political leaders and scientists alike face the challenge of recognizing interrelationships and interactions between ecological, economic, and social factors and taking account of these factors when seeking solution strategies. To meet this challenge, decision-makers require interdisciplinary approaches and strategies that cut across political lines. Environmental discussions must become more objective, and this includes, especially, debates about the risks of new technologies, which are often ideologically charged. In light of the complex issues involved in sustainable development, we need clearer standards for orienting and assessing our environmental policies. In this context I consider the current work on indicator models as a means to assess and monitor the success of sustainability strategies, to be of great significance.

Sustainable development can succeed only if all areas of the political sector, of society, and of science accept the concept and work together to implement it. A common basic understanding of environmental ethics is needed to ensure that protection of the natural foundation of life becomes a major consideration in all political and individual action. A dialogue among representatives of all sectors of society is needed if appropriate environmental policies are to be devised and implemented.

66. Biotechnology _____.
   A. can help save energy and integrate industry and agriculture
   B. can rid humans of diseases and solve food problems
   C. can treat pollution and protect environment
   D. all of the above

67. Wastewater can be treated _____.
   A. in genetic engineering
   B. by means of biotechnology
   C. in agriculture as well as in industry
   D. without the need for breaking down pollutants

68. When he says approaches and strategies that cut across political lines, the author means that they _____.
   A. involve economic issues   B. observe ecological criteria
   C. are politically significant   D. overcome political barriers

69. It can be inferred from the passage that the complexity of sustainable development _____.
   A. makes it necessary to improve the assessing standards
   B. renders environmental discussion possible
   C. charges new technologies risks
   D. requires simplification

70. The success of sustainable development lies in _____.
   A. its concept to be of great significance
   B. good social teamwork
   C. appropriate environmental policies
   D. the representatives of all sectors of society

Passage Three

Folk wisdom holds that the blind can hear better than people with sight. Scientists have a new reason to believe it.

Research now indicates that blind and sighted people display the same skill at locating a sound's origin when using both ears, but some blind people can <u>home</u> in on sounds more accurately than their sighted counterparts when all have one ear blocked. Canadian scientists describe the work in the Sept. 17 *Nature*.

Participants in the study were tested individually in a sound-insulated room. They faced 16 small, concealed loudspeakers arrayed in a semicircle a few feet away. With a headrest keeping their heads steady, the participants pointed to the perceived origins of the sounds.

The researchers tested eight blind people, who had been completely sightless from birth or since a very early age. They also tested three nearly blind persons, who had some residual vision at the periphery of their gaze; seven sighted people wearing blindfolds; and 29 sighted people without blindfolds. All participants were tested beforehand to ensure that their hearing was normal.

When restricted to one-ear, or monaural, listening, four of the eight blind people identified sound sources more accurately than did the sighted people, says study coauthor Michel Pare, a neuroscientist at the University of Montreal. The sighted people showed especially poor localization of sounds from the speakers on the side of the blocked ear.

In sighted people who can hear with both ears, "The brain learns to rely on binaural [stereo] cues. These data suggest that blind people haven't learned that and keep monaural cues as the dominant cues," says Eric I. Knudsen, a neurobiologist at Stanford University School of Medicine. "I find it surprising."

71. One thing is sure that participants in the study _____.
   A. had normal hearing
   C. wore blindfolds
   B. were born blind
   D. were divided into two groups

72. Under what conditions, according to Pare, did the blind testers perform better than their sighted counterparts?
   A. When both used one ear.
   B. When the speakers were concealed.
   C. When the sounds were tuned down.
   D. When both were restricted to blindfolds.

73. Knudsen explained the better hearing on the part of the blind in term of _____.
   A. cognitive psychology
   C. binaural cues
   B. visual images
   D. monaural cues

74. The Canadian scientists did their test to answer the question whether _____.
   A. the blind can hear as well as the sighted
   B. the blind have hearing capabilities
   C. blind people track sounds better

D. folk wisdom is educational

75. What folk wisdom holds in the passage _____.
    A. has been scientifically tested in Canada and U.S., with different results produced
    B. has been scientifically verified
    C. merits further investigation
    D. is surprising to everyone

Passage Four

It used to be that a corporation's capital consisted of tangible assets such as buildings, machines, and finished goods. But, in the information economy, value has shifted rapidly from tangible to intangible assets, such as management skills and customer loyalty. But how do you measure intangible assets?

Karl Erik Sveiby began trying to answer that question as a magazine publisher in Sweden and went to become Scandinavia's leading authority on knowledge-based businesses. In his latest book, *The New Organizational Wealth*, he offers insights into valuing and managing intangible assets.

Noting that Microsoft Corporation, the world's largest software firm, once traded at an average share price of $70 at a time when its book value was $7, Sveiby asks: "What is it about Microsoft that makes it worth 10 times the value of its recorded assets? What is the nature of that additional value that is perceived by the market but not recorded by the company?"

Sveiby's answer is intangible assets, which he defines as employee competence, internal structures (systems, patents, etc.), and external structures (customer and supplier relationships and the organization's image). Because of these factors, it follows that owners hold a kind of intangible equity in the company, in addition to tangible assets such as cash and accounts receivable.

Since knowledge is a key intangible asset, the ability to transfer knowledge from one employee to another, or from outside sources to employees, is a key business capacity, in Sveiby's view. The greater the transfer of knowledge, the more overall employee competence improves. The best method for transferring knowledge, says Sveiby, is through direct experience with a subject rather than simply listening to someone or reading about it.

Experience enables learning more than overt teaching because people acquire knowledge tacitly, by observation and listening in an unstructured environment. And, he adds, people will more readily learn from an activity if they enjoy it.

Once the flow of information within an organization is managed properly, the competence of the organization increases, and the relations with customers improve. But

Sveiby also points out that knowledge and information are not the same thing. Information has no value until it becomes integrated knowledge and therefore useful.

76. In the information economy, it is a challenge _____.
   A. to place a high value on intangible assets
   B. to transfer tangible into intangible assets
   C. to change the concept of assets
   D. to quantify intangible assets

77. Microsoft Corporation, in Sveiby's view _____.
   A. is skillful at managing intangible assets
   B. creates most intangible assets in the world
   C. does not hold any tangible, but much intangible assets
   D. possesses much additional intangible assets recognized by the market

78. The transfer of knowledge which is a key intangible asset, according to Sveiby _____.
   A. has much to do with overall employee competence
   B. is best done through hands-on experience
   C. reflects business capacity
   D. all of the above

79. Integrated knowledge, information _____.
   A. begins to spread within an organization
   B. will lose much of its value
   C. will remain useful forever
   D. is an intangible asset

80. Which of the following can be the best title for the passage?
   A. Knowledge as Capital.   B. Exploding Knowledge.
   C. The Power of Knowledge.   D. Information and Knowledge.

Passage Five

High-speed living has become a fact of life, and the frantic pace is taking its toll, according to science writer James Gleick. It's as if the old "Type A" behaviour of a few has expanded into the "hurry sickness" of the many.

"We do feel that we're more time-driven and time-obsessed and generally rushed than ever before," writes Gleick in *Faster: The Acceleration of Just About Everything*, a survey of fast-moving culture and its consequences. We may also be acting more hastily, losing control, and thinking superficially because we live faster.

Technology has conditioned us to expect instant results. Internet purchases arrive by next-day delivery and the microwave delivers a hot meal in minutes. Faxes, e-mails, and cell phones make it possible and increasingly obligatory — for people to work faster. Gleick cites numerous examples of fast-forward changes in our lives: stock trading and news cycles are shorter; sound bites of presidential candidates on network newscasts dropped from 40 seconds in 1968 to 10 seconds in 1988; and some fast-food restaurants have added express lanes.

High expectations for instant service make even the brief wait for an elevator seem interminable（漫长的）. "A good waiting time is in the neighborhood of 15 seconds. Sometime around 40 seconds, people start to get visibly upset," writes Gleick. We're dependent on systems that promise speed but often deliver frustration. Like rush-hour drivers fuming when a single accident halts the evening commute, people surfing the Internet squirm if a Web page is slow to load or when access itself is not instantaneous. And the concept of "customer service" can become an oxymoron（逆喻） for consumers waiting on hold for a telephone representative.

Uptempo living has turned people into multitaskers — eating while driving, writing an e-mail while talking on the phone, or skimming dozens of television programs on split screen. Gleick suggests that human beings may be capable of adjusting to these new levels of stimuli as high-speed culture challenges our brains "in a way they were not challenged in the past, except perhaps in times of war". We may gain the flexibility to do several things at once but lose some of our capacity to focus in depth on a single task.

81. With living pace getting quicker and quicker, the number of those of "Type A" behaviour is _____.
   A. on the rise
   B. out of control
   C. on the decline
   D. under investigation

82. High-speed living brings about the following consequences, exclusive of _____.
   A. superficial thinking
   B. loss of control
   C. waste of time
   D. more haste

83. The best conclusion can be drawn from the 3rd paragraph is that _____.
   A. technology is building a fast-moving culture
   B. we are living in the age of information
   C. economy is booming with technology
   D. the frantic pace is taking its toll

84. As the author implies, the faster we live _____.
   A. the less we do
   B. the less patient we are
   C. the more time we save
   D. the more efficient we have

85. Living faster and faster, the multitaskers tend _____.

A. to scratch the surface of a thing

B. to do things better at the same time

C. to be flexible with their time schedules

D. to have intense concentration on trivial things

Passage Six

Eating is related to emotional as well as physiologic needs. Sucking, which is the infant's means of gaining both food and emotional security, conditions the association of eating with well-being or with deprivation. If the child is breast-fed and has supportive body contact as well as good milk intake, if the child is allowed to suck for as long as he or she desires, and if both the child and mother enjoy the nursing experience and share their enjoyment, the child is more likely to thrive both physically and emotionally. On the other hand, if the mother is nervous and resents the child or cuts him or her off from the milk supply before either the child's hunger or sucking need is satisfied, or handles the child hostilely during the feeding, or props the baby with a bottle rather than holding the child, the child may develop physically but will begin to show signs of emotional disturbance at an early age. If, in addition, the infant is further abused by parental indifference or intolerance, he or she will carry scars of such emotional deprivation throughout life.

Eating habits are also conditioned by family and other psychosocial environments. If an individual's family eats large quantities of food, then he or she is inclined to eat large amounts. If an individual's family eats mainly vegetables, then he or she will be inclined to like vegetables. If mealtime is a happy and significant event, then the person will tend to think of eating in those terms. And if a family eats quickly, without caring what is being eaten and while fighting at the dinner table, then the person will most likely adopt the same eating pattern and be adversely affected by it. This conditioning to food can remain unchanged through a lifetime unless the individual is awakened to the fact of conditioning and to the possible need for altering his or her eating patterns in order to improve nutritional intake. Conditioning spills over into and is often reinforced by religious beliefs and other customs so that, for example, a Jew, whose religion forbids the eating of pork, might have guilt feelings if he or she ate pork. An older Roman Catholic might be conditioned to feel guilty if he or she eats meat on Friday, traditionally a fish day.

86. A well-breast-fed child _____.

A. tends to associate foods with emotions

B. is physiologically and emotionally satisfied

C. cannot have physiologic and emotional problems

D. is more likely to have his or her needs satisfied in the future

87. While sucking, the baby is actually _____.

   A. conscious of the impact of breast-feeding

   B. interacting with his or her mother

   C. creating a nursing environment

   D. impossible to be abused

88. A bottle-fed child _____.

   A. can be healthy physiologically, but not emotionally

   B. cannot avoid physiologic abuse throughout life

   C. is deprived of emotional needs

   D. is rid of physiological needs

89. From the list of eating habits, we learn that _____.

   A. everyone follows his or her eating pattern to death

   B. one's eating pattern varies with his or her personality

   C. there are no such things as psychosocial environments

   D. everybody is born into a conditioned eating environment

90. A Jew or an older Roman Catholic _____.

   A. takes an eating habit as a religious belief

   B. is conditioned to feel guilty of eating pork in his or her family

   C. cannot have a nutritional eating habit conditioned by religious beliefs

   D. observes an eating pattern conditioned by his or her psychosocial environment

答案及解析

Passage One

61.【答案】C

【解析】题目为：作者在第 1 段向人们暗示了什么？A. 没有科学我们无法生存下去；B. 把科学带来的便利视为理所当然；C. 通过科学我们可以提高生活水平；D. 因为科学进步人们不再被疾病困扰。结合第 1 段最后一句话可知：没有科学，我们的生活将改变得非常缓慢，故 A 项不成立；最后一句话前半部分提到，我们在生活中无视科学带来的便利，故 B 项非暗示；结合第 1 段第 2 句话：没有……所带来的巨大进步，我们的生活水平会下降……人们将会遭受无法治愈的病痛。由此可知，D 项非暗示，而且意思过于绝对，故 C 项为正确答案。

62.【答案】B

【解析】题目为：作者使用医疗以及疫苗为了阐述什么？A. 科学是如何发展起来的；B. 科学对于社会意味着什么；C. 科学的本质是什么；D. 疾病如何影响社会。此题解题时要联系全文主旨，通篇文章讲述科学对我们生活方方面面的影响和作用。因而第 2 段中的这两个例子也是为了例证文章的中心思想，因而 B 为正确选项。

63.【答案】C

【解析】题目为：根据作者观点，在哪个方面没有任何东西可以与计算机的发明相媲美？此题解题要点在第 3 段最后一句话，这句话的关键词为 convenience "便利"，所以近义选项为 C。

64.【答案】B

【解析】题目为：作者对于什么感到不满？ A．人们对文化的无知；B．人们忽视科学的便利设施；C．人们对社会毫无贡献；D．人们对科学进步的误解。此题出处在第 4 段第 1 句。

65.【答案】C

【解析】此题问作者的语气。A 项 critical "批判的"；B 项 cognizant "认知的"；C 项 appreciative "感激的"；D 项 paradoxical "荒谬的"。全文提到没有科学的进步和发展，人类生活的方方面面就会受到影响，因而作者对于科学以及科学发展持感激的态度。

Passage Two

66.【答案】D

【解析】此题问生物技术的作用和影响，解题出处在第 1 段。

67.【答案】B

【解析】此题问污水如何处理。第 1 段第 4 行 "Genetically altered microorganisms can break down a wide range of pollutants by being used, for example, in bio-filters and wastewater-treatment facilities, and in the clean-up of polluted sites." 提到了污水的治理，而这句话体现了生物科技的作用和影响，因而正确选项为 B，意为"通过生物科技手段"。

68.【答案】D

【解析】题目中的原句是在第 2 段的第 5 行。这句话的前一句话阐述了政治家和科学家同样面临识别生态、经济和社会因素之间相互关系和相互作用的挑战，并且当他们寻求解决办法的时候，他们同样面临考虑这些因素的挑战。题目出处进一步阐述了为了迎接这一挑战，决策者们需要跨学科的且冲破政治界限的方法和技巧。答案为 D。

69.【答案】A

【解析】答案出处为第 2 段最后一句话。

70.【答案】B

【解析】此题解题出处为最后一段的第 1 句话，即各方面要合作执行。

Passage Three

71.【答案】A

【解析】此题出处为第 4 段最后一句话。

72.【答案】A

【解析】此题原文出处为第 5 段第 1 句话。

73. 【答案】**D**

【解析】首先根据人名确定答案在最后一段，然后根据这个专家的话语可以得出正确选项。

74. 【答案】**C**

【解析】Canadian scientists 的出处在第 2 段，他们的这个试验就是要证明第 1 段的说法，并且第 1 段最后一句话也说明他们的试验就是要证明上述观点。

75. 【答案】**B**

【解析】根据不同科学家和专家的论证，这一观点得到了科学试验的证实。

Passage Four

76. 【答案】**D**

【解析】题目为：在信息经济中，什么是挑战？原文第 1 段第 2 行提到 B 选项，但这是一个事实，而不是要面临的挑战。此题解题的原文信息在第 1 段的最后一句话。measure 与 D 项中 quantify 为近义词，因此 D 项为近义改写。

77. 【答案】**D**

【解析】此题是关于 Sveiby 对微软公司的阐述。与解题有关的原文信息是此段落中 Sveiby 的话：什么使得微软公司市值达到其记录在案的资产价值的十倍？由市场认定但不是公司记录的额外价值的性质是什么？根据这句话只有 D 项符合原文信息。

78. 【答案】**D**

【解析】此题为细节题，解题的原文信息在第 5 段，从第 2 句话开始。

79. 【答案】**D**

【解析】原文信息在最后一段的最后一句话，大意是：信息直到成为整合型的知识，才有价值，因而才是有用的。

80. 【答案】**A**

【解析】此题为主旨题。全文第一段提到如何衡量无形资产，接下来以微软公司为例，最后进一步讨论知识作为无形资产……，故全文而是在讲知识和资产。

Passage Five

81. 【答案】**A**

【解析】此题解题信息在第 1 段最后一句话：…the old "Type A" behavior of a few…into…of the many.

82. 【答案】**C**

【解析】题目为：高速生活给我们带来的结果，除了以下选项中哪一个？第 2 段最后一句话讲述因为生活节奏加快，我们会有什么样的结果。对比原文信息，只有 C. 选项原文没提到，故 C 项为正确选项。

83. 【答案】**A**

【解析】题目是测试第 3 段大意。此段落的第 1 句话为段落的主旨句，科技使得我们更希望即时的结果。对比原文信息，A 为正确选项。

84.【答案】B

【解析】原文信息在第 4 段。这个段落提到了由于想得到快速服务的期望使得我们等电梯的短短的时间都显得很漫长。上网时页面打开得慢，也会使得上网人心情烦躁，坐立不安。这些事例都在说明，生活节奏加快，人们的耐心随之减少。B 为正确选项。

85.【答案】A

【解析】根据题干关键词，相关原文信息在最后一段的最后一句：我们可以立刻十分灵活地做几件事情，但我们失去了在一件事情上面的深入关注。A 项 scratch the surface of a thing 的含义为"只触及某事的表面"，是原文信息的近义改写。

Passage Six

86.【答案】B

【解析】根据题干重要关键词在第 1 段第 3 行开始提到母乳喂养的婴儿。对比相关信息：the child is more likely to thrive both physically and emotionally，选项 B 为近义改写。

87.【答案】B

【解析】原文信息在第 1 段 3 句话，其大意是：如果婴儿可以喝多久就喝多久，而且婴儿和妈妈都在享受这个过程，分享他们彼此的快乐，那么孩子就很可能在身心上都得到很好的发展。这说明喂奶的过程是和妈妈交流的过程，故选项 B 正确。

88.【答案】A

【解析】原文信息在第 1 段 "…will begin to show signs of emotional disturbance at an early age."。

89.【答案】D

【解析】原文信息在最后一段，第 1 句为主题句。

90.【答案】D

【解析】原文信息在最后一段，最后两句话。这道题属于例证处命题，本题出现在例子中，故应该直接找到例子要证明的观点。文章最后一段第 1 句就是主旨句，故选项 D 正确。

三、阅读理解所需语法知识及专项训练

（一）语法基础知识

在阅读理解测试部分，有些考生无法理解作者原意，而且文章中的长难句经常成为考生理解文章的最大障碍。对此，考生的单词量是一个重要因素。另外很重要的一点就是语法知识的欠缺，它使得考生在基本上每个单词都认识的情况下，还是无法弄懂句子、段落甚至文章的含义。概括来说，影响阅读理解的语法知识可归纳为：非谓语动词、复合句以及特殊句式。下面将这三个方面的相关语法知识总结如下：

1. 非谓语动词

在英语语法中，按照动词在句中充当的成分，分为谓语动词和非谓语动词。在阅读理解中，解开长难句复杂关系的难点之一就是如何判断句中的动词是谓语动词还是非谓语动词。考生可通过下面的自测题来检测自己对非谓语动词语法知识的掌握情况。

1. —The last one _____ pays the meal.

   —Agreed!

   A. arrived　　　B. arrives　　　　C. to arrive　　　　D. arriving

2. I smell something _____ in the kitchen. Can I call you back in a minute?

   A. burning　　B. burnt　　　　C. being burnt　　　D. to be burnt

3. At the beginning of class, the noise of desks _____ could be heard outside the classroom.

   A. opened and closed　　　　B. to be opened and closed

   C. being opened and closed　　D. to open and close

4. After a knock at the door, the child heard his mother's voice _____ him.

   A. calling　　　B. called　　　　C. being called　　　D. to call

5. There is nothing more I can try _____ you to stay, so I wish you good luck.

   A. being persuaded　　　　B. persuading

   C. to be persuaded　　　　D. to persuade

6. The Town Hall _____ in the 1800's was the most distinguished building at that time.

   A. to be completed　　　　B. having been completed

   C. completed　　　　　　　D. being completed

7. The country has already sent up three unmanned spacecraft, the most recent _____ at the end of last March.

   A. has been launched　　　B. having been launched

   C. being launched　　　　　D. to be launched

8. John received an invitation to dinner, and with his work _____, he gladly accepted it.

   A. finished　　B. finishing　　　C. having finished　　D. was finished

9. "Things _____ never come again!" I couldn't help talking to myself.

   A. lost　　　　B. losing　　　　C. to lose　　　　D. have lost

10. —Can I smoke here?

    —Sorry. We don't allow _____ here.

    A. people smoking　　　　B. people smoke

    C. to smoke　　　　　　　D. smoking

11. He is very popular among his students as he always tries to make them _____ in his

lectures.

    A. interested   B. interesting   C. interest   D. to interest

12.   that she didn't do a good job, I don't think I am abler than her.

    A. To have said   B. Having said   C. To say   D. Saying

13. She wants her paintings   in the gallery, but we don't think they would be very popular.

    A. display   B. to display   C. displaying   D. displayed

14. The flowers his friend gave him will die unless   every day.

    A. watered   B. watering   C. water   D. to water

15. The children went home from the grammar school, their lessons   for the day.

    A. finishing   B. finished   C. had finished   D. were finished

16. Because air pollution has been greatly reduced, this city is still   .

    A. a good place to live   B. a good place for living in

    C. a good place to be lived in   D. a good place to live in

17. Did you smell something   ?

    A. having burnt   B. to have burnt   C. burning   D. to be burning

18. I don't mind   the decision as long as it is not too late.

    A. you to delay making   B. your delaying making

    C. your delaying to make   D. you delay to make

19.   from the outer space, our earth looks like a water-covered ball.

    A. Having seen   B. Seeing

    C. Seen   D. Having been seen

20.   in an atmosphere of simple living was what her parents wished for.

    A. The girl was educated   B. The girl educated

    C. The girl's being educated   D. The girl to be educated

答案：1-5　CACAD　　6-10　CBAAA　　11-15　ABDAB　　16-20　DCBCD

非谓语动词语法知识重点简要回顾

I.   非谓语动词的形式

	不定式	动名词	现在分词	过去分词
肯定式	to do	doing	doing	done
否定式	not to do	not doing	not doing	not done
完成式	to have done	having done	having done	done
被动式	to be done	being done	being done	done

例如：

I have many things to do. 不定式做定语修饰 things

Seeing these pictures, he thought of those days in Beijing. 现在分词 seeing 做状语

Cheating should be banned thoroughly in exams. 动名词 cheating 做主语

The teacher came into the room, followed by two students. 过去分词 followed 做伴随状语

He is a man loved by all. 过去分词 loved 做定语修饰 man

II. 非谓语动词所做的成分

	主语	宾语	表语	定语	状语	补语（宾）
不定式	√	√	√	√	√	√
动名词	√	√	√	√		
现在分词			√	√	√	√
过去分词			√	√	√	√

III. 不定式

（1）做主语

To complete the 24-storied building in 10 months was a great achievement.

在 10 个月内建成一座 24 层的大楼是个伟大的成就。

不定式做主语时常把 it 放在句首做形式主语，而将不定式移到谓语后面；

It was a great achievement to complete the 24-storied building in 10 months.

不定式的逻辑主语（for / of + 代词 / 名词），意义有所差别；

It was brave of him to dive from the cliff. (=He was brave to dive from the cliff.)

It is necessary for you to listen to other people's advice. (=It is necessary that you listen to other people's advice.)

常用 of 的形容词：careless, clever, considerate, foolish, good, impolite, kind, naughty, nice, silly, stupid。

（2）做动词宾语

I hope to improve my English gradually.

I promised not to tell anyone about it.

They asked how to get to the railway station.

后接不定式做宾语的常用动词（往往表示请求、要求、选择、决定、打算、企图等）：

afford	agree	ask	attempt	beg	bother	care	choose
claim	consent	decide	demand	desire	expect	fail	fear
hesitate	intend	plan	manage	learn	pretend	offer	pledge
prepare	refuse	resolve	determine	threaten	undertake	wish	hope

（3）做宾语补足语

His mother advised him not to go out at night.

I asked him to give me a hand.

（4）做后置定语

I never think that I can get the opportunity to work abroad one day.

（5）做表语

The task is to clear up these dishes.

（6）做表语补足语

The water is unfit to drink.

Ann is easy to get along with.

（7）做目的状语

He stopped twice, and leaned on his cane to rest.

He moved to the front row so as to hear the speaker better.

（8）做结果状语

He returned home after the long journey only to find that his house had been broken into.

IV. 动名词

（1）做主语

Milking for once is not a hard job.

It's no use crying over spilt milk.

（2）做宾语

I don't mind telling you the truth.

Let's stop arguing.

① 只能接动名词做宾语的常用动词如下，可通过下列口诀辅助记忆：

喜欢考虑与避免（enjoy, consider, avoid）

停止放弃太危险（stop, quit, risk）

承认理解很值得（admit, understand, be worth）

幻想想象莫拖延（fancy, imagine, delay, postpone）

要求完成时期望（require, finish, look forward to）

建议继续勤操练（suggest, keep on, practice）

不禁原谅是坚持（can't help, excuse, insist on）

继续成功不弃嫌（go on, succeed in, mind）+ deny

② 下列特殊句型中要用动名词的形式

It is no use（no good, no point, no sense, a waste of time 等名词）+ (in) doing sth.

It is good（nice, interesting, useless 等形容词）+(in) doing sth.

There is no point（use, sense, good 等名词）+ (in) doing sth.

have difficulty (trouble, problem, pleasure, a difficult time) + (in) doing sth.

例如：

It's simply a waste of time and money seeing that movie.

There is no point in my going out to date someone.

I find it no good advising him to go with us.

③ 有些动词后既可以接 doing 也可以接 to do，但有区别，如下所示：

> forget to do / forget doing

Don't forget to bring pen and paper for the quiz. 考试时别忘了带笔和纸。
I'll never forget meeting you the first time. 我永远不会忘记我们的第一次见面。

> remember to do / doing

Remember to take the medicine after dinner. 记得饭后吃药。
I remember switching off the light before I left. 我记得我走前关灯了。

> regret to do / doing

I regret to tell you that you failed the exam. 我很遗憾告诉你你考试不及格。
I regret having said that rude word to him. 我后悔对他说了粗话。

> stop doing / to do

He stopped writing and had a talk with me. 他停下笔，和我聊起天来。
He stopped to have a rest. 他停下来，休息一下。

> mean doing / to do

His nodding means agreeing. 他点头意味着同意了。
He meant to do that work by himself. 他打算自己做那份工作。

> try doing / to do

We try to finish the task on time. 我们试图按时完成任务。
She tried making a dress by herself, but she failed.
她试着自己做衣服，但没成功。

> like / dislike doing / to do

I like watching TV every night, but I don't like to watch TV this evening because
I am busy. 每天晚上我都喜欢看电视，但今晚我不想看了，因为太忙。

V. 分词

（1）做宾补

Do you see the dark cloud hovering over the surface of the earth?
The shop girl's good intention left the old man feeling better than before.

（2）做定语

All people involved have been questioned.
The factory making trucks is located at the foot of the mountain.

（3）做状语

> 表时间

Turning around, she saw Tom in tears.

↘ 表原因

Being ill, he couldn't go to class.

Seriously injured, Allen was rushed to the hospital.

↘ 表让步，由 although / though, even if / though 引入放句首

Even if coming by the subway, you'll need 45 minutes to get here.

Although given the best medical care, he died.

↘ 表条件

Unless asked to answer questions, the pupils were not supposed to talk in Mrs Smith's class.

If going there by plane, we'll have to pay twice as much.

↘ 表伴随

Singing and laughing, the pupils came into the room.

He sat in an armchair, watching TV.

↘ 固定短语

generally (strictly, etc.) speaking	judging from / by
talking of	allowing for
considering	taken as a whole
barring	assuming / supposing
according to	owing to
taking everything into consideration	leaving … on one side
generally / frankly / roughly /strictly / honestly speaking	

（4）分词的独立主格结构

① 分词可有其独立的逻辑主语

② 常是名词或代词主格置于分词前

③ 常做句子状语，置于句首或句尾

The river having risen in the night, the crossing was impossible.

Weather permitting, we'll have the match tomorrow.

The work done, we went home.

2. 名词性从句

根据名词性从句所充当的成分，可以分为主语从句、宾语从句、表语从句、同位语从句。

 自测题

1. Although there are many predictions about the future, no one knows for sure _____ the world would be like in 50 years.

   A. how   B. that   C. which   D. what

2. I don't think Mr. Watson will come here again today. Please give the ticket to _____

comes here first.

    A. whomever   B. whom   C. who   D. whoever

3. Undoubtedly, _____ wins the election is going to have a tough job getting the economy back on its feet.

    A. anyone   B. who   C. whoever   D. everyone

4. It is a great pity for _____ to be any quarrel in the school board meeting.

    A. where   B. here   C. there   D. why

5. They want to know _____ do to help us.

    A. what can they   B. what they can

    C. how they can   D. how can they

6. These photographs will show you _____.

    A. what does our village look like   B. what our village looks like

    C. how does our village look like   D. how our village looks like

7. Can you make sure _____ the gold ring?

    A. where Alice had put   B. where did Alice put

    C. where Alice has put   D. where has Alice put

8. Go and get your coat. It's _____ you left it.

    A. there   B. where   C. there where   D. where there

9. _____ the 2012 Olympic Games will be held in London is not known yet.

    A. Whether   B. If   C. Whenever   D. That

10. It worried her a bit _____ her hair was turning grey.

    A. while   B. that   C. if   D. for

11. _____ he said at the meeting astonished everyone present.

    A. When   B. What   C. How   D. That

12. _____ we cannot get seems better than _____ we have.

    A. What; what   B. What; that   C. That; that   D. That; what

13. The fact _____ he has made great progress in this term is quite clear.

    A. why   B. if   C. what   D. that

答案：1-5 D D C C B   6-10 B C B A B   11-13 B A D

名词性从句语法知识重点简要回顾

I. 主语从句

    分为由 that 引导的主语从句（that 不可省）和由 wh- 引导的主语从句。例如：

    What they are after is profit.

    That he is a rich man is known to all.

    When we shall have our sports meeting is still a question.

Whether we'll go outing depends on the weather.

II. 宾语从句

分为由 that 引导的宾语从句（that 可以省）和由 wh- 引导的宾语从句。例如：

Let's see how we can raise our efficiency.

I don't doubt that they'll be able to overcome the difficulty.

She was never satisfied with what she had achieved.

III. 表语从句

分为 that 引导的表语从句（that 不可省）和 wh- 引导的表语从句。例如：

This is what I want to say.

The fact is that she pretended to be ill yesterday.

IV. 同位语从句

that 引导的同位语从句（that 不可省）

wh- 引导的同位语从句

（1）同位语从句在句中做名词的同位语，用以说明名词所表示的具体内容。例如：

An order came that all villagers must leave the village.

（2）同位语从句与定语从句的区别：如果从句所修饰的名词在从句中充当成分，就是定语从句，反之就是同位语从句。例如：

The order that you gave us is right.（定语从句）

He has the hope that he'll become a college student.（同位语从句）

3. 定语从句

 自测题

1. All of the plants now raised on farms have been developed from plants _____ in the wild.

    A. once they grew   B. that once grew

    C. they grew once   D. once grew

2. Scientists can predict regions _____ new species are most likely to be found.

    A. where   B. when   C. why   D. how

3. The only thing _____ really matters to the parents is how soon their children can return home.

    A. what   B. that   C. which   D. this

4. The *Mona Lisa*, _____ in Italy, is now in the Louvre, a museum in Paris.

    A. who painted   B. who was painted

    C. which painted   D. which was painted

5. The parents were much kinder to their youngest child than they were to the

others, _____, of course, made the others jealous.

    A. which   B. that   C. what   D. who

6. The symbols of mathematics _____ we are most familiar are the signs of addition, subtraction, multiplication, division and equality.

    A. to which   B. which   C. with which   D. in which

7. _____ is often the case with a new idea, much initial activity and optimistic discussion produce no concrete proposal.

    A. It   B. Which   C. As   D. That

答案：1-5　B A B D A　　6-7　C C

 定语从句语法知识重点简要回顾

I. 定语从句的定义

修饰名词的从句（修饰名词的句子成分是定语）。例如：

He is a man who is loved by all.

定语从句修饰名词 man

II. 定语从句的分类

定语从句分为限制性定语从句和非限制性定语从句（主句和从句之间用逗号隔开）。例如：

She is the nurse who looks after my sick mother.（限制性定语从句）

Football, which is a very interesting game, is played all over the world.（非限制性定语从句）

III. 定语从句的组成部分

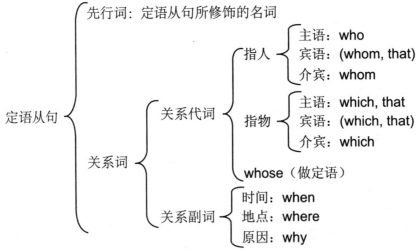

注：关系词所起的作用：

    ① 引导从句

    ② 代替先行词在从句中充当成分

    关系代词与关系副词的关系：介词 + 关系代词 = 关系副词

请拆分下面的定语从句

① <u>She is the nurse</u> <u>who looks after my sick mother</u>.

           主句   从句

先行词为 nurse, who 为关系代词并且代替 nurse 在从句中充当主语。

② Do you know the man I spoke to?

③ Do you know the man to whom I spoke?

④ Football, which is a very interesting game, is played all over the world.

⑤ The book you lent me is very interesting.

⑥ The knife with which I used to cut the bread is very sharp.

⑦ She is the student whose mother is a teacher.

⑧ I've lost the dictionary whose cover is blue.

⑨ The day will come when the people all over the world will win liberation.

⑩ I visited the school where my mother taught English ten years ago.

⑪ Do you know the reason why he left here?

4. 状语从句

自测题

1. You can arrive in Beijing earlier for the meeting _____ you don't mind taking the night train.
   A. if   B. unless   C. though   D. until

2. _____ pollution control measures tend to be money-consuming, many industries hesitate to adopt them.
   A. Although   B. However   C. When   D. Since

3. _____ urgent the situation may be, you will need to make one change at a time, and then move on.
   A. As   B. Whenever   C. However   D. Whatever

4. _____ I admit that the problems are difficult, I don't agree that they cannot be solved.
   A. When   B. Where   C. While   D. Why

5. The ATMs enable bank customers to access their money 24 hours a day and seven days a week _____ ATMs are located.
   A. wherever   B. whenever   C. however   D. whatever

6. It was _____ good weather that we all want to go out for a traveling.
   A. so   B. such   C. because   D. /

7. Although it was raining, _____ still worked in the fields.
   A. but they   B. and they   C. they   D. and yet they

8. I haven't decided _____ I should attend that meeting or not.

    A. if   B. that   C. whether   D. why

9. _____ the weather is fine, I open all the windows.

    A. As   B. For   C. Because of   D. Since that

10. You can also do something great _____ you work very hard at it.

    A. as long as   B. as far as   C. whether   D. so that

11. _____ you have promised him, you should keep your promise.

    A. Now that   B. When   C. After   D. For

12. I was speaking to Ann on the phone about our tour plan _____ suddenly we were cut off.

    A. that   B. while   C. before   D. when

答案：1-5　A D C C A　　6-10　B C C A A　　11-12　A D

📖 状语从句语法知识重点简要回顾

I.　状语从句的分类

分为时间状语从句、地点状语从句、原因状语从句、目的状语从句、结果状语从句、让步状语从句、比较状语从句、方式状语从句、条件状语从句。

II.　时间状语从句

（1）引导时间状语从句的连词：when, while, as, before, after, until, till, as soon as, no sooner… than, since, hardly… when, scarcely… when

    ① when 引导的时间状语从句的动词既可以是延续性动词，又可以是瞬间动词。

        It was 9 o' clock when I got home.

        The doorbell rang when my mother was cooking in the kitchen.

    ② while 所引导的时间状语从句的动词只能是延续性动词。

        While we were watching TV, he came in.

    ③ as 所引导的时间状语从句中的动词可以是延续性动词，或是侧重两个动作的同步，"一边，一边"。

        意为：

        As the children walked along the street, they sang happily.

    ④ when 的特殊用法：when = at that time something happened suddenly 正在那时突然……

        I had just started back for the house to change my clothes when I heard the strange noise.

    ⑤ while 的特殊用法：表示对比，译成"而"。

        She likes pop music, while her brother likes light music.

        while，译为"虽然"。

        While I understand your viewpoint, I don't agree with you.

（2）since & before

① It is + 一段时间　since　　表示一段时间的起始点，"自从"
It is + 一段时间　before　表示一段时间的终止点
It is three years since I began to study here.
It was three years before we met again.

② 如果 since 引导的时间状语从句中的动词是延续性动词，意为否定。
It's a long time since Jack lived here. 杰克早不在这儿住了。
It's a year since I smoked. 我已经有一年不吸烟了。
It's been years since I enjoyed myself so much as last night. 我已经有很多年没有像昨晚那么痛快了。

③ before, 译为"就，才"。
It wasn't long before the fire went out. 没过多久，火就熄灭了。
I hadn't gone much farther before I caught up with her. 没走多远，我就赶上了。

（3）hardly… when, no sooner… than, scarcely… when 一……就……
We had hardly got into the village when it began to rain.
我刚一进村子就下雨了。
= Hardly <u>had we got into</u> the village when it began to rain. 否定词置句首，部分倒装。
He had no sooner arrived home than he was asked to start on another journey.
= No sooner had he arrived home than he was asked to start on another journey.

（4）not… until 直到……才……
She didn't stop crying until her mother came back.
① 强调句型
It was not until her mother came back that she stopped crying.
② 倒装结构
Not until her mother came back did she stop crying.

（5）其他
Directly I had done it, I knew I had made a mistake.
The moment (that) I saw you, I knew you were angry with me.
Immediately he saw the police, he ran away.

III.　地点状语从句

Make a mark where you have any doubt or question.
区分定语从句和地点状语
Put the book where it used to be.（地点状语从句）
I visited the factory where my father worked before.（定语从句，先行词 the factory 在从句中充当地点状语）

IV.　原因状语从句

（1）引导原因状语从句的连词：because, as, since, now that
　　because：回答 why, 不与 so 连用

since = as = now that 表示众所周知、显而易见的理由，在彼此已知道的事做理由陈述时使用，意为"既然"。

Since / As / Now that you are here, let's start the meeting.

（2）其他

Considering that they are just beginners, they are doing quite a good job.（考虑到）

Seeing he refused to help us, there is no reason why we should now help him.（鉴于）

（3）for（并列连词），表原因时，意在解释说明。

I caught a cold, for I had been walking around in the rain.

V. 目的状语从句

（1）引导目的状语从句的连词：so that, in order that, in case, for fear that, etc.

Let's take the front seats so that / in order that we may see more clearly.

You'd better take more clothes in case it is cold.（以免，以防）

He hid his jewelry for fear that it would be stolen.（唯恐）

（2）表目的的其他说法

to do, in order to do, so as to do（不能放在句首）

So as to catch the bus, he got up early.（×）

He got up early so as to catch the bus.（√）

VI. 结果状语从句

（1）引导结果状语从句的连词：so... that..., such... that..., so ... as to do

（2）such... that... & so... that...

① 含义：如此……以至于……

② 引导结果状语从句

③ 句型：such + a / an + a. + 名词单数 + that ... = so + a. + a / an + 名词单数 + that...

such + a. + 名词复数 +that ...

such + a. + 不可数名词 + that...

so + a. + that...

The teacher set such a difficult examination question that none of us worked it out.

= The teacher set so difficult an examination question that none of us worked it out.

特别关注：注意区分结果状语从句和定语从句。

It is so cold outside that I don't want to go out.

④ 当名词前有 many, much, few, little 修饰时，用 so 而不用 such。

The house cost so much money that we didn't buy it.

VII. 让步状语从句

（1）引导让步状语从句的连词：though, although, even if, even though, -ever, no matter wh-, as, while

① though = although "虽然"，不与 but 连用，可以与 yet, still 连用

He still went there, though he didn't feel very well.

② no matter wh- & -ever

No matter where you are, you should work out.

However late he is, his mother will wait for him to have a dinner together.

= No matter how late he is, …

（2）as 引导的让步状语从句

① *a. / ad.*

Clever as he is, he never works hard.

Much as I admire his courage, I don't think he acted wisely.

② *v.*

Try as he does, he never seems able to do the work beautifully.

③ *n.*

Child as he is, he has a lot of knowledge.

VIII. 比较状语从句

同级比较 as… as… 或 so… as…（多用于否定句中）。例如：

Jim is not quite as good a student as his sister.

She is almost as happy here as she was at home.

The horse is getting old and can't run as / so fast as did.

IX. 方式状语从句

as 意为"按照，像"。例如：

Please do it as I tell you to.

As Americans like baseball, the British like soccer.

X. 条件状语从句

（1）引导条件状语从句的连词：if, unless, as long as（只要），注意从句的将来动作用一般现在时表示。

As long as you study hard, you'll get good results.

Unless he comes, I won't come here.

（2）其他

We'll let you use the room on condition that / provided that you keep it clean and tidy.

5．虚拟语气

 自测题

1. If they had sent a check to the telephone company last week, their telephone _____ out of service at this moment.

   A. will not be   B. will not have been

   C. would not be   D. would not have been

2. _____ before we departed last weekend, we would have had a wonderful dinner party.
   A. Had they arrived   B. Would they arrive
   C. Were they arriving   D. Were they to arrive

3. Had Paul received six more votes in the last election, he _____ our chairman now.
   A. must be   B. would have been
   C. shall be   D. would be

4. Both approaches require that the actor _____ his or her own personal values as well as the character's.
   A. must understand   B. should understand
   C. has to understand   D. need to understand

5. It is requested that all the students _____ present at the meeting tomorrow.
   A. were   B. will be   C. are   D. be

6. The extensive survey suggested that their assumptions _____ totally wrong.
   A. were   B. be   C. was   D. would be

7. A recent survey suggested that if money were not an issue, most mothers _____ not to work at all.
   A. should prefer   B. prefer
   C. would prefer   D. preferred

8. We are sure that _____ to do this face to face, he would find it difficult to express himself without losing his temper.
   A. were he to try   B. would he try
   C. was he trying   D. if he tries

9. Had I been you, I _____ an umbrella with me.
   A. would take   B. had taken
   C. would have taken   D. will take

10. This result suggested that his plan _____ something wrong.
    A. should have   B. have
    C. has   D. has had

11. _____ today, he would get there by Friday.
    A. Would he leave   B. Was he leaving
    C. Were he to leave   D. If he leaves

12. The law requires that everyone _____ his car checked at least once a year.
    A. has   B. had

C. have   D. have to have

答案：1-5 C A D B D   6-10 A C A C C   11-12 A C

📖 虚拟语气语法知识重　点简要回顾

I.　虚拟语气在条件句中的应用

条件句的分类 { 真实条件句：假设的情况有可能发生
            { 虚拟条件句：纯然假设的情况或是发生的可能性不大

II.　虚拟条件句的应用

	主　句		从　句	
与现在事实相反	would should could might	+ do	动词的过去式	{ did { were
与过去事实相反	would should could might	+ have done	had + 过去分词	
与将来事实相反	would could should might	+ do	动词的过去式	{ did { were { were to do { should do

（1）一般情况

　　① 与现在事实相反。例如：

　　　　If I had much money, I would buy a house.

　　　　If you were me, how would you deal with the problem?

　　② 与过去事实相反。例如：

　　　　If the hurricane had happened during the daytime, there would have been many more deaths.

　　③ 与将来事实相反。例如：

　　　　If I failed / should fail / were to fail, I would try again.

（2）错综复杂时间条件句：有时条件从句所表示的动作与主句动作发生的时间不一致。例如：

　　If the weather had been more favorable, the crops would be growing still better.

　　注：从句为过去的动作，主句是现在的动作

　　Amy would be alive today if the doctor had come sooner last night.

　　注：从句为过去的动作，主句是现在的动作

（3）if 条件句中 if 的省略（部分倒装）。例如：

　　If we had made enough preparations, we would have succeeded.

→ Had we made enough preparations, we would have succeeded.

If there would be a flood, what should we do?

→ Should there be a flood, what should we do?

（4）表示假设的其他方式。例如：

Without music, the world would be a dull place.

We could have done better under more favorable conditions.

III. wish 的名词从句的虚拟语气

（1）用法：退后一个时态

现在→过去

过去→过去的过去

将来→过去的将来

I wish I remembered the address.

We wish we had paid more attention to our pronunciation.

I wish he would try again.

（2）同样用法的其他句型

as if = as though 似乎，好像……

if only 要是……就好了

They talked as if they had been friends for years.

The teacher has loved students as if they were her children.

If only I had listened to your advice.

If only I hadn't lost it.

IV. (should) + do

（1）suggest, order, demand, propose, command, request, desire, insist（建议、命令、要求、坚持）的名词性从句

I suggest that he（should）give up smoking.

My suggestion is that he (should) give up smoking.

It is suggested that he (should) give up smoking.

My suggestion that he (should) give up smoking was supported by his parents.

特例：suggest "建议" 用虚拟语气 (should) do

　　　　　 "暗示" 不用虚拟语气

Her surprised impression suggested she didn't know that.

insist "要求" 用虚拟语气 (should) do

　　　 "坚持认为" 不用虚拟语气

I insist that I'm right.

（2）It's a pity, It's a shame, It's incredible, It's strange, It's no wonder, It's natural 等主语从句中

It is a great pity that he should be so conceited.

It's incredible that he should have finished the work so soon.

6. 倒装

 自测题

1. Not until recent years _____ a popular means of communication.
   A. e-mail became
   B. e-mail has become
   C. did e-mail become
   D. will e-mail become

2. _____ shall we forget the day when we received the admission into Harvard University.
   A. No time
   B. Never
   C. No sooner
   D. Nonetheless

3. Scarcely _____ those words when suddenly the monster was transformed into a very handsome youth.
   A. had he uttered
   B. did he utter
   C. he had uttered
   D. he did utter

4. Only by understanding the Web deeply _____ hope for people to grasp its full potential.
   A. can there be
   B. can be there
   C. be there can
   D. there can be

5. _____ will Mr. Forbes be able to regain control of the company.
   A. With hard work
   B. As regards his hard work
   C. Only if he works hard
   D. Despite his hard work

6. The price here is much higher than in some other stores. Never again _____ here.
   A. I will shop
   B. will I shop
   C. shop I
   D. I do shop

7. Only _____ solve this problem.
   A. I can
   B. can I
   C. am I
   D. I am

8. Not only _____ face it, but also _____ try to conquer it.
   A. we should; we should
   B. should we; should we
   C. we should; should we
   D. should we; we should

9. Under his arm _____ a pair of shoes which he had bought from the shop.
   A. is
   B. are
   C. were
   D. was

答案：1-5 C B A A C 6-9 B A D D

倒装语法知识重点简要回顾

I. 倒装语序
完全倒装（主语和谓语倒装，主谓→谓主）
部分倒装（只是谓语相应的助动词提前）

II. 完全倒装

（1）由引导词 there 引起的句子（there be 句型中）。例如：

There are many people in the park.

（2）由 there, here 等词引起，谓语为 come, go 的句子。例如：

There comes the bus.

特例：当句子的主语为代词时，不倒装。例如：

Here you are.

There he comes.

（3）由 then 引起，谓语为 come 等词的句子。例如：

Then came a new difficulty.

特例：当句子的主语为代词时，不倒装。

（4）以 out, in, up, down, away 等副词在句首表强调。例如：

Up went the arrow into the air.

特例：当句子的主语为代词时，不倒装。例如：

Down it flew.

Away they went.

（5）表语置于句首"表语 + 系动词 + 主语"。例如：

表语可以是：

① 介词短语

On either side were rows of trees.

② 形容词

Very important in students' life is hard-working.

③ 副词

Below is a restaurant.

④ 过去分词

Seated on the ground are a group of young men.

⑤ 现在分词

Watching the performance were mostly foreign guests.

（6）以 so, nor, neither 开头的句子，谓语所表示的情况也适合于另一个人，注意助动词的选择。例如：

He went swimming yesterday. So did I.

He has learned English for 4 years. So have I.

He can't drive a car. Nor / Neither can I.

特例：如果只是重复前面一句话的意思，不倒装。例如：

It was cold yesterday. So it was.

III. 部分倒装

（1）省略了 if 的虚拟条件句（had, were, should 开头）。例如：

Were she here, she would support the plan.

Had I been informed earlier, I could have done something.

Should anyone call, tell him to wait for me here.

（2）某些表示祝愿的句子。例如：

May you succeed.

（3）as 的让步状语从句。例如：

Angry as he was, he managed to speak calmly.

（4）表示"一……就"的特殊句型

No sooner… than…

Hardly… when…

Scarcely… when…

（5）Not until 的句型。例如：

Not until I began to work did I realize how much time I had wasted.

（6）含有否定意义的词放在句首。例如：

Never shall I forget it.

Little did he know who she was.

（7）做状语的 only 短语位于句首时。例如：

Only in this way can you work out the problem.

特例：当 only 修饰主语时不倒装。例如：

Only a teacher can do it.

（8）So…that 句型中的 so + a. / ad. 位于句首时。例如：

So loudly did he speak that even people in the next room could hear him.

7．强调句型

（1）强调句型只有 it is / was 两种形式。

（2）区分强调句型和 it 为形式主语的主语从句。例如：

It is important that we should get good command of English.

It is English that we should get good command of.

（二）长难句分析

在正式医学博士英语统考中，很多考生虽然有很好的单词基础，但对于阅读理解，尤其是长难句感到无所适从，进而影响对篇章的理解以及正确解题。这是因为这类考生运用语法背景知识的综合能力欠佳。具备一定的语法知识，考生应付简单句或者单一型的复合句还有信心，但是当语句综合了多种语法现象后，考生就无能为力了。这部分就这一问题给予考生一些启示和帮助。

总的说来，长难句之所以又长又难，是因为在语句中综合运用了如下结构：并列平行结构、非谓语动词、复合句以及特殊句型。下面请考生运用上面所掌握的基本语法知识分析下面的长难句，并且进行翻译。

1. Sveiby's answer is intangible assets, which he defines as employee competence, internal structures (systems, patents, etc.), and external structures (customer and supplier relationships and the organization's image).

_____

_____

【单　　词】intangible asset 无形资产；competence 能力。

【结构分析】由 which 引导非限制性定语从句，在定语从句中，由 and 连接两个并列成分。

【参考译文】Sveiby 的答案是无形资产，他将无形资产界定为员工能力、内部结构（制度、专利品等）以及外部结构（顾客和厂商的关系以及企业形象）。

2. Since knowledge is a key intangible asset, the ability to transfer knowledge from one employee to another, or from outside sources to employees, is a key business capacity, in Sveiby's view.

_____

_____

_____

【单　　词】capacity 能力；transfer...from...to... 将……从……转移到……

【结构分析】since 引导一个原因状语从句，在主句中，由不定式修饰名词 ability。在不定式中有一个由 or 连接的并列成分。

【参考译文】按照 Sveiby 的观点来看，既然知识是个关键的无形资产，将知识从一个员工传递给另一个员工，或者从外部资源传递给员工的能力就是企业的一个重要能力。

3. Like rush-hour drivers fuming when a single accident halts the evening commute, people surfing the Internet squirm if a Web page is slow to load or when access itself is not instantaneous.

_____

_____

_____

【单　　词】fume 发怒；halt 停止；commute 交通；squirm 蠕动；instantaneous 瞬间的。

【结构分析】fuming 现在分词做定语修饰 driver；when 引导时间状语从句；surfing 现在分词做定语修饰 people；if 引导的条件状语从句与 when 引导的时间状语从句并列。

【参考译文】就像因事故而被堵在晚间高峰路上发怒的司机一样，如果网页打开很慢或者当不能很快进入网页时，上网的人就会坐立不安。

4. Sucking, which is the infant's means of gaining both food and emotional security, conditions the association of eating with well-being or with deprivation.

_____

_____

【单　　词】sucking 吸吮；condition 是动词，意为"决定，为……条件"；deprivation 剥夺。

【结构分析】which 引导非限制性定语从句修饰 sucking。

【参考译文】作为婴儿获得食物和情感安全的一个手段，吸吮决定了吃东西与健康之间的联系或者与剥夺之间的联系。

5. If the child is breast-fed and has supportive body contact as well as good milk intake, if the child is allowed to suck for as long as he or she desires, and if both the child and mother enjoy the nursing experience and share their enjoyment, the child, is more likely to thrive both physically and emotionally.

_____

_____

_____

【单　　词】thrive 茁壮成长。

【结构分析】此语句是由 and 连接三个并列 if 引导的条件状语从句。

【参考译文】如果孩子是母乳喂养并且既能喝到优质的奶水，又可以享受有益的身体接触，如果允许孩子想吸吮多久就多久，并且如果母婴都能享受哺乳过程并且分享快乐，那么孩子就有可能身心都能茁壮健康地成长。

6. On the other hand, if the mother is nervous and resents the child or cuts him or her off from the milk supply before either the child's hunger or sucking need is satisfied, or handles the child hostilely during the feeding, or props the baby with a bottle rather than holding the child, the child may develop physically but will begin to show signs of emotional disturbance at an early age.

_____

_____

_____

【单　　词】resent 愤恨；hostilely 敌对地；prop 支撑；disturbance 扰乱。

【结构分析】在由 if 引导的条件状语从句中，由 or 连接一共 5 个并列成分。

【参考译文】另一方面，如果母亲很紧张并且怨恨孩子或者在孩子仍旧很饿或还没吃够的时候不让孩子吃奶了，再或者在喂奶时对待孩子充满敌意，或者用奶瓶支撑孩子而不是抱着孩子，这个孩子可能身体发育但是将会在早期开始出现情绪障碍的迹象。

7. This conditioning to food can remain unchanged through a lifetime unless the individual is awakened to the fact of conditioning and to the possible need for altering his or her

eating patterns in order to improve nutritional intake.

_____

_____

_____

【单　　词】conditioning 训练，熏陶，使习惯于；alter 改变；nutritional 有营养的。

【结构分析】在由 unless 引导的条件状语从句中，altering 为现在分词做介词 for 的宾语，并且 in order to do 为不定式短语做目的状语。

【参考译文】这种取得食物的习惯可能一生都不会有任何改变，除非一个人对这种熏陶的事实有所醒悟，为了改进营养的摄入而改变他或她的饮食方式。

8. Without the vast advances made by chemists, physicists, biologists, geologists, and other diligent scientists, our standards of living would decline, our flourishing, wealthy nation might come to an economic depression, and our people would suffer from disease that could not be cured.

_____

_____

_____

【单　　词】diligent 勤奋的；decline 下降；flourishing 繁茂的；economic depression 经济衰退。

【结构分析】此句为一种特殊句型：虚拟语气。Without the vast advances made by chemists, physicists, biologists, geologists, and other diligent scientists… 相当于 if 引导的虚拟条件句，即 if there were not the vast advances made by chemists, physicists, biologists, geologists, and other diligent scientists… 在虚拟条件句的主句中，that 引导的定语从句修饰 disease。

【参考译文】如果没有由化学家、物理学家、生物学家、地质学家以及其他勤奋的科学家所取得的巨大进步，我们的生活水平就会下降，我们繁荣而富有的国家就可能出现经济衰退，我们的人民就会患上无法治愈的疾病。

9. Despite the greatness of present-day innovators and scientists and their revelations, it is requisite to examine the amenities of science that our culture so blatantly disregards.

_____

_____

_____

【单　　词】innovators 创新者；revelation 启示；requisite 必不可少的；amenity 便利设施，舒适；blatantly 明目张胆地，公开地；disregard 忽视。

【结构分析】that 引导的定语从句修饰 amenity。

【参考译文】尽管当今创新者、科学家以及他们的启示很伟大，但还是有必要审视被我们的文化如此公开漠视的科学带给我们的便利和愉快。

10. Political leaders and scientists alike face the challenge of recognizing interrelationships and interactions between ecological, economic, and social factors and taking account of these factors when seeking solution strategies.

_____

_____

_____

_____

【单　　词】challenge 挑战；interaction 相互作用；take account of 考虑。

【结构分析】recognizing 与 taking account of 为并列成分，都做介词 of 的宾语。interrelationships 与 interactions 为并列成分，都做动词 recognizing 的宾语。seeking 为现在分词做时间状语。

【参考译文】政治家和科学家同样面临识别生态、经济和社会因素之间相互关系和相互作用的挑战，并且当他们寻求解决办法的时候，他们同样面临考虑这些因素的挑战。

（三）长难句专项练习

1. A person may relay his or her feelings, thoughts, and reactions through body positioning, body contact, body odors, eye contact, responsive actions, habits, attitudes, interests, state of health, dress and grooming, choice of lifestyle, and use of talents — in fact, through everything the individual says or does.

_____

_____

_____

_____

【单　　词】relay 传递；body odors 体味；grooming 打扮，装束。

【结构分析】此句较长的原因在于 through 后面的并列宾语内容较多。句子主干为：A person relay his or her feelings, thoughts and reactions through everything the individual says or does.

【参考译文】一个人可以通过身体姿势、身体接触、体味、眼神的交流、回应举动、习惯、态度、兴趣、身体状况、衣着服饰、生活方式的选择以及才能的运用，实际上通过所有这个人的所做所说来传递他或她的感受、看法以及反应。

2. The degree to which a person is able to communicate depends upon the extent of his or her conscious awareness, priority of need, and control of this process.

_____

_____

_____

【单　　词】conscious awareness 意识知觉。

【结构分析】此句中 which 引导的定语从句使句子主干的主语与谓语分开，主谓应该为：the degree depends on…

【参考译文】一个人能够交流的程度取决于他或她意识觉知的内容、需要的优先以及对于这个过程的控制。

3. The person often projects fears and fantasies onto others, so that no matter what the real content is of the messages that others relay, the messages received are threatening ones.

【单　　词】project 投掷，发送；project sth. onto sb. 将……加诸……；fantasy 幻想。

【结构分析】so that 引导结果状语从句，在该结果状语从句中 no matter what 引导状语从句，这个状语从句中 that others relay 是定语从句，修饰 messages。

【参考译文】一个人经常将恐惧和幻想加诸别人身上，这样无论别人传递的信息真正内容是什么，这个人接收到的信息都是感到有威胁性的。

4. Unless such a block is removed shortly after happening, it can have profound and complicating effects that will distort emotional and mental growth and arrest the development potential of the individual.

【单　　词】block 妨碍；profound 深远的；complicating 复杂的；distort 扭曲，歪曲；arrest 阻止。

【结构分析】unless 引导条件状语从句，在主句中 that will distort…and arrest… 为定语从句，修饰 effect。

【参考译文】除非这样的障碍在其发生后不久就被消除，否则它会产生深远且复杂的影响。这样的影响将会扭曲情感和心理方面的成长，也会阻碍一个人潜能的开发。

5. Without the vaccines created by doctors, disease such as polio, measles, hepatitis, and the flu would post a threat to our citizens, for although some of these diseases may not be deadly, their side effects can be a vast detriment to an individual affected with the disease.

【单　　词】vaccine 疫苗；polio 小儿麻痹症；measles 麻疹；hepatitis 肝炎；detriment 损害。

【结构分析】without 引导的介词短语相当于由 if 引导的虚拟条件句。such as 后面为并列列举 diseases。for 引导表原因的并列句。在这个并列句中 although 引导让步状语从句。an individual affected 中的 affected 为过去分词做定语修饰 individual。

【参考译文】如果没有医生们发明的疫苗，疾病例如小儿麻痹症、麻疹、肝炎以及流感将会威胁到我们的公民。因为尽管这些疾病可能不致命，但它们的副作用对患病人却造成莫大的伤害。

6. Without the presence of this machine, our world could exist, but the conveniences brought into life by the computer are unparalleled.

【单　　词】unparalleled 空前的，无比的。

【结构分析】without 引导的介词短语相当于由 if 引导的条件虚拟句，brought into life... 不是谓语动词，而是过去分词做 conveniences 的定语。

【参考译文】如果没有这个机器的出现，我们的世界或许还存在，但计算机带给我们生活的便利是史无前例的。

7. Research now indicates that blind and sighted people display the same skill at locating a sound's origin when using both ears, but some blind people can home in on sounds more accurately than their sighted counterparts when all have one ear blocked. Canadian scientists describe the work in the Sept. 17 *Nature*.

【单　　词】indicate 指出；counterpart 配对物；home in on sth. 把（注意力等）集中于……

【结构分析】在 that blind and sighted people display 引导的宾语从句中，using 为现在分词做状语，when all have one ear blocked 为状语从句。

【参考译文】如今，研究表明：当使用两只耳朵定位声源时，盲人和有视力的人显示出同样的技能，但是当他们的一只耳朵被堵住时，一些盲人的注意力要比同样测试的有视力的人更能准确地集中在声音上。加拿大科学家在 9 月 17 日《自然》杂志上对此有所描述。

8. A survey of news stories in 1996 reveals that the antiscience tag has been attached to many other groups as well, from authorities who advocated the elimination of the last remaining stocks of smallpox virus to Republicans who advocated decreased funding for basic research.

_____

_____

_____

_____

【单　　词】antiscience tag 反科学的标签；attached to 将……系在……；elimination 消除；smallpox 天花。

【结构分析】主句主干结构为：A survey… reveals。that 引导 reveal 的宾语从句。宾语从句的主干为 the antiscience tag has been attached to many other groups… from authorities… to Republicans... 在宾语从句中，who advocated the elimination... 是定语从句，修饰 authorities；而 who advocates decreased... 是另一个定语从句修饰 Republicans。

【参考译文】1996 年的一篇新闻报道调查显示，反科学的标签也可以贴在许多其他团体上，从鼓吹要消灭最后残留的天花病毒的组织机构到主张削减基础研究经费的共和党人。

9. The great interest in exceptional children shown in public education over the past three decades indicates the strong feeling in our society that all citizens, whatever their special conditions, deserve the opportunity to fully develop their capabilities.

_____

_____

_____

_____

【单　　词】exceptional children 特殊儿童；deserve to 值得，应受。

【结构分析】句子主语为 great interest，谓语为 indicates。shown 为过去分词修饰 interest。the strong feeling... 为 indicate 的宾语从句。在宾语从句中，that all citizens... 为同位语从句，whatever their special conditions 为插入语。

【参考译文】在过去 30 年间，公共教育对特殊儿童的极大兴趣表明我们社会中人们的一种强烈感受，即无论公民处于多么特殊的境地，所有人都应该有充分发挥自身才能的机会。

10. Even the folk knowledge in social systems on which ordinary life is based in earning, spending, organizing, marrying, taking part in political activities, fighting and so on, is not very dissimilar from the more sophisticated images of the social system derived from the social sciences, even though it is built upon the very imperfect samples of personal experience.

_____

_____

_____

_____

【单　　词】dissimilar 相异的；sophisticated 久经世故的；derive from 从……由来。

【结构分析】主句主语为 folk knowledge, 谓语为系表结构 is not very dissimilar from…, derived from 为过去分词短语做定语修饰 images。even though 为让步状语从句。

【参考译文】甚至在基于普通生活的社会体系中，在挣钱、花钱、结社、结婚、参加政治活动及战争等方面的大众知识与那些从社会学衍生而来的社会体系中更高深的描绘并没有很大的不同，尽管这一结论基于个人经历中那些极不完美的例子。

11. Foods and medicine, also classified according to their reputed intrinsic nature as Yin (cold) and Yang (hot), may be taken therapeutically to correct the imbalance resulting from ill health, or to correct imbalance due to the overindulgence in a food manifestly excessively "hot" or "cold", or due to age or changed physiological status (for example, pregnancy).

_____

_____

_____

_____

【单　　词】reputed 有名气的；intrinsic 内在的；therapeutically 治疗地；overin-dulgence 过度嗜好；manifestly 明白地。

【结构分析】主语为 food and medicine, 这个主语由过去分词短语 classified... 修饰；谓语为 may be taken therapeutically…，两个不定式 to correct... 为并列结构，做目的状语；两个 due to... 为介词短语，表原因，且由 or 连接。

【参考译文】根据其普遍认可的内在性质，食物和药品也被分为"阴"（凉性）和"阳"（热性）；在治疗学上，它们可以用来治疗由疾病引起的失调，也可治疗因过度嗜好过热或过冷食品而引发的身体失衡，或治疗因年龄或生理变化（如怀孕）所带来的身体失调。

12. It is information systems that affect the scope and quality of health care, make social services more equitable, enhance personal comfort, provide a greater measure of safety and mobility, and extend the variety of leisure forms at one's disposal.

_____

_____

_____

_____

【单　　词】scope 范围；equitable 公正的；mobility 活动性；at one's disposal 任某人支配。

【结构分析】此句为强调句型,强调的内容为 information system, affect、make、enhance、provide、extend 为并列谓语。

【参考译文】正是信息系统影响着人们医疗保健的范围和质量,它使社会服务更加公正,它提高了个人的舒适度,为安全和自由行动采取更多的措施,并根据个人的意愿增加闲暇活动的多样性。

13. While larger banks can afford to maintain their own data-processing operations, many smaller regional and community banks are finding that the costs associated with upgrading data-processing equipment and with the development and maintenance of new products and technical staff are prohibitive.

_____

_____

_____

_____

【单　　词】maintenance 维护;prohibitive 禁止的。

【结构分析】while 引导让步状语从句,主句主干为 banks are finding,后面紧跟一个由 that 引导的宾语从句,在该宾语从句中,主语为 costs, associated with 为过去分词做定语,且为多个并列结构,谓语为 are prohibitive。

【参考译文】尽管大银行有能力花钱来保持它们自己的数据处理正常运行,但是许多小的地区银行和社区银行却发现:与更新数据处理设备、发展和维护新产品以及技术人员费用等有关的成本费用高不可攀;而且技术人员的费用也非常昂贵。

14. The point at which tool using and tool making acquire evolutionary significance is surely when an animal can adapt its ability to manipulate objects to a wide variety of purposes, and when it can use an object spontaneously to solve a brand-new problem that without the use of a tool would prove insoluble.

_____

_____

_____

_____

【单　　词】evolutionary 进化的;manipulate 操纵,使用;spontaneously 自然地,本能地;insoluble 无法解决的。

【结构分析】句子的框架是 "The point...is...when...and when..."。两个 when 引导的从句为并列的表语从句。at which tool using and tool making acquire evolutionary significance 为定语从句修饰主语 the point;第二个 when 引导的表语从句中也有 that 引导的定语从句修饰 a brand-new problem。ability to manipulate objects 译为"操纵物体的能力";"...a brand-new problem that without the use of a tool would prove insoluble"中 without

和 insoluble 为双重否定，可译成肯定句。

【参考译文】当动物能够使自己操纵物体的能力适用于更广泛的目标范围，并且能够自发地使用物体解决只有通过工具才能解决的崭新问题时，工具的使用和制造就一定达到了具有进化意义的阶段。

15. At the same time, the American Law Institute — a group of judges, lawyers, and academics whose recommendations carry substantial weight — issued new guidelines for tort law stating that companies need not warn customers of obvious dangers or bombard them with a lengthy list of possible ones.

_____

_____

_____

_____

【单　　词】substantial 实质的；tort law 民事侵权法；bombard 炮轰，轰击。

【结构分析】主语为 the American Law Institute，谓语为 issued，"a group of…"为插入语。stating 为现在分词，"that companies need not…"为 state 的宾语从句。

【参考译文】与此同时，美国法律研究所—— 由一群法官、律师和理论专家组成，他们的建议分量极重，发布了新的民事伤害法令指导方针，宣称公司不必提醒顾客注意显而易见的危险，也不必连篇累牍地一再提请他们注意一些可能会出现的危险。

四、考查内容及相应的应试技巧

（一）主要测试题型

1. 主旨题

此类考题主要测试考生对全文中心思想的理解和把握，常用提问方式有：

The main idea of this passage is _____.

The best title of this passage is _____.

The passage mainly discusses _____.

The main purpose of the article is _____.

The general idea of the passage is _____.

当考生根据题目特点判断考题为主旨题时，先不要急于解题。在完成其他细节题后，会对文章有比较深入的了解，这样解题会比较省时省力。另外，解题时，应该重点阅读文章的首段和末段，看是否出现文章的主题句。如果没有，则阅读每一段的主题句，然后总结出大意，对比选项。

2. 细节题

此类考题在考试中比重较大，主要有以下几种方式：细节排除题、细节辨析题、细节判断题。细节题是测试考生对文章某个特性信息的掌握和理解。如果细节题与某一具体细节有关，则根据线索词在原文寻找答案。如果测试事例作者对这一现象的看法，就要联系本段落的主题句解题，考虑段落所体现的逻辑关系。往往在文章中能够找到解题看法的线索词，如：

表示列举的线索词：first, second, finally, next, then, meanwhile, besides, also, in addition to 等；

表示因果关系的线索词：because, as a result of, due to, for, since, now that, thus, therefore, consequently, hence, accordingly, on account of, lead to, result in, result from 等；

表示比较的线索词：unlike, like, in comparison, likewise, similarly 等；

表示转折的线索词：but, yet, however, on the other hand, though, although, while, nevertheless, on the contrary, in spite of, despite 等；

表示举例的线索词：for instance, such as, for example, that is, namely 等。

3. 解释题或猜词题

这类考题测试考生对某一个词语、短语或语句的正确理解，通常包括单词释义、短语释义、句子释义。常用提问方式有：

By…the author means / refers to _____.

In this paragraph, the word "…" probably means _____.

The first sentence in Paragraph 5 means _____.

According to the passage, … can be best defined as _____.

The line…that author uses the word "…" to indicate _____.

这类考题的解题关键在于，一定要在原文信息中理解单词或短语的含义。

4. 态度题

这类考题考查考生对作者针对某现象的看法、观点等。常用提问方式有：

The author's attitude towards something is _____.

What's the writer's attitude to _____?

What's the tone of the passage?

5. 推理题

推理就是对文章的引申义或比喻义进行逻辑推理，从字面理解上升到对文章的宏观把握。题干常见词汇：imply, suggest, infer, assume。这类题型较难。

We can infer from the passage that _____.

It can be assumed that _____.

The passage suggests that _____.

The next paragraph would probably discuss _____.

From the passage, we can see the author feels that _____.

（二）应试技巧提示

1．先看题目，再看文章

由于医学博士英语考试时间很紧，而且这部分一共有六篇较长的文章，因而考生必须在短时间内，既快速又准确地解题。在这种情况下，建议考生先看题目，根据题目设置以及题干的关键词直接在文章中找到相应的原文信息，这样能够缩短阅读时间以及阅读量。

2．一切解题来源于原文信息

无论是上述哪类题型，所有解题都必须依据原文信息。避免"想当然"的好办法就是在原文解题出处做标注，根据原文做出正确选择。

3．培养快速阅读能力

在 65 分钟内，要完成 6 篇文章的阅读以及 30 道阅读理解的题目，对考生来说，是一个巨大的挑战。而这一挑战的最大障碍就是时间有限。因而考生要考虑如何在有限时间内完成这部分测试。在这种情况下，建议考生根据题目阅读，并且只阅读与题目有关的相关信息，换句话说，没有设置考题的原文部分略读或者不读，这样就能大大减少文章阅读量。

4．注重不同题型不同解题方法

在英语阅读理解中，常用的阅读方法有：

skimming（快速浏览法）用于找出文章的主旨大意；

scanning（找读法）用于快速查找所需特定信息，用于细节题；

intensive reading（精读法）用于无法立即从文章中找到答案，需要一定的判断、推理以及参考上下文信息的情况。

考生要根据不同的题型，使用恰当的阅读方法，灵活运用，在备考阶段要在阅读技巧和阅读方法方面多加练习。在下面的专项练习部分，本书将根据不同题型给予更加细致的分析。

5．认真揣摩错误选项的方式

在近几年的医学博士考试中，出题方式使得题目本身的难度增加，再加上四个选项的设置也更加混淆考生的理解，极容易出现错误。因而在平时训练备考时，应着重注意混淆项的设置，提高自身"去伪存真"的能力。

五、阅读理解专项练习及最新真题解析

Passage One

By almost every measure, Paul Pfingst is an unsentimental prosecutor. Last week the San Diego County district attorney said he fully intends to try to suspect Charles Andrew Williams, 15, as an adult for the Santana High School shootings. Even before the tragedy, Pfingst had stood behind the controversial California law that mandates treating murder suspects as young as 14 as adults.

So nobody would have wagered that Pfingst would also be the first D.A. in the U.S. to launch his very own Innocence Project. Yet last June, Pfingst told his attorneys to go back over old murder and rape convictions and see if any unravel with newly developed DNA-testing tools. In other words, he wanted to revisit past victories — this time playing for the other team. "I think people misunderstand being conservative for being biased," says Pfingst. "I consider myself a pragmatic guy, and I have no interest in putting innocent people in jail."

Around the U.S., flabbergasted defense attorneys and their jailed clients cheered his move. Among prosecutors, however, there was an awkward pause. After all, each DNA test costs as much as $5,000. Then there's the unspoken risk: if dozens of innocents turn up, the D.A. will have indicted his shop.

But nine months later, no budgets have been busted or prosecutors ousted. Only the rare case merits review. Pfingst's team considers convictions before 1993, when the city started routine DNA testing. They discard cases if the defendant has been released. Of the 560 remaining files, they have re-examined 200, looking for cases with biological evidence and defendants who still claim innocence.

They have identified three so far. The most compelling involves a man serving 12 years for molesting a girl who was playing in his apartment. But others were there at the time. Police found a small drop of saliva on the victim's shirt — too small a sample to test in 1991. Today that spot could free a man. Test results are due any day. Inspired by San Diego, 10 other counties in the U.S. are starting DNA audits.

1. How did Pfingst carry out his own Innocence Project?
   A. By getting rid of his bias against the suspects.
   B. By revisiting the past victories.
   C. By using the newly developed DNA-testing tools.
   D. By his cooperation with his attorneys.

2. Which of the following can be an advantage of Innocence Project?
   A. To help correct the wrong judgments.
   B. To oust the unqualified prosecutors.
   C. To make the prosecutors in an awkward situation.
   D. To cheer up the defense attorneys and their jailed clients.

3. The expression "flabbergasted" (Paragraph 3) most probably means _____.
   A. excited   B. competent   C. embarrassed   D. astounded

4. Why was Pfingst an unsentimental prosecutor?
   A. He intended to try a fifteen-year old suspect.

B. He had no interest in putting the innocent in jail.

C. He supported the controversial California law.

D. He wanted to try suspect as young as fourteen.

5. Which of the following is NOT true according to the text?

A. Pfingst's move didn't have a great coverage.

B. Pfingst's move had both the positive and negative effect.

C. Pfingst's move didn't work well.

D. Pfingst's move greatly encouraged the jailed prisoners.

 本文话题

　　第一段指出芬斯特作为一位铁面无私的检察官的一些做法；第二段指出芬斯特实施"清白计划"的打算及做法；第三段指出实施"清白计划"造成的反应以及可能存在的问题；第四段和第五段是实施"清白计划"的结果和影响。

 难词译注

prosecutor ['prɔsikjuːtə(r)] n.	检察官，检察员，起诉人，原告
controversial [kɔntrə'vəːʃ(ə)l] a.	争论的，争议的
mandate ['mændeit] v.	批准制定一个训令，如通过法律；发布命令或要求
wager ['weidʒə(r)] v.	下赌注，保证
conviction [kən'vikʃ(ə)n] n.	定罪，宣告有罪
unravel [ʌn'ræv(ə)l] v.	阐明，解决
flabbergast ['flæbəgɑːst; (US) -gæst] v.	<口> 使大吃一惊，哑然失色，使目瞪口呆
indict [in'dait] v.	起诉，控告，指控，告发
bust [bʌst] v.	破产或缺钱
oust [aust] v.	剥夺，取代，驱逐
discard [di'skɑːd] v.	抛开，遗弃，废弃
molest [mə'lest] v.	骚乱，困扰，调戏
saliva [sə'laivə] n.	口水，唾液

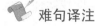 难句译注

1. Even before the tragedy, Pfingst had stood behind the controversial California law that mandates treating murder suspects as young as 14 as adults.

　　【分析】主体句式：...Pfingst had stood behind ...

结构分析：even before the tragedy 是本句的时间状语；主句是 Pfingst had stood behind...；that 引导的宾语从句修饰 law；在从句中，as...as 是词组，意思是"和……一样"；出现的第三个 as 是介词，意思是"作为"。

【译文】甚至在这场悲剧发生之前芬斯特就支持加利福尼亚州的一项颇有争议的法律。这项法律规定，以成人身份受审的谋杀嫌疑犯的最低年龄可以降到 14 岁。

答案及解析

1. 【问题】芬斯特是如何开展他的"清白计划"的？

A．通过消除他对嫌疑人的偏见。　　B．通过重访过去的成功。

C．通过使用新的 DNA 检测工具。　　D．通过和律师合作。

【答案】C

【解析】事实细节题。文中对应信息 "Pfingst told his attorneys to go back over old murder and rape convictions and see if any unravel with newly developed DNA-testing tools." 是对第二段第一句的补充说明。

2. 【问题】下列哪一个是"清白计划"的优势？

A．纠正过去错判的案件。　　B．驱逐不合格的检察官。

C．使得检察官处于尴尬的境地。　　D．鼓励辩护律师和入狱的犯人。

【答案】A

【解析】推理判断题。从上下文我们可以得知，实施"清白计划"就是使用先进的 DNA 技术来重新审理过去的案件当中可能存在的冤案和错案。

3. 【问题】第三段中 flabbergasted 的意思是_____。

A．兴奋的　　B．胜任的

C．尴尬的　　D．惊讶的

【答案】D

【解析】猜词题。从第二段第一句话得知，芬斯特可能是美国第一个实施非常独特的"清白计划"的人，因此他的做法很可能是令人感到吃惊的，从而可猜出该词的含义。

4. 【问题】为什么芬斯特是个铁血检察官？

A．他曾经审判过一个 15 岁的嫌疑人。　　B．他无意将清白的人错判入监。

C．他支持有争议的加州法律。　　D．他想审判小至 14 岁的嫌疑人。

【答案】B

【解析】推理判断题。从第一段和第二段给出的事例可以看出，芬斯特不愿放过任何一个犯罪的人，即便他的年龄还不算大；他也不愿使无辜者蒙冤，即便案件已经审理。

5. 【问题】根据文章，下列哪一个不正确？

A．芬斯特的行动覆盖面不大。

B．芬斯特的行为有正面和负面的效果。

C. 芬斯特的行为见效不大。

D. 芬斯特的行为很大程度鼓舞了入狱的犯人。

【答案】C

【解析】推理判断题。正因为"Pfingst's move works well",美国才又有"ten other counties are starting DNA audits",而且"no budgets have been busted or prosecutors ousted"。

Passage Two

As you read this, nearly 80,000 Americans are waiting for a new heart, kidney or some other organ that could save their life. Tragically, about 6,000 of them will die this year — nearly twice as many people as perished in the Sept. 11 attacks — because they won't get their transplant in time. The vast majority of Americans (86%, according to one poll) say they support organ donation. But only 20% actually sign up to do it. Why the shortfall?

Part of the problem is the way we handle organ donations. Americans who want to make this sort of gift have to opt in — that is, indicate on a driver's license that when they die, they want their organs to be made available. Many European and Asian countries take the opposite approach; in Singapore, for example, all residents receive a letter when they come of age informing them that their organs may be harvested unless they explicitly object. In Belgium, which adopted a similar presumed-consent system 12 years ago, less than 2% of the population has decided to opt out.

Further complicating the situation in the U.S. is the fact that whatever decision you make can be overruled by your family. The final say is left to your surviving relatives, who must make up their minds in the critical hours after brain death has been declared. There are as many as 50 body parts, from your skin to your corneas, that can save or transform the life of a potential recipient, but for many families lost in grief, the idea of dismembering a loved one is more than they can bear.

The U.S., like all medically advanced societies, has struggled to find a way to balance an individual's rightful sovereignty over his or her body with the society's need to save its members from avoidable deaths. Given America's tradition of rugged individualism and native distrust of Big Brotherly interference, it's not surprising that voters resisted attempts to switch to a presumed-consent system when it was proposed in California, Oregon, Minnesota, Pennsylvania and Maryland. Health Secretary Tommy Thompson last spring announced plans for a new initiative to encourage donations — including clearer consent forms — but its impact is expected to be modest. Given the crying need for organs, perhaps it's time we considered shifting to something closer to the presumed-consent model.

Meanwhile, if you want to ensure that your organs are donated when you die, you should say so in a living will or fill out a Uniform Donor Card (available from the American

Medical Association). Make sure your closest relatives know about it. And if you don't want to donate an organ, you should make your wishes equally explicit.

6. According to the author, one of the reasons for a shortage of organs in America is that _____.

A. most Americans are reluctant to donate their organs after death

B. the information about organ donation is not popular in America

C. the ways to handle organ donation is far from perfect

D. people waiting for transplant are rapidly increasing in America

7. What is most Americans' attitude towards the organ donation?

    A. Indifferent.   B. Indignant.   C. Detached.   D. Supportive.

8. It can be inferred from Paragraph 4 that _____.

A. Americans have a long tradition of weak individualism

B. all the states in America resist the presumed-consent system

C. it's not easy to find a way to serve the society's need and at the same time to protect the individual's right in the matter of organ donation

D. the government is not active in solving the problem

9. The term "presumed-consent" probably means _____.

A. one's organs should be donated whether they agree or not

B. one is supposed to agree that their organ will be donated after death unless they explicitly object

C. dismembering a dead body is inhuman

D. one is assumed to be happy after they decide to donate their organs

10. From the text, we can see the author's attitude towards organ donation is _____.

    A. supportive   B. indignant   C. indifferent   D. negative

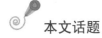 本文话题

    本篇文章在提出了一个解决美国国内捐献器官严重紧缺问题的办法。第一段以人们的良好愿望和严峻现实的强烈对比开始，第二段找出了产生这一问题的一个原因——运作方式有待提高，第三段找出了产生这一问题的另一个原因—— 人们的心理承受能力。第四段说明美国必须解决这个问题。最后一段指明目前捐献器官的方式及注意事项。

 难词译注

perish ['periʃ] v.	死，暴卒，毁灭
donation [dəu'neiʃən] n.	捐赠
shortfall ['ʃɔːtfɔːl] n.	不足之量，短缺的数额
opt [ɔpt] v.	（常与 for 连用）决定做；选择，选取

consent [kən'sent] *n & v.*	同意
overrule [ˌəuvə'ruːl] *v.*	驳回，否决
cornea ['kɔːniə] *n.*	角膜
dismember [dis'membə] *v.*	肢解
sovereignty ['sɔvrinti] *n.*	完全独立和自我统治，主权
rugged ['rʌgid] *a.*	粗犷的

 难句译注

1. There are as many as 50 body parts, from your skin to your corneas, that can save or transform the life of a potential recipient, but for many families lost in grief, the idea of dismembering a loved one is more than they can bear.

   【分析】主体句式：There are…, but the idea…is…

   结构分析：这句是由 but 做连接词的两个分句。第一个分句中包含一个由 that 引导的定语从句修饰 body parts；第二个分句的主语是 the idea。

   【译文】人身上有 50 种可捐献的器官，皮肤和角膜都包括在内。每种都可能救活一个人或改变他们的命运。但对正沉浸在丧失亲人之痛的人来说，把逝去的亲人大卸八块是他们承受不了的。

2. The U.S., like all medically advanced societies, has struggled to find a way to balance an individual's rightful sovereignty over his or her body with the society's need to save its members from avoidable deaths.

   【分析】主体句式：The U.S. … has struggled to find a way to balance …with…

   结构分析：其中短语"balance…with…"的含义是"使……和……相平衡"。

   【译文】像其他医学发达的国家一样，美国也在努力寻求个人和国家之间的最佳平衡点。即让个人对自己的身体有合法的拥有权，又能满足社会救死扶伤的需要。

答案及解析

6. 【问题】根据本文作者，美国器官短缺的原因之一是 _____ 。

   A．大多数美国人不愿意在死后捐献器官

   B．关于器官捐献的信息在美国不流行

   C．处理器官捐献的方式远远不够完善

   D．等待移植的人在美国迅速增加

   【答案】C

   【解析】事实细节题。从第一、二段可以读出，绝大多数美国人愿意捐出自己的器官，只是运作方式还有待提高。

7. 【问题】大多数美国人对器官捐献的态度是什么？

   A．冷漠的。　　　　　　　　B．愤怒的。

   C．不关注的。　　　　　　　D．支持的。

【答案】D

【解析】推理判断题。从第一段"The vast majority of Americans say they support organ donation"可以看出答案。

8. 【问题】从第四段可以推理得知 _____。

    A. 美国人的脆弱的个人主义历史悠久

    B. 美国所有的州都抵制假定捐献人同意的制度

    C. 在器官捐献方面找到满足社会需求，同时保护个人权益的方法是不容易的

    D. 政府在解决问题方面不积极

【答案】C

【解析】属事实细节题。政府也想改变目前这种状况，只不过措施不那么有效。

9. 【问题】术语"presumed-consent"的意思是 _____。

    A. 无论他们是否同意，他们的器官都应该被捐献

    B. 人们被认为同意在死后捐出自己器官，除非他们明确地反对

    C. 解剖尸体是不人道的

    D. 人们在决定捐献器官后应该感到高兴

【答案】B

【解析】属猜测词义题。从第二段对新加坡和比利时的描述中可以得出结论。

10. 【问题】从文中可以看出，作者对器官捐献的态度是 _____。

    A. 支持的   B. 愤怒的

    C. 冷淡的   D. 否定的

【答案】A

【解析】推理判断题。作者认为解决器官短缺这个难题，应该向新加坡和比利时学习，采取新的强有力的措施。最后一段作者给出了想捐献器官的做法以及应注意的问题，这也可以看出作者支持的态度。

Passage Three

Many theories concerning the causes of juvenile crime focus either on the individual or on society as the major contributing influence. Theories centering on the individual suggest that children engage in criminal behavior because they were not sufficiently penalized for previous delinquent acts or that they have learned criminal behavior through interaction with others. A person who becomes socially alienated may be more inclined to commit a criminal act. Theories focusing on the role of society in juvenile delinquency suggest that children commit crimes in response to their failure to rise above their socioeconomic status, or as a repudiation of middle-class values.

Most theories of juvenile delinquency have focused on children from disadvantaged families, ignoring the fact that children from affluent homes also commit crimes. The latter may commit crimes because of the lack of adequate parental control, delays in achieving adult status, and hedonistic tendencies. All theories, however, are tentative and are subject to criticism.

Changes in the American social structure may indirectly affect juvenile crime rates. For example, changes in the economy that lead to fewer job opportunities for youth and rising unemployment in general make gainful employment increasingly difficult for young people to obtain. The resulting discontent may in turn lead more youths into criminal behavior.

Families have also experienced changes within the last several decades. More families are one-parent households or have two working parents; consequently, children are likely to have less supervision at home than was common in the traditional family structure. This lack of parental supervision is thought to be an influence on juvenile crime rates.

Other identifiable causes of delinquent acts include frustration or failure in school, the increased availability of drugs, alcohol, and guns, and the growing incidence of child abuse and child neglect. All these conditions tend to increase the probability of a child committing a criminal act, although a direct causal relationship has not yet been established.

No specific treatment has been proven the most effective form. Effectiveness is typically measured by recidivism rates — that is, by the percentage of children treated who subsequently commit additional criminal acts. The recidivism rates for all forms of treatment, however, are about the same. A large percentage of delinquent acts are never discovered, which further complicates this measurement. Thus, an absence of subsequent reported delinquent acts by a treated child may mean nothing more than that the child was not caught.

11. Which of the following is NOT the factor of juvenile crimes according to the theories focusing on individuals?

A. Insufficient punishment.　　　　B. Less parental supervision.

C. Isolation from others.　　　　D. Lack of self-control.

12. According to the theories centering on society, which of the following is true?

A. Juveniles could not find his status in the society.

B. Unemployment leads to juvenile crimes.

C. Child abuse leads children to engaging in crimes.

D. Children's discontent with the changes in social structure causes juvenile crimes.

13. The sentence "All theories, however, are tentative and are subject to criticism." implies that _____.

A. all theories didn't disclose the true reasons for juvenile crimes

B. contributing factors these theories indicate are not comprehensive and convincing

C. these theories misled people's attention to the juvenile delinquency

D. these theories didn't supply the answers for the juvenile crimes

14. What can we know about recidivism rates?

    A. They are used to measure the effectiveness of treatments of juvenile delinquency.

    B. They indicate that children's criminal percentage.

    C. They simplified the measurement of treatments.

    D. They are modified in accordance with the specific treatment.

15. What is the tone of the passage?

    A. Critical.   B. Supportive.   C. Objective.   D. Indifferent.

 本文话题

青少年犯罪。

 难词译注

juvenile [ˈdʒuːvinail] *n.*	青少年
delinquent [diˈliŋkwənt] *a.*	违法的
repudiation [riˌpjuːdiˈeiʃən] *n.*	批判
alienate [ˈeiljəneit] *v.*	疏远
affluent [ˈæfluənt] *a.*	富裕的
recidivism [riˈsidivizəm] *n.*	累犯

 难句译注

1. Theories centering on the individual suggest that children engage in criminal behavior because they were not sufficiently penalized for previous delinquent acts or that they have learned criminal behavior through interaction with others.

    【分析】centering 现在分词做定语修饰 theories；that 引导宾语从句；because 引导原因状语从句；or 连接两个并列宾语从句。

    【译文】侧重个人的理论认为，儿童因为上一次的犯错没有受到足够的惩罚而参与犯罪，另外，认为儿童通过和他人的交往而学坏。

2. Theories focusing on the role of society in juvenile delinquency suggest that children commit crimes in response to their failure to rise above their socioeconomic status, or as a repudiation of middle-class values.

    【分析】focusing 现在分词做定语修饰 theories；or 连接两个并列成分，即 in response to... 和 as a repudiation...

    【译文】侧重在青少年犯罪中社会所处角色的理论认为，儿童犯罪是由于他们在社会经济中无法摆脱命运而引起的，或者是作为对中产阶级价值观的批判而产生。

3. ...changes in the economy that lead to fewer job opportunities for youth and rising

unemployment in general make gainful employment increasingly difficult for young people to obtain.

【分析】that 引导定语从句修饰 changes。

【译文】经济上的变革导致年轻人工作机会减少、失业增加，这使年轻人找到工作的机会变得越来越困难。

答案及解析

11. 【问题】根据个人理论，下面哪一个不是青少年犯罪的原因？

A. 惩罚不够。 B. 缺乏父母管教。

C. 孤僻。 D. 缺少自控能力。

【答案】D

【解析】细节题。A 项原文信息在第 1 段 "…because they were not sufficiently penalized for previous delinquent acts…"；B 项原文信息在第 2 段 "…because of the lack of adequate parental control…" 以及第 4 段 "…children are likely to have less supervision…"；C 项原文信息在第 1 段 "A person who becomes socially alienated may be more inclined to commit a criminal act."。由此可知只有 D 项未提及。

12. 【问题】根据社会理论，下面哪一个是正确的？

A. 青少年在社会上无法找到他们的地位。

B. 失业导致青少年犯罪。

C. 儿童受虐促使孩子们参与犯罪。

D. 孩子对社会结构变化不满导致青少年犯罪。

【答案】D

【解析】细节题。D 项原文信息在第 3 段，最后一句话提到，孩子们对因经济变化导致的就业机会少或失业不满，这导致他们的犯罪行为。

13. 【问题】"所有这些理论都是尝试性的，容易遭受批评"这句话暗示我们_____。

A. 所有理论都没有揭示青少年犯罪的真正原因

B. 这些理论提出的原因不够全面，也缺乏说服力

C. 这些理论误导了人们对青少年犯罪的关注

D. 这些理论没能为青少年犯罪提供答案

【答案】B

【解析】推断题。根据全文，这些理论有一定道理，但不能涵盖所有的原因，各自都有不足。故 B 含义与之最为接近。

14. 【问题】关于累犯率我们知道什么？

A. 被用于衡量针对青少年犯罪解决办法的有效程度。

B. 表明儿童犯罪的百分比。

C. 简化解决办法。

D. 被根据特定的解决办法进行修改。

【答案】A

【解析】关于累犯率的信息在原文最后一段。

15. 【问题】这篇文章的语气是什么？

      A. 批评的。   B. 支持的。   C. 客观的。   D. 漠不关心的。

【答案】C

【解析】态度题。综观全文，作者只是在客观地罗列各种理论，没有体现任何个人的偏爱和喜好，因而 C 为正确答案。

Passage Four

Most office workers assume that the messages they send to each other via electronic mail are as private as a telephone call or a face-to-face meeting. That assumption is wrong. Although it is illegal in many areas for an employer to <u>eavesdrop</u> on private conversations or telephone calls—even if they take place on a company-owned telephone—there are no clear rules governing electronic mail. In fact, the question of how private electronic mail transmissions should be has emerged as one of the more complicated legal issues of the electronic age.

People's opinions about the degree of privacy that electronic mail should have vary depending on whose electronic mail system is being used and who is reading the messages. Does a government office, for example, have the right to destroy electronic messages created in the course of running the government, thereby denying public access to such documents? Some hold that government offices should issue guidelines that allow their staff to delete such electronic records, and defend this practice by claiming that the messages thus deleted already exist in paper versions whose destruction is forbidden. Opponents of such practices argue that the paper versions often omit such information as who received the messages and when they received them, information commonly carried on electronic mail systems. Government officials, opponents maintain, are civil servants; the public should thus have the right to review any documents created during the conducting of government business.

Questions about electronic mail privacy have also arisen in the private sector. Recently, two employees of an automotive company were discovered to have been communicating disparaging information about their supervisor via electronic mail. The supervisor, who had been monitoring the communication, threatened to fire the employees. When the employees field a grievance complaining that their privacy had been violated, they were let go. Later, their court case for unlawful termination was dismissed; the company's lawyers successfully argued that because the company owned the computer system, its supervisors had the right to read anything created on it.

In some areas, laws prohibit outside interception of electronic mail by a third party without proper authorization such as a search warrant. However, these laws do not cover "inside" interception such as occurred at the automotive company. In the past, courts have ruled that interoffice communications may be considered private only if employees have a "reasonable expectation" of privacy when they send the messages. The fact is that no absolute guarantee of privacy exists in any computer system. The only solution may be for users to scramble their own messages with encryption codes; unfortunately, such complex codes are likely to undermine the principal virtue of electronic mail: its convenience.

16. The underlined word "eavesdrop" refers to _____.
    A. spy   B. overhear   C. watch over   D. wiretap

17. According to the passage, which of the following statements is true?
    A. There is a general consensus among people about the privacy of electronic mails.
    B. There are clear regulations supervising the privacy of electronic mails.
    C. There is no absolute guarantee of privacy in the computer system.
    D. The best solution is to use complex code to protect mails.

18. Based on the passage, the author's attitude towards interception of electronic mail can most accurately be described as _____.
    A. outright disapproval of the practice
    B. support for employers who engage in it
    C. support for employees who lose their jobs because of it
    D. intellectual interest in its legal issues

19. The example of automotive company is used to imply _____.
    A. in the private sector, it is natural to violate employees' privacy
    B. there is no law covering such interception
    C. determining whether the eavesdrop violate privacy depends on whose electronic mail system is being used and who is reading the messages
    D. employees should be careful with their communication in the computer system

20. The author's primary purpose in writing the passage is to _____.
    A. demonstrate that the individual right to privacy has been eroded by advances in computer technology
    B. compare the legal status of electronic mail in the public and private sectors
    C. draw an extended analogy between the privacy of electronic mail and the privacy of telephone conversations or face-to-face meetings
    D. illustrate the complexities of the privacy issues surrounding electronic mail in the workplace

本文话题

电子邮件的私密性。

难词译注

grievance ['griːvəns] *n.*	委屈
interception [ˌintəˈsepʃən] *n.*	拦截，侦听
scramble ['skræmbl] *v.*	搅乱
encryption [inˈkripʃən] *n.*	编密码
undermine [ˌʌndəˈmain] *v.*	破坏

难句译注

1. Although it is illegal in many areas for an employer to <u>eavesdrop</u> on private conversations or telephone calls — even if they take place on a company-owned telephone — there are no clear rules governing electronic mail.

    【分析】Although 引导让步状语从句，even if 引导从句作为插入语。

    【译文】尽管在很多地方，上司窃听员工私人谈话或电话通话——哪怕是公司的公用电话——是非法的，但是还没有明确的法规来监管电子邮件的隐私窥探。

2. Opponents of such practices argue that the paper versions often omit such information as who received the messages and when they received them, information commonly carried on electronic mail systems.

    【分析】that 引导宾语从句。

    【译文】这一做法的反对者认为：纸质的文件经常遗漏信息，如谁接收到这些信息，什么时间接到的，而这些信息是电子邮件系统一般都提供的。

答案及解析

16. 【问题】画线词"eavesdrop"的含义是_____。

    A. 侦察　　　　B. 无意中听到　　　　C. 监督　　　　D. 窃听

    【答案】D

    【解析】猜词题。画线词 eavesdrop 的含义为"窃听"，故选项 D 意思最接近。

17. 【问题】根据文章，下面哪一项是正确的？

    A. 人们对电子邮件的私密性有共识。

    B. 有很明确的规定监管电子邮件的私密性。

    C. 计算机系统的私密性没有绝对的保证。

    D. 最好的办法就是使用复杂的编码保护邮件。

    【答案】C

    【解析】细节题。根据第 2 段可以判断人们对这个话题有不同的看法，故 A 项认为人们有一致看法，不正确。再看 B 项，第 1 段中的"there are no clear rules governing electronic mail"说明还没有法规监管电子邮件。C 项原文信息在最后一段：The fact is that no absolute guarantee of privacy exists in any computer system. 最后看 D 项，最后一段提到唯一的办法是使用复杂的编码，但也提到这破坏了电子邮件的便捷特性，因而不是最好的解决办法，综上可知，C 正确。

18. 【问题】根据文章所述，作者关于对电子邮件监听的态度可以被最准确地描述为：

    A. 完全不赞成这一做法。   B. 支持这样做的雇主。

    C. 支持因此丢工作的员工。   D. 对这类法律问题知识上的兴趣。

【答案】D

【解析】态度题。此题用排除法比较容易解题。综观全文，没有体现作者对不同观点的任何态度，没有支持哪一方。

19. 【问题】汽车制造公司的例子被用来暗示：

    A. 在私企，侵犯员工的隐私很正常。

    B. 尚无法律对监听对象有专门规定。

    C. 决定偷听是否违背隐私取决于用的是谁的电子邮件系统，以及谁看到信息。

    D. 员工应该小心在计算机系统上的聊天。

【答案】B

【解析】推断题。原文相关信息在最后一段：these laws do not cover "inside" interception such as occurred at the automotive company，故 B 正确。

20. 【问题】作者写这篇文章的目的是_____。

    A. 表明个人隐私权已经随着计算机技术的进步遭受践踏

    B. 对比在公共部门和私人部门中电子邮件的法律地位

    C. 将电子邮件的私密性与个人电话或面对面交谈的私密性做比较

    D. 阐述职场电子邮件私密性的复杂性

【答案】D

【解析】推断题。根据主旨以及各段大意可以解题。

Passage Five

There's a species of smoker among us that is common yet poorly understood. Their habitat consists of parties, barbecues, and the sidewalks outside bars and restaurants. They prefer to scrounge for their cigarettes, and if they do buy a pack, they're apt to nurse it for a week or more. You may hear them say, "I'm not a smoker," or "Only on weekends." These are "social smokers" — and there are more of them than you might think.

Smoking is often characterized as an all-or-nothing activity — on doctor's office questionnaires it's usually a yes-or-no question, for instance — but by some estimates, anywhere from one-fifth to one-third of adults who smoke don't light up every day. While some of these so-called nondaily smokers smoke regularly but sparingly, up to 30% likely fall into the social-smoker category.

Hard numbers are difficult to come by, in part because the definition of a social smoker is so vague. A 2007 study of social smoking among college students — one of very few that have been published on the subject — found the term was used "loosely and inconsistently", even among researchers. But most people know a social smoker when they see one. They smoke occasionally, almost always in groups, and more often than not while drinking alcohol. By definition, they do not consider themselves addicted to nicotine. Many started smoking casually in high school or college but never graduated to a daily habit.

While the overall number of smokers in the United States is dropping, the proportion of occasional smokers appears to be on the rise. News reports and studies have also provided anecdotal（传闻的）evidence that social smoking is increasing, especially among young people.

The reasons for this apparent trend haven't been fully explained. Some suggest that the growing awareness of health risks, the stigma surrounding smoking (which may explain why the smokers interviewed for this article didn't want their full names used), and the smoking bans in public places are causing heavy smokers to cut back. Vickie, for instance, wouldn't be caught dead smoking around her two young children, and the restrictions against smoking at work or inside bars and restaurants are often enough to extinguish her urges, she says — especially in the wintertime.

Another popular theory is that social smokers, unlike social drinkers, don't really exist. Social smokers, the thinking goes, are low-level addicts either in denial or on the brink of addiction. It's a bit like the old saying about there being two types of motorcyclists: those who have had accidents and those who are going to. And research indicates that there may be something to this: In the recent study of college students, 60% of the students surveyed who denied that they were smokers did identify themselves as social smokers; roughly 10% of these alleged nonsmokers in fact smoked at least every other day.

21. What can be known about social smokers?
    A. They tend to light up on weekends.
    B. They are not real smokers.
    C. They tend to nurse a pack for several days or more.
    D. They only appear in parties or restaurants.

22. Which of the following words is closest in meaning with the underlined word "sparingly" in Paragraph 2?
    A. Economically.   B. Prudently.
    C. Extravagantly.   D. Indulgently.

23. What can be inferred from the phrase "loosely and inconsistently" in Paragraph 3?
    A. Researchers are not convinced of the reasons for social smokers.

B. There is no consensus about the definition of social smokers.

C. Social smokers are hard to be characterized by people.

D. There is no definite standard for distinguishing social smokers from others.

24. According to the passage, what may be the explanation for the trend that occasional smokers are on the rise while the overall number of smokers are decreasing?

A. The growing awareness of health.

B. Bans on smoking at home.

C. Advice from medical professionals.

D. The increasing self-discipline.

25. What can be implied from the old saying about there being two types of motorcyclists?

A. Social smokers are in danger of addiction to nicotine.

B. Social smokers don't addict to smoking at all.

C. Social smokers don't consider themselves as smokers.

D. Social smokers either deny their addiction or are at the risk of addiction.

 本文话题

社交型吸烟者。

 难词译注

habitat ['hæbitæt] *n.*	聚集处
scrounge [skraundʒ] *v.*	白要，白拿
vague [veig] *a.*	含糊的
nicotine ['nikəti:n] *n.*	尼古丁

 难句译注

In the recent study of college students, 60% of the students surveyed who denied that they were smokers did identify themselves as social smokers; roughly 10% of these alleged nonsmokers in fact smoked at least every other day.

【分析】surveyed 是过去分词做定语，修饰 students；that 引导宾语从句。

【译文】在最近针对大学生的研究中，60% 被调查的学生否认自己是烟民，同时视自己为社交型吸烟者；事实上，那些声称自己为非烟民的人中，约 10% 的人每隔一天会吸一次烟。

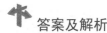 答案及解析

21. 【问题】有关社交吸烟者我们可以知道什么？

　　A. 他们总是在周末吸烟。

B. 他们不是真正的吸烟者。

C. 他们总是几天或更长的时间吸一包（烟）。

D. 他们只出现在聚会和餐馆。

【答案】C

【解析】细节题，选项 C 相关原文信息在第一段 "…they're apt to nurse it for a week or more…"。

22. 【问题】下面哪一个词的意思和画线词 "sparingly" 最接近？

A. 节约地。　　　B. 谨慎地。　　　C. 挥霍无度地。　　　D. 放任地。

【答案】A

【解析】猜词题。画线词的含义为"节俭地"。根据上下文信息也可以得出答案。

23. 【问题】从 "loosely and inconsistently" 这个词组可以推断出什么？

A. 研究者们不相信社交吸烟者的理由。

B. 关于社交吸烟者的定义没有一致看法。

C. 人们很难定义社交吸烟者。

D. 没有区分社交吸烟者和其他吸烟者确定的标准。

【答案】B

【解析】推断题。根据本段第 1 句话 "Hard numbers are difficult to come by, in part because the definition of a social smoker is so vague…"就可以解题，这句话是这一段的主题句。vague 的含义为"含糊的，不清楚的"。

24. 【问题】根据文章所述，针对偶尔吸烟者人数在上升而整体吸烟者人数在下降这一趋势的解释是什么？

A. 健康意识的增强。　　　　　B. 家中禁烟。

C. 医学专业人士的建议。　　　D. 自律增强。

【答案】A

【解析】细节题。在文章第 4 段提到题目所说的这一现象，虽然第 5 段第一句话中没有完整的解释，但是人们健康意识的增强可以作为一个解释，因而答案为 A。

25. 【问题】从那个有关两种骑摩托车者的古老谚语中可以得到什么暗示？

A. 社交吸烟者处于尼古丁上瘾的危险中。

B. 社交吸烟者对吸烟根本不会上瘾。

C. 社交吸烟者自认为不是吸烟者。

D. 社交吸烟者要么否认他们上瘾，要么否认他们处于上瘾的危险中。

【答案】D

【解析】推断题。这个比喻出现在最后一段，根据对这一比喻的解释和最后一段有关 social smokers 的相关信息可以解题。

Pasage Six

Scientists have known for more than two decades that cancer is a disease of the genes. Something scrambles the DNA inside a nucleus, and suddenly, instead of dividing in a measured fashion, a cell begins to copy itself furiously. Unlike an ordinary cell, it never stops. But describing the process isn't the same as figuring it out. Cancer cells are so radically different from normal ones that it's almost impossible to untangle the sequence of events that made them that way. So for years researchers have been attacking the problem by taking normal cells and trying to determine what changes will turn them cancerous—always without success.

Until now, according to a report in the current issue of *Nature*, a team of scientists based at M.I.T. 's Whitehead Institute for Biomedical Research has finally managed to make human cells malignant—a feat they accomplished with two different cell types by inserting just three altered genes into their DNA. While these manipulations were done only in lab dishes and won't lead to any immediate treatment, they appear to be a crucial step in understanding the disease. This is a "landmark paper", wrote Jonathan Weitzman and Moshe Yaniv of the Pasteur Institute in Paris, in an accompanying commentary.

The dramatic new result traces back to a breakthrough in 1983, when the Whitehead's Robert Weinberg and colleagues showed that mouse cells would become cancerous when spiked with two altered genes. But when they tried such alterations on human cells, they didn't work. Since then, scientists have learned that mouse cells differ from human cells in an important respect: they have higher levels of an enzyme called telomerase. That enzyme keeps caplike structures called telomeres on the ends of chromosomes from getting shorter with each round of cell division. Such shortening is part of a cell's aging process, and since cancer cells keep dividing forever, the Whitehead group reasoned that making human cells more mouselike might also make them cancerous.

The strategy worked. The scientists took connective-tissue and kidney cells and introduced three mutated genes—one that makes cells divide rapidly; another that disables two substances meant to rein in excessive division; and a third that promotes the production of telomerase, which made the cells essentially immortal. They'd created a tumor in a test tube. "Some people believed that telomerase wasn't that important," says the Whitehead's William Hahn, the study's lead author. "This allows us to say with some certainty that it is."

Understanding cancer cells in the lab isn't the same as understanding how it behaves in a living body, of course. But by teasing out the key differences between normal and malignant cells, doctors may someday be able to design tests to pick up cancer in its earliest stages. The finding could also lead to drugs <u>tailored</u> to attack specific types of cancer, thereby lessening our dependence on tissue-destroying chemotherapy and radiation. Beyond that, the Whitehead research suggests that this stubbornly complex disease may have a simple origin, and the identification of that origin may turn out to be the most important step of all.

26. From the first paragraph, we learn that _____.
   A. scientists had understood what happened to normal cells that made them behave strangely
   B. when a cell begins to copy itself without stopping, it becomes cancerous
   C. normal cells do not copy themselves
   D. the DNA inside a nucleus divides regularly

27. Which of the following statements is TRUE according to the text?
   A. The scientists traced the source of cancers by figuring out their DNA order.
   B. A treatment to cancers will be available within a year or two.
   C. The finding paves way for tackling cancer.
   D. The scientists successfully turned cancerous cells into healthy cells.

28. According to the author, one of the problems in previous cancer research is that _____.
   A. enzyme kept telomeres from getting shorter
   B. scientists didn't know there existed different levels of telomerase between mouse cells and human cells
   C. scientists failed to understand the connection between a cell's aging process and cell division
   D. human cells are mouselike

29. Which of the following best defines the word "tailored" (Line 4, Para. 5)?
   A. Made specifically.   B. Used mainly.
   C. Targeted.   D. Aimed.

30. The Whitehead research will probably result in _____.
   A. a thorough understanding of the disease
   B. beating out cancers
   C. solving the cancer mystery
   D. drugs that leave patients less painful

本文话题

癌症研究新突破。

 难词译注

nucleus ['njuːklɪəs] *n.*   细胞核
untangle [ʌn'tæŋgl] *v.*   解开
malignant [mə'lɪgnənt] *a.*   恶性的

manipulation [mə,nipjuˈleiʃən] *n.*	处理，操作
spike [spaik] *n.*	穿刺
telomerase [ˈteləmiəˈreiz] *n.*	端粒酶
telomere [ˈteləmiə] *n.*	端粒（在染色体端位上的着丝点）
chromosome [ˈkrəuməsəum] *n.*	染色体
mutate [mjuːˈteit] *v.*	变异
chemotherapy [,keməuˈθerəpi] *n.*	化疗

 答案及解析

26. 【问题】从第 1 段我们可以知道：

A. 科学家们已经完全明白那些行为古怪的正常细胞出了什么问题。

B. 当一个细胞不停地复制自己时，它就是癌细胞。

C. 正常细胞不会复制自己。

D. 细胞核内的 DNA 定期分裂。

【答案】B

【解析】细节题。根据原文第 1 段第 1 句话可以得知，癌症是一种基因变异。而随后又进一步阐释这种基因变异：Something scrambles the DNA inside a nucleus, and suddenly, instead of dividing in a measured fashion, a cell begins to copy itself furiously. Unlike an ordinary cell, it never stops. 这句话的含义是：细胞核内的 DNA 被某种物质打乱，并且细胞突然不再有规则地分裂，而开始大量复制自身。不同于普通细胞的是，这种复制活动永无休止。故 B 正确。

27. 【问题】根据文章所述，下面哪一个是正确的？

A. 科学家们通过知道癌症 DNA 的次序追踪到癌症的源头。

B. 一两年内将会有治疗癌症的方法。

C. 研究结果为解决癌症铺平了道路。

D. 科学家们成功地将癌细胞转化为健康细胞。

【答案】C

【解析】 细节题。见原文第 2 段：While these manipulations were done only in lab dishes and won't lead to any immediate treatment, they appear to be a crucial step in understanding the disease. 这句话告诉我们，尽管这些操作仅仅是在实验室的器皿中完成的，不会立刻形成任何治疗手段，但这些都是了解这一疾病的重要一步。同时后面的一句 "This is a landmark paper" 更说明这项研究是在为彻底治愈癌症铺路。

28. 【问题】根据作者的观点，上一个癌症研究存在的问题之一是_____。

A. 酶使得端粒无法变短

B. 科学家们不知道鼠细胞和人体细胞之间有不同的端粒酶

C. 科学家们不知道一个细胞的衰老过程与细胞分裂的关系

D．人类细胞类似鼠细胞

【答案】B

【解析】细节题。题目中提到的实验出现在第 3 段，本段第 2 句话告诉我们这个实验失败了，下一句告诉我们失败的原因：Since then，scientists have learned that mouse cells differ from human cells in an important respect: they have higher levels of an enzyme called telomerase.

29．【问题】下面哪一个能最好地定义 "tailor"？

A．专门制作。　　　B．主要使用。　　　C．定向的。　　　D．瞄准的。

【答案】A

【解析】猜词题。根据 tailor 所在的最后一段的句子："The finding could also lead to drugs tailored to attack specific types of cancer…" 可知这个要针对特定的癌症，因而 tailor 的含义就是 A。

30．【问题】Whitehead 的研究将可能导致_____。

A．对这种病的彻底认识　　　　B．打败癌症

C．解决癌症之谜　　　　　　　D．使病人减少痛苦的药

【答案】D

【解析】推理题。文中最后一段第 3 句提到，这项研究可能发明一些专门用于特定类型癌症的药物，因此减少我们对化疗和辐射的依赖，可见癌症患者在治疗时有可能不再像以前那样痛苦。

Passage Seven

Is there any beverage that's more versatile than beer? The malted barley brew can provide a way to bond with buddies, celebrate victories, mourn defeats, and is almost a prerequisite for watching sports. However, if your waistline has started to expand into the stereotypical beer belly zone, you may be looking with disdain at that pint in your hand.

It's commonly assumed that there is a direct correlation between the amount of beer men consume and the size of their beer bellies, but how accurate is this perception? We've investigated the connection between beer and beer bellies, so read on to learn the truth.

Despite the common "beer belly" moniker, excess belly flab is not always caused by swigging too many pints of liquid bread. Beer, at around 140 calories per 12-ounce bottle, is high in calories and frequent imbibing can result in the extra calories that lead to a distended waistline. So, in this case, there is a link. However, like fat that appears in other areas of the body, it has more to do with how many overall calories you consume versus how many you're burning through regular exercise. Your body can't tell the difference between beer-related calories and extra calories from any other food. So, the answer is also, no.

Calories certainly hold part of the answer, but so does age: metabolism slows down after the age of 35, so you may find that the further the calendar advances, the more trouble you have keeping a trim figure. Another part of the reason has to do with your gender. While most women tend to keep their extra flab on their hips, thighs and buttocks, men commonly store fat around the waist. So combine your age and gender with an excess of calories, and the result can be a charming pot belly.

Not only is it an unattractive accessory, belly fat — or visceral fat — is now getting extra attention as one of the riskiest kinds of extra flab a person can sport. People with excess belly fat have a tendency to develop nasty conditions such as insulin resistance, diabetes, high blood pressure, heart disease, and high cholesterol over and above the already increased risk a person receives from other forms of obesity.

So, how do you know if your spare tire is overinflated? Use a measuring tape. Keeping in mind that everybody is different, a general guideline some doctors use for men is a maximum waist measurement of 40 inches. Anything over that and your chances of developing nasty health problems will escalate. To see how you compare, wrap a tape measure around the area above your hipbone. Make sure the tape is level all the way around your midsection, hold it snug, breathe out, and see what the damage is.

31. According to the passage, which of the following statements is true?
    A. Beer belly is in proportion to the amount of beer consumed.
    B. The excess belly flab is not caused by beer.
    C. A complex factor along with age and gender may lead to distended waistline.
    D. Compared with women, men store more fat around the waist.

32. Which of the following statements is true about reasons for fat deposited in the belly?
    A. Age correlates with fat stored in the belly.
    B. Males tend to store fat around the waist.
    C. Extra calories lead to a distended waistline.
    D. All of the above.

33. According to the passage, as a risk of health, beer belly may develop some diseases EXCEPT _____.
    A. diabetes   B. hepatitis
    C. hypertension   D. cardiovascular disease

34. According to the passage, the way to know how much belly is too much is _____.
    A. measuring the waistline
    B. blood routine
    C. urine routine

D. consult medical professionals

35. The next paragraph would probably discuss _____.
    A. how to give up drinking beer
    B. how to get rid of beer belly
    C. how to know whether you are addicted to beer
    D. how to deal with the diseases in relation to beer belly

 本文话题

啤酒肚。

 难词译注

versatile ['və:sətail] *a.*	通用的，万能的
malted barley	麦芽
prerequisite [ˌpriːˈrekwizit] *n.*	先决条件
stereotypical [ˈstiəriəˌtaipikəl] *a.*	模式化观念的
pint [paint] *n.*	品脱
moniker [ˈmɔnikə(r)] *n.*	绰号
flab [flæb] *n.*	松弛
swig [swig] *v.*	痛饮
imbibe [imˈbaib] *v.*	吸收
distend [disˈtend] *v.*	使扩大
metabolism [meˈtæbəlizəm] *n.*	新陈代谢
visceral fat	内脏脂肪
insulin [ˈinsjulin] *n.*	胰岛素
cholesterol [kəˈlestərəul] *n.*	胆固醇
obesity [əuˈbiːsəti] *n.*	肥胖

 难句译注

1. Beer, at around 140 calories per 12-ounce bottle, is high in calories and frequent imbibing can result in the extra calories that lead to a distended waistline.
   【分析】that 引导定语从句修饰 calories。
   【译文】啤酒含有很高的热量，每 12 盎司的瓶装啤酒大约含有 140 卡路里的热量，经常喝啤酒会使腰围增大。

2. However, like fat that appears in other areas of the body, it has more to do with how many overall calories you consume versus how many you're burning through regular exercise.

【分析】that 引导定语从句修饰 fat。versus 是介词，此处意为"相对，相比"。

【译文】然而，与身体其他部位的脂肪一样，腹部脂肪的多少更取决于你摄入的热量与通过锻炼而燃烧掉的热量的差值。

答案及解析

31. 【问题】根据文章，下面哪一个表述是正确的？

    A．啤酒肚和喝的啤酒量成正比。

    B．大啤酒肚不是由啤酒造成的。

    C．包括年龄和性别在内的复杂因素可能导致腰围增大。

    D．与女性相比，男性在腰上囤积更多的脂肪。

【答案】C

【解析】细节题。原文第 3 段和第 4 段提到造成啤酒肚的原因：卡路里摄入、年龄以及性别等。

32. 【问题】下面哪一个关于腹部脂肪堆积的原因是正确的？

    A．年龄与腹部脂肪堆积相关。   B．男性总是在腰上囤积脂肪。

    C．热量过多可能导致腰围增大。   D．以上都是。

【答案】D

【解析】细节题。解题信息依然在原文第 3 段和第 4 段。

33. 【问题】根据文章，作为一个健康的危险因素，啤酒肚可能导致疾病，除了_____。

    A．糖尿病   B．肝炎

    C．高血压   D．心血管疾病

【答案】B

【解析】细节题。原文信息在第 5 段最后一句话：…develop nasty conditions such as insulin resistance, diabetes, high blood pressure, heart disease, and high cholesterol over and above the already increased risk a person receives from other forms of obesity.

34. 【问题】根据文章，知道多大的肚子算超标的方法是_____。

    A．量腰围   B．血常规

    C．尿常规   D．咨询医学专业人士

【答案】A

【解析】细节题。原文相关信息在最后一段。

35. 【问题】下一个段落可能讨论_____。

    A．如何戒啤酒   B．如何消除啤酒肚

    C．如何知道你是否对啤酒上瘾   D．如何应对和啤酒肚相关的疾病

【答案】B

【解析】推理题。综观全文，提到啤酒肚的成因、危害以及如何判断腹部腰围。按照逻辑推理，下一个段落应该讲述如何消除啤酒肚。

Passage Eight

Can the Internet help patients jump the line at the doctor's office? The Silicon Valley Employers Forum, a sophisticated group of technology companies, is launching a pilot program to test online "virtual visits" between doctors at three big local medical groups and about 6,000 employees and their families. The six employers taking part in the Silicon Valley initiative, including heavy hitters such as Oracle and Cisco Systems, hope that online visits will mean employees won't have to skip work to tend to minor ailments or to follow up on chronic conditions. "With our long commutes and traffic, driving 40 miles to your doctor in your hometown can be a big chunk of time," says Cindy Conway, benefits director at Cadence Design Systems, one of the participating companies.

Doctors aren't clamoring to chat with patients online for free; they spend enough unpaid time on the phone. Only 1 in 5 has ever e-mailed a patient, and just 9 percent are interested in doing so, according to the research firm Cyber Dialogue. "We are not stupid," says Stirling Somers, executive of the Silicon Valley employers group. "Doctors getting paid is a critical piece in getting this to work." In the pilot program, physicians will get $20 per online consultation, about what they get for a simple office visit.

Doctors also fear they'll be swamped by rambling e-mails that tell everything but what's needed to make a diagnosis. So the new program will use technology supplied by Healinx, an Alameda, Calif.-based start-up. Healinx's "Smart Symptom Wizard" questions patients and turns answers into a succinct message. The company has online dialogues for 60 common conditions. The doctor can then diagnose the problem and outline a treatment plan, which could include e-mailing a prescription or a face-to-face visit.

Can e-mail replace the doctor's office? Many conditions, such as persistent cough, require a stethoscope to discover what's wrong — and to avoid a malpractice suit. Even Larry Bonham, head of one of the doctor's groups in the pilot, believes the virtual doctor's visits offer a "very narrow" sliver of service between phone calls to an advice nurse and a visit to the clinic.

The pilot program, set to end in nine months, also hopes to determine whether online visits will boost worker productivity enough to offset the cost of the service. So far, the Internet's record in the health field has been underwhelming. The experiment is "a huge roll of the dice for Healinx," notes Michael Barrett, an analyst at Internet consulting firm Forester Research. If the "Web visits" succeed, expect some HMOs (Health Maintenance Organizations) to pay for online visits. If doctors, employers, and patients aren't satisfied, figure on one more e-health start-up to stand down.

36. The Silicon Valley employers promote the e-health program for the purpose of _____ .
    A. rewarding their employees
    B. gratifying the local hospitals
    C. boosting worker productivity
    D. testing a sophisticated technology

37. What can be learned about the on-line doctors' visits?
    A. They are a quite promising business.
    B. They are funded by the local government.
    C. They are welcomed by all the patients.
    D. They are very much under experimentation.

38. According to Paragraph 2, doctors are _____ .
    A. reluctant to serve online for nothing
    B. not interested in Web consultation
    C. too tired to talk to the patients online
    D. content with $20 paid per Web visit

39. "Smart Symptom Wizard" is capable of _____ .
    A. making diagnoses
    B. producing prescriptions
    C. profiling patients' illness
    D. offering a treatment plan

40. It can be inferred from the passage that the future of online visits will mostly depend on whether _____ .
    A. the employers would remain confident in them
    B. they could effectively replace office visits
    C. HMOs would cover the cost of the service
    D. new technologies would be available to improve the e-health project

本文话题

虚拟网上问诊。

难词译注

sophisticated [səˈfistikeitid] *a.*	老练的；复杂巧妙的
ailment [ˈeilmənt] *n.*	疾病
chunk [tʃʌŋk] *n.*	大块
clamor [ˈklæmə] *v.*	大声要求
swamp [swɔmp] *v.*	淹没
rambling [ˈræmbliŋ] *a.*	凌乱的；不切题的；蔓生的
succinct [səkˈsiŋkt] *a.*	简洁的
stethoscope [ˈsteθəskəup] *n.*	听诊器

dice [dais] *n.*   骰子

malpractice ['mælpræktis] *n.*   玩忽职守

offset ['ɔ:fset] *v.*   抵消

答案及解析

36. 【问题】硅谷的老板们推广电子医疗项目有什么目的?

    A. 奖励员工。   B. 使当地医院满意。

    C. 提高工人生产力。   D. 测试一个复杂的技术。

【答案】C

【解析】细节题。原文信息首先出现在第 1 段:…hope that online visits will mean employees won't have to skip work to tend to minor ailments of to follow up on chronic conditions. 这句话告诉我们,这些参与其中的老板们希望网上问诊,这意味着他们的员工不必翘班去看病。在最后一段第 1 句话也提到:The pilot program, set to end in nine months, also hopes to determine whether online visits will boost worker productivity enough to offset the cost of the service. 此句意为:这一试验项目九个月后就将结束,同样希望能确定网上问诊是否能提高工人生产力,以抵消这项服务的费用。故选 C。

37. 【问题】有关网上问诊我们可以知道什么?

    A. 这是很有前景的生意。   B. 由当地政府资助。

    C. 深受所有患者的欢迎。   D. 还处于试验阶段。

【答案】D

【解析】细节题。此题用排除法较容易解题。文章第 4 段和第 5 段阐述这一项目的不足和担心,很多参与者还持观望态度,无法判断这个项目是否有发展前途,故 A 错。B 为错误选项,文章没有提到该项目由政府资助;C 为错误选项,理由与 B 相同。最后一段提到该项目是 pilot program,意思就是"试验性的,试点的"。故 D 正确。

38. 【问题】在第 2 段,医生们对网上问诊的态度是_____。

    A. 不愿意免费进行网上问诊

    B. 对网上会诊不感兴趣

    C. 太疲劳了,以至于不愿意在网上和患者交流

    D. 对每次网上会诊 20 元费用感到满意

【答案】A

【解析】段落大意。根据第 2 段的内容,可以首先排除 C 和 D,因为没有相关信息。第 2 段第 1 句话 "Doctors aren't clamoring to chat with patients online for free." 意思是医生们不情愿在网上和患者免费交流。因而选项 A 为正确答案。

【问题】SSW 能够做什么?

A. 进行诊断。 B. 开处方。

C. 扼要介绍病人病情。 D. 提供治疗方案。

39. 【答案】C

【解析】细节题。有关 SSW 的原文信息在第 3 段。第 3 段提到，这个项目使用称为 SSW 的新技术。该技术可以询问病人，并将病情简要记录下来，然后由医生诊断病情，确定治疗方案。这个方案可以是将处方发邮件给病人或者面对面的问诊。

40. 【问题】从文章中可以推断网上问诊的前景主要依靠什么？

A. 老板们是否对它有信心。

B. 是否能有效取代面对面的问诊。

C. HMOs 是否负担费用。

D. 新的技术是否能改进该项目。

【答案】B

【解析】推断题。根据全文内容以及上面几道细节题可知：硅谷老板们推广电子医疗为了提高工人的生产力，但医生们对于网上问诊的态度很不情愿，因而可以推断，网上问诊在今后前景，就取决于是否能有效地取代面对面的问诊，故选项 B 正确。

Passage Nine

Can electricity cause cancer? In a society that literally runs on electric power, the very idea seems preposterous. But for more than a decade, a growing band of scientists and journalists has pointed to studies that seem to link exposure to electromagnetic fields with increased risk of leukemia（白血病）and other malignancies（恶性肿瘤）. The implications are unsettling, to say the least, since everyone comes into contact with such fields, which are generated by everything electrical, from power lines and antennas to personal computers and micro-wave ovens. Because evidence on the subject is inconclusive and often contradictory, it has been hard to decide whether concern about the health effects of electricity is legitimate or the worst kind of paranoia（妄想狂）.

Now the alarmists have gained some qualified support from the U.S. Environmental Protection Agency. In the executive summary of a new scientific review, released in draft form late last week, the EPA has put forward what amounts to the most serious government warning to date. The agency tentatively concludes that scientific evidence "suggests a casual link" between extremely low-frequency electromagnetic fields — those having very long wave-lengths and leukemia, lymphoma and brain cancer. While the report falls short of classifying ELF fields as probable carcinogens（致癌物质）, it does identify the common 60-hertz magnetic field as "a possible, but not proven, cause of cancer in humans".

The report is no reason to panic or even to lost sleep. If there is a cancer risk, it is a small one. The evidence is still so controversial that the draft stirred a great deal of debate within the Bush Administration, and the EPA released it over strong objections from the Pentagon and the White House. But now no one can deny that the issue must be taken seriously and that much more research is needed.

At the heart of the debate is a simple and well-understood physical phenomenon: When an electric current passes through a wire, it generates an electromagnetic field that exerts forces on surrounding objects. For many years, scientists dismissed any suggestion that such forces might be harmful, primarily because they are so extraordinarily weak. The ELF magnetic field generated by a video terminal measures only a few milligauss（磁场强度单位）, or about one-hundredth the strength of the earth's own magnetic field. The electric fields surrounding a power line can be as high as 10 kilovolts per meter, but the corresponding field induced in human cells will be only about 1 millivolt per meter. This is far less than the electric fields that the cells themselves generate.

How could such minuscule forces pose a health danger? The consensus used to be that they could not, and for decades scientists concentrated on more powerful kinds of radiation, like X-rays, which pack sufficient wallop to knock electrons out of the molecules that make up the human body. Such "ionizing" radiations have been clearly linked to increased cancer risks and there are regulations to control emissions.

But epidemiological studies, which find statistical associations between sets of data, do not prove cause and effect. Though there is a body of laboratory work showing that exposure to ELF fields can have biological effects on animal tissues, a mechanism by which those effects could lead to cancerous growths has never been found.

The Pentagon is far from persuaded. In a blistering 33-page critique of the EPA report, Air Force scientists charge its authors with having "biased the entire document" toward proving a link. "Our reviewers are convinced that there is no suggestion that (electromagnetic fields) present in the environment induce or promote cancer," the Air Force concludes. "It is astonishing that the EPA would lend its imprimatur on this report." Then Pentagon's concern is understandable. There is hardly a unit of the modern military that does not depend on the heavy use of some kind of electronic equipment, from huge ground-based radar towers to the defense systems built into every warship and plane.

41. The main idea of this passage is _____.
    A. studies on the cause of cancer
    B. controversial viewpoints in the cause of cancer
    C. the relationship between electricity and cancer

D. different ideas about the effect of electricity on cancer

42. The viewpoint of the EPA is _____.
   A. that there is casual link between electricity and cancer
   B. that electricity really affects cancer
   C. controversial
   D. that low frequency electromagnetic field is a possible cause of cancer

43. Why did the Pentagon and White House object to the release of the report?
   A. Because it may stir a great deal of debate among the Bush Administration.
   B. Because every unit of the modern military has depended on the heavy use of some kind of electronic equipment.
   C. Because the Pentagon's concern was understandable.
   D. Because they had different arguments.

44. It can be inferred from physical phenomenon _____.
   A. the force of the electromagnetic field is too weak to be harmful
   B. the force of the electromagnetic field is weaker than the electric field that the cells generate
   C. electromagnetic field may affect health
   D. only more powerful radiation can knock electron out of human body

45. What do you think ordinary citizens may do after reading the different arguments?
   A. They are indifferent.
   B. They are worried very much.
   C. They may exercise prudent avoidance.
   D. They are shocked.

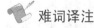 本文话题

电是否致癌。

难词译注

preposterous [priˈpɔstərəs] a.	荒谬的
legitimate [liˈdʒitimit] a.	合法的，合理的
tentatively [ˈtentətivli] ad.	试验性地，暂时性地
lymphoma [limˈfəumə] n.	淋巴瘤
minuscule [miˈnʌskjuːl] a.	很小的，很不重要的
consensus [kənˈsensəs] n.	一致同意
wallop [ˈwɔləp] v. /n.	乱窜，猛冲

epidemiological [ˌepiˌdemiˌɔ'lədʒikɔl] *a.*	流行病学的
blistering ['blistəriŋ] *a.*	愤怒的，猛烈的
critique [kri'tiːk] *n.*	评论，批评
imprimatur [ˌimpri'meitə] *n.*	出版许可（官方审查后的），批准

 难句译注

1. The evidence is still so controversial that the draft stirred a great deal of debate within the Bush Administration, and the EPA released it over strong objections from the Pentagon and the White House.

   【分析】so...that 如此……以至于。

   【译文】证据很有争议，以至于报告草案在布什政府内引起激辩，而环保署无视五角大楼和白宫的强烈反对，公布了这份报告。

2. ...and for decades scientists concentrated on more powerful kinds of radiation, like X-rays, which pack sufficient wallop to knock electrons out of the molecules that make up the human body.

   【分析】which 引导定语从句，修饰 powerful kinds of radiation；that 引导定语从句修饰 molecules。

   【译文】而且几十年来，科学家专注于更为强大的辐射类别，如 X 光射线，其聚合的冲击力足以把电子从组成人体的分子中撞出来。

答案及解析

41. 【问题】这篇文章的主题是_____。
    A. 有关癌症原因的研究　　　　B. 有关癌症原因的有争议的观点
    C. 电和癌症的关系　　　　　　D. 电对产生癌症所起的作用的不同观点

    【答案】D

    【解析】主旨题。根据每段的段落大意可以总结出文章的主旨。第 1 段提出文章讨论的话题，电是否会致癌，科学家们进行研究，觉得似乎是如此。紧接着文章阐述 EPA 组织针对这一问题的报告，似乎认为二者之间存在关系，但未经科学证实。尽管如此，危险性很微小，不过仍应认真对待。但空军方面的科学家不认同这一观点。至此，我们可以得出结论：文章对电是否能致癌这一话题阐述了不同的观点。

42. 【问题】EPA 的观点是_____。
    A. 电和癌症间的关联不紧密
    B. 电的确影响癌症
    C. 很有争议
    D. 电子磁场的低频率可能是导致癌症的一个原因

    【答案】A

【解析】细节题。原文信息为第 3 段第 1 句话。该句意为：无需对这个报告产生恐慌甚至寝食难安。就算是癌症的一个危险因素，也是很小的一个。故说明二者关系不紧密。

43. 【问题】为什么五角大楼和白宫反对这个报告的发表？
    A. 因为这可能在布什政府内部引起很多争论。
    B. 因为现代军事的每一个部门都完全依赖这种电子设备的使用。
    C. 因为五角大楼的关注是可以理解的。
    D. 因为他们有不同的观点。

【答案】B

【解析】推断题。A 项不是原因，而是结果。C 项与题目不符，答非所问。文中没有 D 项的相关信息。

44. 【问题】从物理现象可以推断出_____。
    A. 电子磁场的威力很弱，不会有害
    B. 电子磁场的威力比细胞产生的电场要弱
    C. 电子磁场可能影响健康
    D. 只有更强大的射线才可以将人体内的电子敲出来

【答案】A

【解析】推断题。原文信息在第 5 段：For many years, scientists dismissed any suggestion that such forces might be harmful, primarily because they are so extraordinarily weak. 此句意为"多年以来，科学家认为这样的强度不会有害，因为其威力太弱了。"

45. 【问题】你认为普通市民在读了这些不同的观点后可能做什么？
    A. 他们无所谓，漠不关心。　　　　B. 他们十分担心。
    C. 他们可能谨慎避免。　　　　　　D. 他们很震惊。

【答案】C

【解析】推断题。文章针对电是否致癌的阐述告诉我们，对于这个问题还没有一个定性的结论，因而不选 B 和 D 两项；虽然没有定性，但是这个问题毕竟与人的生命有关，故读者不会对此漠不关心，故不选 A。

Passage Ten

A rapid pace of technological advance has been accepted by many manufacturing industries for some time now, but for the office worker, who has led a sheltered existence in comparison, radical changes are a new experience. With the advent of electronic data processing techniques and, especially, computers, this situation has altered very swiftly. Office staff are suddenly finding themselves exposed to the traumatic consequences of scientific progress.

Research into the social and organizational problems of introducing computers into offices has been in progress in the social science department in Liverpool University for the past four years. In the firms we have been studying, change has usually been seen simply as a technical problem to be handled by technologists. The fact that the staff might regard the introduction of a computer as a threat to their security and status has not been anticipated. Company directors have been surprised when, instead of cooperation, they encountered anxiety and hostility.

Once the firm has signed the contract to purchase a computer, its next step, one might expect, would be to "sell" the idea to its staff, by giving reassurances about redundancy, and investigating how individual jobs will be affected so that displaced staff can be prepared for a move elsewhere. In fact, this may not happen. It is more usual for the firm to spend much time and energy investigating the technical aspects of the computer, yet largely to ignore the possibility of personnel difficulties. This neglect is due to the absence from most firms of anyone knowledgeable about human relations. The personnel manager, who might be expected to have some understanding of employee motivation, is in many cases not even involved in the changeover.

Again, because the changeover is seen only as a technical problem, little thought is given to communication and consultation with staff. Some firms go so far as to adopt a policy of complete secrecy, telling their staff nothing. One director told us: "If we are too frank, we may create difficulties for ourselves." This policy was applied to managers as well as clerks because, it was explained, "our managers will worry if they find out they will lose workers and so have their empires reduced". Several months after the arrival of the computer, the sales manager in this firm had still not been given full information on the consequences of this change.

The real bogey of the computer is that it is likely or even intended to displace staff. So it constitutes a major threat to staff security, and for this reason alone is likely to be resisted. An important part of the preparations for a machine must be, therefore, the estimating of the number of redundancies, and identifying jobs which will be eliminated or reduced in scope by the machine.

46. According to the research conducted by social science department in Liverpool University, which of the following is true?
    A. Company directors welcome new technologies.
    B. New technologies promote employees' teamwork.
    C. Workers feel threatened by the introduction of technologies.
    D. Technologies lead to workers' psychological diseases.

47. Employees are worried about the adoption of technologies because _____.
    A. they have no ideas on how to use them
    B. they have not been given full information on the consequences of this change
    C. firms are likely to adopt a policy of complete secrecy

D. probably employees will be replaced by them

48. According to the passage, once the firm purchase computers, what problems do they encounter?

A. Workers are prepared for a move.

B. Personnel difficulties will be ignored.

C. Personnel managers have no insights into employee motivation.

D. How much does individual job will be affected.

49. The underlined word "bogey" is closest in meaning to _____.

A. fear B. ghost C. cause D. revenant

50. According to the passage, which of the following is the author's opinion?

A. Employers should be discreet about the introduction of new technologies.

B. Workers are replaced inevitably by technologies.

C. With the advent of new technologies, firms are likely to get into difficulties with new technologies.

D. Employers should require technologists to handle technical problems instead of employees.

 本文话题

新科学技术的引进对员工的影响。

 难词译注

advent ['ædvənt] n.	到来
traumatic [trɔː'mætik] a.	创伤的
anticipate [æn'tisipeit] v.	预期，期望
reassurance [ˌriːə'ʃuərəns] n.	放心
redundancy [ri'dʌndənsi] n.	冗余

 难句译注

1. A rapid pace of technological advance has been accepted by many manufacturing industries for some time now, but for the office worker, who has led a sheltered existence in comparison, radical changes are a new experience.

【分析】who 引导定语从句，修饰 office worker。

【译文】科学技术的飞速发展被许多制造业所接受已经有一段时间了，但相比之下对于生活在庇护下的办公室文员来说，彻底的变化却是一种全新的经历。

2. The fact that the staff might regard the introduction of a computer as a threat to their

security and status has not been anticipated.

【分析】that 引导同位语从句。

【译文】员工可能把计算机的引进视为对自身安全和地位的威胁，这个事实没有被预料到。

答案及解析

46.【问题】根据利物浦大学社会科学部的研究，哪一个是正确的？

　　　　A．公司主管欢迎新科学技术。

　　　　B．科学技术促进员工的团队合作。

　　　　C．工人们感觉新技术的引进是对他们的威胁。

　　　　D．科学技术导致员工心理疾病。

【答案】C

【解析】细节题。原文信息在第 2 段：The fact that the staff might regard the introduction of a computer as a threat to their security and status has not been anticipated. 这句话告诉我们出现了员工感到威胁的事实。

47.【问题】员工担心新技术的引进，因为_____。

　　　　A．他们不知道如何使用

　　　　B．他们没有被详细告知这种变化会带来什么结果

　　　　C．公司很可能采取完全保密的政策

　　　　D．员工很有可能被新技术所取代

【答案】D

【解析】细节题。根据文章的阐述，员工的担心来自于对自身地位和安全的威胁。

48.【问题】一旦公司购买计算机，他们就可能遇到什么麻烦？

　　　　A．员工准备调动。

　　　　B．人事困难将被忽视。

　　　　C．人事经理对员工动机没有深入了解。

　　　　D．个人工作将会在多大程度上受到影响。

【答案】B

【解析】细节题。原文信息在第三段：It is more usual for the firm to spend much time and energy investigating the technical aspects of the computer, yet largely to ignore the possibility of personnel difficulties. 对于公司来说通常会花时间和精力调查计算机技术方面的问题，而大大忽略了人事问题的可能性。

49.【问题】画线词"bogey"和_____意思最接近。

　　　　A．恐惧　　　　B．幽灵　　　　C．缘由　　　　D．亡魂

【答案】A

【解析】猜词题。根据画线词所在的最后一段和语句，可以推测出计算机对于员工最大的危险就是会取代他们的位置。故与画线词所在语句意思最接近的就是 A。

50.【问题】哪一项是作者的观点？

A．雇主要谨慎引进新技术。

B．员工势必要被科学技术所取代。

C．随着新的科学技术的到来，公司很可能陷入新科技所带来的问题中。

D．雇主应该要求技术人员解决技术问题，而不是要求员工。

【答案】C

【解析】细节题。A 项在原文中无相关信息；B 项也没有；D 项有相关信息，但不是作者观点；故 C 正确。

Passage Eleven

Biologically, there is only one quality which distinguishes us from animals: the ability to laugh. In a universe which appears to be utterly devoid of humor, we enjoy this supreme luxury. And it is a luxury, for unlike any other bodily process, laughter does not seem to serve a biologically useful purpose. In a divided world, laughter is a unifying force. Human beings oppose each other on a great many issues. Nations may disagree about systems of government and human relations may be plagued by ideological factions and political camps, but we all share the ability to laugh. And laughter, in turn, depends on that most complex and subtle of all human qualities: a sense of humor. Certain comic stereotypes have a universal appeal. This can best be seen from the world-wide popularity of Charlie Chaplin's early films. The little man at odds with society never fails to amuse no matter which country we come from. As that great commentator on human affairs, Dr. Samuel Johnson, once remarked, "Men have been wise in very different modes; but they have always laughed in the same way."

A sense of humor may take various forms and laughter may be anything from a refined tingle to an earth quaking roar, but the effect is always the same. Humor helps us to maintain a correct sense of values. It is the one quality which political fanatics appear to lack. If we can see the funny side, we never make the mistake of taking ourselves too seriously. We are always reminded that tragedy is not really far removed from comedy, so we never get a lop-sided view of things.

This is one of the chief functions of satire and irony. Human pain and suffering are so grim; we hover so often on the brink of war; political realities are usually enough to plunge us into total despair. In such circumstances, cartoons and satirical accounts of somber political events redress the balance. They take the wind out of pompous and arrogant politicians who have lost their sense of proportion. They enable us to see that many of our most profound actions are merely comic or absurd. We laugh when a great satirist like Swift writes about war in *Gulliver's Travels*. The Lilliputians and their neighbors attack each other because they can't agree which end to break an egg. We laugh because we meant to laugh; but we are meant to weep too. It is too powerful a weapon to be allowed to flourish in totalitarian regimes（极权主义政治制度）.

The sense of humor must be singled out as man's most important quality because it is associated with laughter. And laughter, in turn, is associated with happiness. Courage, determination, initiative — these are qualities we share with other forms of life. But the sense of humor is uniquely human. If happiness is one of the great goals of life, then it is the sense of humor that provides the key.

51. The most important of all human qualities is _____.
    A. a sense of humor
    B. a sense of satire
    C. a sense of laughter
    D. a sense of history

52. The author mentions about Charlie Chaplin's early films because _____.
    A. they can amuse people
    B. human beings are different from animals
    C. they show that certain comic stereotypes have a universal appeal
    D. they show that people have the same ability to laugh

53. One of the chief functions of irony and satire is _____.
    A. to show absurdity of actions
    B. to redress balance
    C. to take the wind out of politicians
    D. to show too much grimness in the world

54. What do we learn from the sentence（Line 9, Para.3）"It is too powerful a weapon to be allowed to flourish in totalitarian regimes."?
    A. It can reveal the truth of political events with satire.
    B. It can arouse people to riot.
    C. It shows tragedy and comedy are related.
    D. It can make people laugh.

55. Who is Swift?
    A. A novelist.   B. A poet.   C. A dramatist.   D. An essayist.

本文话题

幽默感。

难词译注

devoid [di'vɔid] a.　　　　缺乏的
plague [pleig] n.　　　　瘟疫；苦恼
faction ['fækʃən] n.　　　　派别

fanatic [fə'nætik] *n.*		狂热者
hover ['hɔvə] *v.*		盘旋
somber ['sɔmbə(r)] *a.*		阴暗的，阴森的
redress [ri'dres] *v.*		纠正
pompous ['pɔmpəs] *a.*		华而不实的
regime [rei'ʒiːm] *n.*		政体，政权

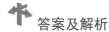 答案及解析

51. 【问题】人类所有素质中最重要的是_____。

    A. 幽默感   B. 讽刺   C. 微笑   D. 历史感

【答案】A

【解析】文章开头就点题：…there is only one quality which distinguishes us from animals: the ability to laugh. 此句意为：人类区别动物的唯一特性就是能够笑。文章后面的内容从不同角度阐述幽默感。故选 A。

52. 【问题】作者提到卓别林的早期电影因为_____。

    A. 这些电影能娱乐大众

    B. 人类不同于动物

    C. 这些电影显示出一定的戏剧模式广受欢迎

    D. 这些电影显示出人们发笑的能力是一样的

【答案】C

【解析】细节题中的例证题。原文信息在第 1 段：…a sense of humor of certain comic stereotypes have a universal appeal. This can best be seen from the world-wide popularity of Charlie Chaplin's early films. 这句话的逻辑关系就是因果，此句意为：某种喜剧形式的幽默感会对全世界都有吸引力。这一点在卓别林的早期电影中有很好的体现。

53. 【问题】讽刺的主要功能之一是_____。

    A. 表现出行为的荒谬   B. 恢复平衡

    C. 挫败政客们   D. 显示世界的严酷

【答案】B

【解析】细节题。原文信息在第 3 段前三句。

54. 【问题】从第 3 段最后一句话中可以知道什么？

    A. 它用讽刺的手法揭示政治事件的真相。

    B. 它可以挑动人们发生暴乱。

    C. 它表明悲剧和喜剧是相关联的。

    D. 它能使人发笑。

【答案】A

【解析】该句意为："讽刺是一种太过强大的武器，不容许在极权主义政治制度下发展

壮大"。

55. 【问题】Swift 是谁？

    A．小说家。   B．诗人。

    C．戏剧家。   D．散文家。

【答案】A

【解析】Swift 是《格列佛游记》的作者。根据原文信息可知，在这本书中有小人国的人和他们邻居的战争情节。因而这本书应该是小说。本题亦可通过常识解答。

Passage Twelve

There is a common perception among many athletes, coaches, and even some sport psychologists that anxiety is a "bad" state, and should be reduced at all costs. Sport psychologists would traditionally most likely begin with teaching an anxious athlete relaxation and deep breathing skills. In my practice, I have found another approach also to be beneficial. Research has found that it is usually the person's perception of their high arousal that may influence performance, not the high arousal itself. If the athlete believes they are anxious, and believe that this anxiety may affect their performance, usually the anxiety increases. Their anxiety can then become out of control, reducing their performance, and completing a self-fulfilling prophecy.

Taking these findings on board, often when an athlete approaches me before a major competition flustered about his or her anxiety, I reply "Great!" After a brief look of confusion, I explain to the athlete that his body is getting ready to compete. The body is pumping blood to his muscles ready for explosive exercise. I may also have a brief chat about evolution, and how the body's flight or fight system is activated during potentially threatening situations.

This response increases heart rate and blood flow to the specific muscles involved in speed, strength, and power that was designed to help us either run away or defend ourselves from potential predators. I liken the body's response to the state they try and achieve in warm-up, with an increase in heart rate, and maybe a light sweat. Then we may have a discussion about the opposite state of total relaxation and boredom, and how this state would not be ideal for competition (of course this approach would not be relevant for sports requiring fine motor control and slow heart rate, such as shooting or archery). Athletes may also find it helpful if their anxiety is reframed as anticipation, passion, and excitement for the upcoming competition.

Although relaxation interventions can be valuable tools for performance enhancement, mental skills probably will be ineffective if the anxiety is out of control, or the source of the athlete's anxiety stems from deeper issues. These deeper concerns may include anxiety about performing in front of a significant other person (e.g., wanting to make Mum or Dad proud), or fear of not living up to a protected image of him or herself (e.g., having to perform well to live up to the image of the perfect athlete).

Relaxation skills can only go so far in helping these athletes, and a more effective approach may be referring these athletes to a sport psychologist with counseling experience. The referral process itself may be a delicate process given the stigma associated with seeing a "shrink" and admitting a perceived "weakness".

56. Which of the following statements is NOT true among athletes and coaches?
    A. Anxiety before the match is unbeneficial to athletes' performance.
    B. Such bad influence as anxiety should be eliminated before the match.
    C. Taking deep breath and relaxation are the most effective ways to alleviate athlete's anxiety.
    D. In some cases, anxiety can boost athlete's performance.

57. The author says "Great" to an anxious athlete for the purpose of _____.
    A. telling him that anxiety is beneficial to the athlete
    B. making the athlete realize that he is ready for competition
    C. implying the athlete's positive perception of his high arousal may boost his performance
    D. intending to make the athlete relaxed

58. According to the author, which of the following statements about the body's response to the anxious state is true?
    A. It is unbeneficial to athlete's performance.
    B. It shows that athletes are ready to achieve in warm-up.
    C. It is suitable for all sorts of sports.
    D. In any case, athletes inevitably find such a response helpful.

59. According to the passage, in some situations, the mental skills probably be ineffective EXCEPT _____.
    A. athletes live in fear of being defeated
    B. athletes strongly wish to live up to his parents' expectation
    C. athletes have too strong anxiety about themselves and they lose self-control
    D. athletes are worried about their performance in front of significant persons

60. The best title for the passage is _____.
    A. Anxiety, a Big Threat to Athletes
    B. Means of Eliminating Athletes' Anxiety
    C. Coping with Athletes' Anxiety Effectively
    D. Influence of Anxiety on Athletes

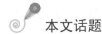 本文话题

如何解决运动员的赛前焦虑。

 难词译注

perception [pə'sepʃən] *n.*	理解，感知
arousal [ə'rauzəl] *n.*	觉醒，激励
prophecy ['prɔfisi] *n.*	预言
activate ['æktiveit] *v.*	刺激，使活动
liken ['laikən] *v.*	把……比作
archery ['ɑ:tʃəri] *n.*	箭术

✝ 答案及解析

56.【问题】关于运动员和教练员，下面哪一个表述不正确？

　　　　A. 赛前的紧张不利于运动员的发挥。

　　　　B. 像焦虑这种负面影响在赛前应该消除。

　　　　C. 深呼吸、放松是缓解运动员焦虑最有效的方法。

　　　　D. 在一些情况下，焦虑可以促进运动员的发挥。

【答案】D

【解析】细节题。原文第 1 段：There is a common perception among many athletes, coaches, and even some sport psychologists that anxiety is a "bad" state, and should be reduced at all costs. 通过对这句话的理解，我们可以得知，在运动员、教练员以及运动心理学家看来，焦虑应该不惜一切代价地消除。故选项 D 不正确。

57.【问题】作者提到他对一个焦虑的运动员说"很好"，其目的是_____。

　　　　A. 告诉他焦虑对运动员有益

　　　　B. 使运动员认识到他为比赛做好了准备

　　　　C. 暗示运动员，对紧张感的积极观点可以促进他的发挥

　　　　D. 打算使运动员放松

【答案】C

【解析】推断题。作者提出他如何与一个焦虑运动员共同处理焦虑的例子是为了进一步例证自己的观点：...it is usually the person's perception of their high arousal that may influence performance, not the high arousal itself.

58.【问题】根据作者的观点，对焦虑状态的身体反应，下面哪种观点是正确的？

　　　　A. 对运动员发挥没好处。

　　　　B. 它表明运动员在热身时做好了准备。

　　　　C. 它适合各类运动项目。

　　　　D. 在任何状况下，运动员必定发觉这一反应很有帮助。

【答案】B

【解析】细节题，排除法解题。A 项不符合作者的观点，其观点在第 1 段有阐述。C 项在原文第 3 段提到：...of course this approach would not be relevant for sports requiring fine motor control and slow heart rate, such as shooting or archery. 即这种方法不适合像射击、射箭等项目。D 项第 4 段也提到：...mental skills probably will be ineffective if the anxiety is out of control, or the source of the athlete's anxiety stems from deeper issues. 此句意为"如果运动员的焦虑失控或者其源自很深层的问题，这种办法就没效了"。故只有 B 正确。

59.【问题】根据本文，除了_____，在某些状况下心理技巧也可能失效。

　　　　A．运动员生活在怕被打败的恐惧中。

　　　　B．运动员强烈希望自己不辜负父母的期望。

　　　　C．运动员的焦虑太严重并且他们无法控制。

　　　　D．运动员担心在重要人物面前的表现。

【答案】A

【解析】推断题。相关原文信息在第 4 段。

60.【问题】文章最好的题目是_____。

　　　　A．焦虑——运动员最大的威胁　　B．消除运动员焦虑的手段

　　　　C．有效处理运动员的焦虑　　　　D．焦虑对运动员的影响

【答案】C

【解析】主旨题。首先确定各个选项的关键词，即威胁、手段、处理、影响，然后根据各段大意可以概括总结文章题目。

Passage Thirteen

There must be few questions on which responsible opinion is so utterly divided as on that of how much sleep we ought to have. There are some who think we can leave the body to regulate these matters for itself. "The answer is easy," says Dr. A. Burton. "With the right amount of sleep you should wake up fresh and alert five minutes before the alarm rings." If he is right many people must be undersleeping, including myself. But we must remember that some people have a greater inertia than others. This is not meant rudely. They switch on slowly, and they are reluctant to switch off. They are alert at bedtime and sleepy when it is time to get up, and this may have nothing to do with how fatigued their bodies are, or how much sleep they must take to lose their fatigue.

Other people feel sure that the present trend is towards too little sleep. To quote one medical opinion, thousands of people drift through life suffering from the effects of too little sleep; the reason is not that they can't sleep. Like advancing colonists, we do seem to be grasping ever more of the land of sleep for our waking needs, pushing the boundary back and reaching, apparently, for a point in our evolution where we will sleep no more. This in itself, of course, need not be a bad thing. What could be disastrous, however, is that we should press too quickly towards this goal, sacrificing sleep only to gain more time in which to <u>jeopardize</u> our civilization by actions and decisions made weak by fatigue.

Then, to complete the picture, there are those who believe that most people are persuaded to sleep too much. Dr. H. Roberts, writing in *Every Man in Health*, asserts: "It may safely be stated that, just as the majority eat too much, so the majority sleep too much." One can see the point of this also. It would be a pity to retard our development by holding back those people who are gifted enough to work and play well with less than the average amount of sleep, if indeed it does them no harm. If one of the trends of evolution is that more of the life span is to be spent in gainful waking activity, then surely these people are in the van of this advance.

61. The author seems to indicate that _____.
    A. there are many controversial issues like the right amount of sleep
    B. among many issues the right amount of sleep is the least controversial
    C. people are now moving towards solving many controversial issues
    D. the right amount of sleep is a topic of much controversy among doctors

62. The author disagrees with Dr. Burton because _____.
    A. few people can wake up feeling fresh and alert
    B. some people still feel tired with enough sleep
    C. some people still feel sleepy with enough sleep
    D. some people go to bed very late at night

63. The underlined word "jeopardize" is closest in meaning to _____.
    A. endeavor   B. endanger   C. endorse   D. endow

64. In the last paragraph the author points out that _____.
    A. sleeping less is good for human development
    B. people ought to be persuaded to sleep less than before
    C. it is incorrect to say that people sleep too little
    D. those who can sleep less should be encouraged

65. We learn from the passage that the author _____.
    A. comments on three different opinions
    B. favours one of the three opinions
    C. explains an opinion of his own
    D. revises someone else's opinion

 本文话题

人们的睡眠长短。

难词译注

jeopardize [ˈdʒepədaiz] v.　　　　　　　　　　　　　危害

答案及解析

61. 【问题】作者似乎要指出_____。

A. 有很多有争议的话题，例如睡眠量

B. 在众多话题中适当的睡眠量是最不具争议的话题

C. 现在人们转向解决许多有争议的问题

D. 多少睡眠量是适当的在医生中很有争议

【答案】D

【解析】此题为主旨题。文章首句揭示主题：There must be few questions on which responsible opinion is so utterly divided as on that of how much sleep we ought to have. 此句意为：很少有问题像我们应该睡多长时间那样引起如此大的分歧。

62. 【问题】作者不同意 Burton 博士的观点，因为_____。

A. 很少有人醒来感到精力充沛并思维敏捷

B. 一些睡得很足的人仍旧感到劳累

C. 一些睡得很足的人仍旧感到困

D. 一些人很晚才上床睡觉

【答案】A

【解析】细节题。原文中能够体现作者对 Dr. Burton 的观点的态度信息在第 1 段：If he is right many people must be undersleeping, including myself. 此句意为：如果他（Dr. Burton）是对的话，许多人都一定是睡眠不足，包括我在内。这句话体现作者与 Dr. Burton 的观点不一致。

63. 【问题】与画线词 "jeopardize" 含义最接近的是_____。

A. 努力　　　　B. 危及　　　　C. 签署　　　　D. 捐赠

【答案】B

【解析】猜词题。由上下文可知，画线词的含义为"危害"。

64. 【问题】在最后一段，作者指出_____。

A. 睡眠不足对人体成长有好处　　　B. 应该劝说人们要比以前睡得少一些

C. 人们睡得太少的说法不正确　　　D. 应该鼓励那些睡眠少的人

【答案】D

【解析】细节题。原文信息为最后一段：It would be a pity to retard our development by holding back those people who are gifted enough to work and play well with less than the average amount of sleep, if indeed it does them no harm. 有些人天生就可以少睡觉，并且不耽误工作和玩乐，如果确实对他们无害，那么因

阻止他们这样做而延误我们整个社会发展的话，就太遗憾了。

65.【问题】从文章中我们可以知道作者_____。

    A．对于三种不同观点进行评论   B．赞成三个不同观点中的一个

    C．解释他自己的一个观点   D．修正其他人的观点

【答案】A

【解析】主旨题。综观全文，作者就对睡眠的三种观点进行阐述，并且针对这三种观点进行了评论，最终提出自己的看法。因而选项 A 为正确答案。

Passage Fourteen

I am one of the many city people who are always saying that given the choice we would prefer to live in the country away from the dirt and noise of a large city. I have managed to convince myself that if it weren't for my job I would immediately head out for the open spaces and go back to nature in some sleepy village buried in the county. But how realistic is the dream?

Cities can be frightening places. The majority of the population live in massive tower blocks, noisy, dirty and impersonal. The sense of belonging to a community tends to disappear when you live fifteen floors up. All you can see from your window is sky, or other blocks of flats. Children become aggressive and nervous, cooped up at home all day, with nowhere to play; their mothers feel isolated from the rest of the world. Strangely enough, whereas in the past the inhabitants of one street all knew each other, nowadays people on the same floor in tower blocks don't even say hello to each other.

Country life, on the other hand, differs from this kind of isolated existence in that a sense of community generally binds the inhabitants of small villages together. People have the advantage of knowing that there is always someone to turn to when they need help. But country life has disadvantages too. While it is true that you may be among friends in a village, it is also true that you are cut off from the exciting and important events that take place in cities. There's little possibility of going to a new show or the latest movie. Shopping becomes a major problem, and for anything slightly out of the ordinary you have to go on an expedition to the nearest large town. The city-dweller who leaves for the country is often oppressed by a sense of unbearable stillness and quiet.

What, then, is the answer? The country has the advantage of peace and quiet, but suffers from the disadvantage of being cut off; the city breeds a feeling of isolation, and constant noise batters the senses. But one of its main advantages is that you are at the centre of things, and that life doesn't come to an end at half past nine at night. Some people have found (or rather bought) a compromise between the two: they have expressed their preference for the "quiet life" by leaving the suburbs and moving to villages within commuting distance of large cities. They generally have about as much sensitivity as the plastic flowers they leave behind — they are polluted with strange ideas about change and improvement which they force on to the unwilling original inhabitants of the villages.

What then of my dreams of leaning on a cottage gate and murmuring "morning" to the locals as they pass by. I'm keen on the idea, but you see there's my cat, Toby. I'm not at all sure that he would take to all that fresh air and exercise in the long grass. I mean, can you see him mixing with all those hearty males down the farm? No, he would rather have the electric imitation-coal fire any evening.

66. We get the impression from the first paragraph that the author _____.
    A. used to live in the country   B. used to work in the city
    C. works in the city   D. lives in the country

67. In the author's opinion, the following may cause city people to be unhappy EXCEPT _____.
    A. a strong sense of fear   B. lack of communication
    C. housing conditions   D. a sense of isolation

68. The passage implies that it is easy to buy the following things in the country EXCEPT _____.
    A. daily necessities   B. fresh fruits
    C. designer clothes   D. fresh vegetables

69. According to the passage, which of the following adjectives best describes those people who work in large cities and live in villages?
    A. Original.   B. Quiet.   C. Arrogant.   D. Insensitive.

70. Do you think the author will move to the country?
    A. Yes, he will do so.   B. No, he will not do so.
    C. It is difficult to tell.   D. He is in two minds.

 本文话题

城乡生活的差异。

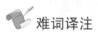 难词译注

aggressive [əˈgresiv] a.	好斗的
coop up	禁闭
compromise [ˈkɔmprəmaiz] n.	妥协，折中
commute [kəˈmjuːt] v.	（乘车）往返
murmur [ˈməːmə] n.	咕哝，低语

难句译注

1. I am one of the many city people who are always saying that given the choice we would prefer to live in the country away from the dirt and noise of a large city.

   【分析】who 引导定语从句，修饰 people。that 引导的宾语从句中，有一个相当于虚拟条件句的特殊句型。

   【译文】很多在城市里生活的人总是说，如果有选择的话我宁愿住在乡下，远离肮脏、喧闹的大城市；我就是他们中的一员。

2. I have managed to convince myself that if it weren't for my job I would immediately head out for the open spaces and go back to nature in some sleepy village buried in the county.

   【分析】if 引导虚拟条件句。

   【译文】我已经让自己相信：如果不是为了工作，我马上就会去一个开阔的地方，在乡村中一个沉睡的小村落中回归大自然。

3. They generally have about as much sensitivity as the plastic flowers they leave behind — they are polluted with strange ideas about change and improvement which they force on to the unwilling original inhabitants of the villages.

   【分析】they leave behind 做定语从句，修饰 flowers；which 引导定语从句，修饰 strange ideas。

   【译文】他们像他们所留下的塑料花一样，他们被有关改变和进步的奇怪思想所污染。而且，他们还将这些思想强加在村庄里的原著居民身上。

答案及解析

66. 【问题】在第 1 段我们形成的印象是，作者_____。

    A. 过去住在乡下　　　　　　　　B. 过去在城里工作

    C. 现在在城里工作　　　　　　　D. 现在住在乡下

    【答案】C

    【解析】细节题。在第 1 段里有两个虚拟语气可以帮助解题："…given the choice we would prefer to live in the country away from the dirt and noise of a large city." 和 "…if it weren't for my job I would immediately head out for the open spaces…"通过这两个句子可以判断，作者现在身处城市。故 C 正确。

67. 【问题】根据作者的观点，除了_____，以下都是城市人不快乐的原因。

    A. 很强烈的恐惧感　　　　　　　B. 缺少交流

    C. 住房条件　　　　　　　　　　D. 孤独感

    【答案】A

    【解析】细节题。相关信息在原文第 2 段。由 "The sense of belonging to a community tends to disappear…people on the same floor in tower blocks don't even say hello to each other." 可知，城市生活 "lack of communication"；由 "The majority of the population live in massive tower blocks, noisy, dirty and impersonal… All you can see from your window is sky, or other blocks of flats. " 可知，城市生活的 "housing conditions" 让人不开心；由 "Children…cooped up at home all day…their mothers feel isolated from the rest of the world. " 可知，城市生活是 "a sense of isolation"。文中没有提及 "a strong sense of fear"，故 A 为正确答案。

68. 【问题】文章暗示除了_____，其他的都很容易在乡下买到。

    A．日用品   B．新鲜水果

    C．设计师的服装   D．新鲜的蔬菜

    【答案】C

    【解析】推理题。相关原文信息是在第 3 段：Shopping becomes a major problem, and for anything slightly out of the ordinary you have to go on an expedition to the nearest large town. 此句意为：购物是个大问题，并且与日常生活相比稍微特别一点的东西，就不得不去最近的大城镇买了。因而可以推知，设计师的服装相比较而言属于特别的物品，故选 C。

69. 【问题】根据文章，下面哪一个形容词形容那些住在乡下但在城市工作的人最贴切？

    A．淳朴的。   B．安静的。   C．傲慢的。   D．麻木不仁的。

    【答案】D

    【解析】推理题。第 4 段：They generally have about as much sensitivity as the plastic flowers they leave behind — they are polluted with strange ideas about change and improvement which they force on to the unwilling original inhabitants of the villages. 这句话中的 they 指代的就是题目中界定的人群。从这句话当中可以得知：这一群人很不敏感，并且他们会把有关变化和进步的奇怪想法强加给那些乡村里的居民。四个备选形容词只有 insensitive 符合原文的描述。

70. 【问题】你认为作者会搬到乡下吗？

    A．是的，他会这样做。   B．不，他不会这样做。

    C．很难讲。   D．他这两个想法都有。

    【答案】B

    【解析】推理题。在最后一段中，从 "I'm keen on the idea, but…" 这个转折关系可以推断出，作者对于这样的想法很有兴趣，但是由于 but 后面的原因而作罢，故 B 为正确选项。

Passage Fifteen

In the world of entertainment, TV talk shows have undoubtedly flooded every inch of space on daytime television. And anyone who watches them regularly knows that each one varies in style and format. But no two shows are more profoundly opposite in content, while at the same time standing out above the rest, than the Jerry Springer and the Oprah

Winfrey shows.

Jerry Springer could easily be considered the king of "trash talk". The topics on his show are as shocking as shocking can be. For example, the show takes the ever-common talk show themes of love, sex, cheating, guilt, hate, conflict and morality to a different level. Clearly, the Jerry Springer show is a display and exploitation of society's moral catastrophes（灾难）, yet people are willing to eat up the intriguing（有迷惑力的）predicaments（困境）of other people's lives.

Like Jerry Springer, Oprah Winfrey takes TV talk show to its extreme, but Oprah goes in the opposite direction. The show focuses on the improvement of society and an individual's quality of life. Topics range from teaching your children responsibility, managing your work week, to getting to know your neighbors.

Compared to Oprah, the Jerry Springer show looks like poisonous waste being dumped on society. Jerry ends every show with a "final word". He makes a small speech that sums up the entire moral of the show. Hopefully, this is the part where most people will learn something very valuable.

Clean as it is, the Oprah show is not for everyone. The show's main target audience are middle-class Americans. Most of these people have the time, money, and stability to deal with life's tougher problems. Jerry Springer, on the other hand, has more of an association with the young adults of society. These are 18- to 21-year-old ones whose main troubles in life involve love, relationship, sex, money and peers. They are the 18- to 21-year-old ones who see some value and lessons to be learned underneath the show's exploitation.

While the two shows are as different as night and day. Both have ruled the talk show circuit for many years now. Each one caters to a different audience while both have a strong following from large groups of fans. Ironically, both could also be considered pioneers in the talk show world.

71. Compared with other TV talk shows, both the Jerry Springer and the Oprah Winfrey are _____.

    A. more family-oriented   B. unusually popular

    C. more profound   D. relatively formal

72. Though the social problems Jerry Springer talks about appear distasteful, the audience _____.

    A. remain fascinated by them   B. are ready to face up to them

    C. remain indifferent to them   D. are willing to get involved in them

73. Which of the following is likely to be a topic of the Oprah Winfrey show?

    A. A new type of robot.   B. Racist hatred.

    C. Family budget planning.   D. Street violence.

74. Despite their different approaches, the two talk shows are both _____.

    A. ironical   B. sensitive   C. instructive   D. cynical

75. We can learn from the passage that the two talk shows _____.

    A. have monopolized the talk show circuit

    B. exploit the weaknesses in human nature

    C. appear at different times of the day

    D. are targeted at different audiences

本文话题

脱口秀。

难词译注

ironically [aiˈrɔnikli] *ad.*   讽刺地

答案及解析

71. 【问题】和其他电视脱口秀相比，杰瑞和奥普拉的节目_____。

    A. 更加面向家庭   B. 非常受人欢迎

    C. 更深刻   D. 相对正式

    【答案】B

    【解析】推断题。第 1 段最后一句话提到 standing out above the rest，说明他们两个的节目与其他节目相比十分出类拔萃。文章最后一段提到：Each one caters to a different audience while both have a strong following from large groups of fans. 此句意为：两个节目都有大量不同的但很固定的支持者。

72. 【问题】尽管杰瑞谈到的社会问题看上去令人不愉快，但是观众_____。

    A. 仍旧被它们所吸引   B. 自愿面对它们

    C. 仍旧漠不关心   D. 自愿牵涉其中

    【答案】A

    【解析】细节题。原文出处在第 2 段最后一句话。原文大意是：无疑，他的节目是展示和挖掘社会的道德灾难，但人们对其他人在生活中令人好奇的困境却很感兴趣。

73. 【问题】下面哪一个可能成为奥普拉节目的题目？

    A. 新型机器人。   B. 种族仇恨。

    C. 家庭预算计划。   D. 街头暴力。

    【答案】C

    【解析】推理题。在第 3 段阐述了她节目的风格，与 Jerry Springer 的截然不同，她的节目致力于改进社会和提高个人生活质量。话题从教育孩子有责任感、安排一周的工作到逐渐了解邻居。从这段可以看出她的节目更关注家庭。因而选 C。

74. 【问题】尽管这两个脱口秀方法不同，但它们都是_____。

    A. 讽刺的   B. 敏感的   C. 有益的   D. 愤世嫉俗的

【答案】C

【解析】推理题。第 4 段和第 5 段的最后一句话分别认为两个节目都会让人有所回味和领悟。

75. 【问题】从文章我们可以知道这两个脱口秀_____。

    A. 独霸脱口秀节目   B. 揭露人性弱点

    C. 出现在白天的不同时段   D. 定位不同的观众

【答案】D

【解析】细节题。此题用排除法比较简单。由最后一段提到两个节目名列前茅但不是独霸，所以排除 A；根据两个节目的风格就可以知道 B 项错误；原文中没有 C 项相关的信息。因而答案为 D。

Passage Sixteen

It is said that in England death is pressing, in Canada inevitable and in California optional. Small wonder. Americans' life expectancy has nearly doubled over the past century. Failing hips can be replaced, clinical depression controlled, cataracts（白内障）removed in a 30-minute surgical procedure. Such advances offer the aging population a quality of life that was unimaginable when I entered medicine 50 years ago. But not even a great health-care system can cure death and our failure to confront that reality now threatens this greatness of ours.

Death is normal; we are genetically programmed to disintegrate and perish, even under ideal conditions. We all understand that at some level, yet as medical consumers we treat death as a problem to be solved. Shielded by third-party payers from the cost of our care, we demand everything that can possibly be done for us, even if it's useless. The most obvious example is late-stage cancer care. Physicians frustrated by their inability to cure the disease and fearing loss of hope in the patient too often offer aggressive treatment far beyond what is scientifically justified.

In 1950, the U.S. spent $ 12.7 billion on health care. In 2002, the cost will be $ 1,540 billion. Anyone can see this trend is unsustainable. Yet few seem willing to try to reverse it. Some scholars conclude that a government with finite resources should simply stop paying for medical care that sustains life beyond a certain age — say 83 or so. Former Colorado governor Richard Lamm has been quoted as saying that the old and infirm "have a duty to die and get out of the way", so that younger, healthier people can realize their potential.

I would not go that far. Energetic people now routinely work through their 60s and beyond, and remain dazzlingly productive. At 78, Viacom chairman Sumner Redstone jokingly claims to be 53. Supreme Court Justice Sandra Day O'Connor is in her 70s, and former surgeon general C. Everett Koop chairs an Internet start-up in his 80s. These leaders are living proof that prevention works and that we can manage the health problems that come naturally with age. As a mere 68-year-old, I wish to age as productively as they have.

Yet there are limits to what a society can spend in this pursuit. Ask a physician, I know the most costly and dramatic measures may be ineffective and painful. I also know that people in Japan and Sweden, countries that spend far less on medical care, have achieved longer, healthier lives than we have. As a nation, we may be overfunding the quest for unlikely cures while underfunding research on humbler therapies that could improve people's lives.

76. What is implied in the first sentence?

   A. Americans are better prepared for death than other people.

   B. Americans enjoy a higher life quality than ever before.

   C. Americans are over confident of their medical technology.

   D. Americans take a vain pride in their long life expectancy.

77. The author uses the example of cancer patients to show that _____.

   A. medical resources are often wasted

   B. doctors are helpless against fatal diseases

   C. some treatments are too aggressive

   D. medical costs are becoming unaffordable

78. The author's attitude toward Richard Lamm's remark is one of _____.

   A. strong disapproval   B. reserved consent

   C. slight contempt   D. enthusiastic support

79. In contrast to the U.S., Japan and Sweden are funding their medical care _____.

   A. more flexibly   B. more extravagantly

   C. more cautiously   D. more reasonably

80. The text intends to express the idea that _____.

   A. medicine will further prolong people's lives

   B. life beyond a certain limit is not worth living

   C. death should be accepted as a fact of life

   D. excessive demands increase the cost of health care

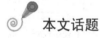 **本文话题**

针对死亡的不同看法。

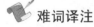 **难词译注**

disintegrate [dis'intigreit] *v.*   使分裂，使解体

perish ['periʃ] v.   凋谢，消亡
extravagantly [ik'strævəgəntli] ad.   奢侈地，挥霍无度地

答案及解析

76.【问题】第一句暗示了什么？
    A. 美国人比其他国家的人更好地为死做好了准备。
    B. 美国人享受了比以前更好的生活质量。
    C. 美国人对他们的医疗技术过于自信。
    D. 美国人对他们的长寿很自负。
【答案】C
【解析】推断题。原文中第 1 句话：It is said that in England death is pressing, in Canada inevitable and in California optional. 此句意为：据说，死亡在英国迫在眉睫，在加拿大不可避免，在加利福尼亚可以选择。从第 1 段后面的阐述中可以得知，美国的医疗技术有了显著的进步，这使美国年纪大的人可以享受更好的生活，这也符合原文信息中的关键词"optional"，人们因为医疗水平的进步可以控制死亡，延缓生命。故选项 C 更接近原文信息。

77.【问题】作者用癌症患者的例子是要说明_____。
    A. 医疗资源总是被浪费   B. 医生对于致命疾病束手无策
    C. 一些治疗方法太激进   D. 医疗成本日益让人支付不起
【答案】A
【解析】细节题中的例证题。癌症的例子出现在第 2 段。这个例子是为证明作者在本段的观点。在第 2 段，作者一开始便提出观点：死亡是很正常的，但人们视死亡为要解决的问题。因而人们要求使用任何方法来解决这一难题，尽管这样做是毫无意义的。根据这些有关观点的原文阐述，对比选项就可以得出答案。

78.【问题】作者对于理查德的评论持何种态度？
    A. 强烈反对。   B. 有所保留地赞成。   C. 有点轻蔑。   D. 大力支持。
【答案】B
【解析】态度题。首先 Richard Lamm's remark 出现在第 3 段最后一句：...the old and infirm "have a duty to die and get out of the way". 含义是年老体衰的人有义务死亡，并且（为年轻健康的人）腾地方。作者对此的态度出现在第 4 段以及第 5 段：第 4 段第 1 句话"I would not go that far.（还以为我不会这么极端）。"第 5 段第 1 句话"Yet there are limits to what a society can spend in this pursuit...（然而，社会在这一追求中的花费是有限制的）。"这一追求指的是追求高质量的老年生活。根据这两个主题句可以推断，作者对 Richard 的观点是不完全赞同的，但与其观点有些近似。故选 B。

79.【问题】与美国作对比，日本和瑞典投资医疗服务_____。
    A. 更灵活   B. 更奢侈
    C. 更谨慎   D. 更合情合理

【答案】D

【解析】细节题。信息在原文第 5 段：I also know that people in Japan and Sweden, countries that spend far less on medical care, have achieved longer, healthier lives than we have. 此句意为：我也知道在日本和瑞典，人们在医疗方面的开销很少，但比我们活得更长更健康。这说明这两个国家的人在医疗方面的开销更为有效，更为合理，不会造成过度的浪费。符合此意的是选项 D。

80.【问题】文章试图表达的想法是_____。

    A. 医药将会进一步延长人们的寿命　　　B. 超过一定限制的生活不值得过

    C. 死亡应该作为生活的事实被人们接受　　D. 过度的需求增加医疗成本

【答案】C

【解析】主旨题。综观全文，作者的观点是：死亡很正常，我们不应该在解决死亡的问题上过分地投入，这样的投入是毫无意义的，换句话说，我们应该坦然地接受死亡。

Passage Seventeen

If you intend to use humor in your talk to make people smile, you must know how to identify shared experiences and problems. Your humor must be relevant to the audience and should help to show them that you are one of them or that you understand their situation and are in sympathy with their point of view. Depending on whom you are addressing, the problems will be different. If you are talking to a group of managers, you may refer to the disorganized methods of their secretaries; alternatively if you are addressing secretaries, you may want to comment on their disorganized bosses.

Here is an example, which I heard at a nurses' convention, of a story which works well because the audience all shared the same view of doctors. A man arrives in heaven and is being shown around by St. Peter. He sees wonderful accommodations, beautiful gardens, sunny weather, and so on. Everyone is very peaceful, polite and friendly until, waiting in a line for lunch, the new arrival is suddenly pushed aside by a man in a white coat, who rushes to the head of the line, grabs his food and stomps over to a table by himself. "Who is that?" the new arrival asked St. Peter. "Oh, that's God," came the reply, "but sometimes he thinks he's a doctor."

If you are part of the group which you are addressing, you will be in a position to know the experiences and problems which are common to all of you and it'll be appropriate for you to make a passing remark about the inedible canteen food or the chairman's notorious bad taste in ties. With other audiences you mustn't attempt to cut in with humor as they will resent an outsider making disparaging remarks about their canteen or their chairman. You will be on safer ground if you stick to scapegoats like the Post Office or the telephone system.

If you feel awkward being humorous, you must practice so that it becomes more natural. Include a few casual and apparently off-the-cuff remarks which you can deliver in a relaxed and unforced manner. Often it's the delivery which causes the audience to smile, so speak slowly and remember that a raised eyebrow or an unbelieving look may help to show that you are making a light-hearted remark. Look for the humor. It often comes from the unexpected. A twist on a familiar quote "If at first you don't succeed, give up" or a play on words or on a situation. Search for exaggeration and understatements. Look at your talk and pick out a few words or sentences which you can turn about and inject with humor.

81. To make your humor work, you should _____.
    A. take advantage of different kinds of audience
    B. make fun of the disorganized people
    C. address different problems to different people
    D. show sympathy for your listeners

82. The joke about doctors implies that, in the eyes of nurses, they are _____.
    A. impolite to new arrivals   B. very conscious of their godlike role
    C. entitled to some privileges   D. very busy even during lunch hours

83. It can be inferred from the text that public services _____.
    A. have benefited many people
    B. are the focus of public attention
    C. are an inappropriate subject for humor
    D. have often been the laughing stock

84. To achieve the desired result, humorous stories should be delivered _____.
    A. in well-worded language   B. as awkwardly as possible
    C. in exaggerated statements   D. as casually as possible

85. The best title for the text may be _____.
    A. Use Humor Effectively   B. Various Kinds of Humor
    C. Add Humor to Speech   D. Different Humor Strategies

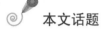 本文话题

如何在发言中使用幽默感。

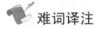 难词译注

stomp [stɔmp] n.	重踏
inedible [in'edibl] a.	不可食用的
notorious [nəu'tɔːriəs] a.	声名狼藉的
off-the-cuff ['ɔfðə'kʌf,] a.	即席的

disparaging [dis'pæridʒiŋ] *a.*   轻视的

scapegoat ['skeipgəut] *n.*   替罪羊

 难句译注

1. Your humor must be relevant to the audience and should help to show them that you are one of them or that you understand their situation and are in sympathy with their point of view.

    【分析】must be relevant to 与 should help 为并列谓语，两个 that 为平行并列的宾语从句。

    【译文】你的幽默要和听众相关，要借助幽默表明你是他们中的一员，或者让他们知道，你理解他们的处境并且同意他们的观点。

2. If you are part of the group which you are addressing, you will be in a position to know the experiences and problems which are common to all of you and it'll be appropriate for you to make a passing remark about the inedible canteen food or the chairman's notorious bad taste in ties.

    【分析】if 引导了一个条件状语从句，which 引导定语从句修饰 group；在主句中 and 连接两个并列句，其中 which are common… 作为定语从句修饰 experiences and problems。

    【译文】如果你是正在听你发言的听众中的一员，你就可以站在他们的角度了解你们共有的经历和存在的问题，也会使你很恰当地对饭厅难以下咽的食物和主席着装的低品位进行评论。

3. Often it's the delivery which causes the audience to smile, so speak slowly and remember that a raised eyebrow or an unbelieving look may help to show that you are making a light-hearted remark.

    【分析】which causes the audience to smile 是定语从句，修饰 delivery。or 连接两个并列主语。

    【译文】通常这是引起观众发笑的话，因而语速要慢，记得挑起眉毛或者一副不相信的面部表情都有助于表明你正在进行一个轻松愉快的发言。

🏆 答案及解析

81.【问题】为了使幽默产生效果，你应该_____。

　　　　A．利用各种听众　　　　　　　　B．取笑无条理的人

　　　　C．有区别地对待不同的听众　　　 D．对听众表现出同情

　　【答案】C

　　【解析】细节题。原文信息在第 1 段。在第 1 段里，作者提到：如果你想在发言中使用幽默，让人发笑，你就必须让你的听众感觉到你是他们中的一分子，针对不同的听众，问题也不同。根据对这些细节的理解，选项中只有 C 项正确。

82.【问题】有关医生的笑话暗示，在护士眼中，医生们_____。

    A. 对新来的人很不礼貌　　　　　B. 很在意他们像上帝一样的角色

    C. 享有特权　　　　　　　　　　D. 很忙，甚至午饭时间也是

【答案】B

【解析】推断题。有关医生的笑话出现在原文第 2 段。既然题目是这个有关医生的笑话给我们什么暗示，因而笑话表面含义的选项都不选。故 B 项为正确选项。

83.【问题】文章暗示公共服务_____。

    A. 造福了很多人　　　　　　　　B. 是公众的焦点

    C. 不适合成为幽默的话题　　　　D. 经常被当作笑料

【答案】D

【解析】推断题。原文中和公共服务有关的信息在第 3 段最后一句话：With other audiences you mustn't attempt to cut in with humor. You will be on safer ground if you stick to scapegoats like the Post Office or the telephone system. 在这句话中 post office 以及 the telephone system 指的就是公共服务。最后一句话的含义是如果你执意拿邮局或电话局这样的替罪羊开玩笑，那么你是安全的。换句话说拿公共服务开玩笑没关系，故选 D。

84.【问题】要想达到想要的结果，幽默的故事应该_____讲述。

    A. 用精辟的语言　　　　　　　　B. 尽可能笨拙地

    C. 用夸张的手法　　　　　　　　D. 尽可能轻松地

【答案】D

【解析】细节题。信息在原文第 4 段第 1 句话：If you feel awkward being humorous, you must practice so that is becomes more natural. 这里的 natural 为关键词，D 项与它相对应。

85.【问题】本文最好的题目是_____。

    A. 有效地使用幽默　　　　　　　B. 多种多样的幽默

    C. 在发言中增加幽默　　　　　　D. 不同的幽默技巧

【答案】A

【解析】主旨题。根据各段的主题句就可以总结概括出文章的主题思想。文章从如何有针对性地使用幽默，到要想达到理想效果，该如何做。这些信息都是围绕如何使用幽默而展开的，故选 A。

Passage Eighteen

Science, in practice, depends far less on the experiments it prepares than on the preparedness of the minds of the men who watch the experiments. Sir Isaac Newton supposedly discovered gravity through the fall of an apple. Apples had been falling in many places for centuries and thousands of people had seen them fall. But Newton for years had been curious about the cause of the orbital motion of the moon and planets. What kept them in place? Why didn't they fall out of the sky? The fact that the apple fell down toward the earth and not up into the tree answered the question he had been asking himself about those larger fruits of the heavens, the moon and the planets.

How many men would have considered the possibility of an apple falling up into the tree? Newton did because he was not trying to predict anything. He was just wondering. His mind was ready for the unpredictable. Unpredictability is part of the essential nature of research. If you don't have unpredictable things, you don't have research. Scientists tend to forget this when writing their <u>cut and dried</u> reports for the technical journals, but history is filled with examples of it.

In talking to some scientists, particularly younger ones, you might gather the impression that they find the "scientific method" a substitute for imaginative thought. I've attended research conferences where a scientist has been asked what he thinks about the advisability of continuing a certain experiment. The scientist has frowned, looked at the graphs, and said "the data are still inconclusive". "We know that," the men from the budget office have said, "but what do you think? Is it worthwhile going on? What do you think we might expect?" The scientist has been shocked at having even been asked to speculate.

What this amounts to, of course, is that the scientist has become the victim of his own writings. He has put forward unquestioned claims so consistently that he not only believes them himself, but has convinced industrial and business management that they are true. If experiments are planned and carried out according to plan as faithfully as the reports in the science journals indicate, then it is perfectly logical for management to expect research to produce results measurable in dollars and cents. It is entirely reasonable for auditors to believe that scientists who know exactly where they are going and how they will get there should not be distracted by the necessity of keeping one eye on the cash register while the other eye is on the microscope. Nor, if regularity and conformity to a standard pattern are as desirable to the scientist as the writing of his papers would appear to reflect, is management to be blamed for discriminating against the "odd balls" among researchers in favor of more conventional thinkers who work well with the team.

86. The author wants to prove with the example of Isaac Newton that _____ .
    A. inquiring minds are more important than scientific experiments
    B. science advances when fruitful researches are conducted
    C. scientists seldom forget the essential nature of research
    D. unpredictability weighs less than prediction in scientific research

87. The author asserts that scientist _____ .
    A. shouldn't replace "scientific method" with imaginative thought
    B. shouldn't neglect to speculate on unpredictable things
    C. should write more concise reports for technical journals
    D. should be confident about their research findings

88. The underlined phrases "cut and dried" in Paragraph 2 is closest in meaning to _____.
    A. run-of-the-mill　　B. outstanding　　C. adoptable　　D. verbatim

89. It seems that some young scientists _____.
    A. have a keen interest in prediction　　B. often speculate on the future
    C. think highly of creative thinking　　D. stick to "scientific method"

90. The author implies that the results of scientific research _____.
    A. may not be as profitable as they are expected
    B. can be measured in dollars and cents
    C. rely on conformity to a standard pattern
    D. are mostly underestimated by management

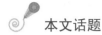
本文话题

在科学领域，什么最重要？

难词译注

conformity [kənˈfɔːmiti] *n.*　　　　　　　　　　　遵守，顺从

难句译注

1.　The fact that the apple fell down toward the earth and not up into the tree answered the question he had been asking himself about those larger fruits of the heavens, the moon and the planets.

　　【分析】that the apple fell down… 做同位语从句；he had been asking himself about those larger fruits of the heavens, the moon and the planets. 为定语从句，修饰 questions。

　　【译文】苹果掉到地上而不是往树上掉，这个事实回答了他一直不解的问题，即有关天地之果实——月球和行星的问题。

2.　If experiments are planned and carried out according to plan as faithfully as the reports in the science journals indicate, then it is perfectly logical for management to expect research to produce results measurable in dollars and cents.

　　【分析】这个主从复合句中的前半部分是 if 引导的条件从句，这个从句中有一个 as… as… 的结构，注意后一个 as 后面跟的是一个句子，其中 the report 谓语是 indicate；后半部分是主句，句中的 it 是形式主语，代替的是后面 for… to… 的结构，这是真正的主语。还需要注意的是 results 后面跟的形容词短语说明的是 results 的衡量方式。

　　【译文】如果按照科学杂志上的报告所指出的那样进行实验，按照计划去实施，那么对于管理者来说，期望研究产生可以用钱来衡量的结果就是完全合乎逻辑的。

3. It is entirely reasonable for auditors to believe that scientists who know exactly where they are going and how they will get there should not be distracted by the necessity of keeping one eye on the cash register while the other eye is on the microscope.

【分析】这个简单句的主语用的是形式主语 it，真正的主语是动词不定式短语。believe 后面跟的是一个 that 引导的宾语从句；who know exactly where they are going and how they will get there should not be distracted by the necessity of keeping one eye on the cash register while the other eye is on the microscope 为定语从句修饰 scientists。while 引导时间状语从句。

【译文】审计人员也完全有理由相信，确切知道自己的目标并知道如何实现这一目标的科学家们根本没必要在用一只眼睛盯着显微镜的同时，还要用另一只眼睛盯着现金计数器。

4. Nor, if regularity and conformity to a standard pattern are as desirable to the scientist as the writing of his papers would appear to reflect, is management to be blamed for discriminating against the "odd balls" among researchers in favor of more conventional thinkers who work well with the team.

【分析】首先，注意这个句子是个倒装句，原因是否定词 nor 在句首，后面紧跟的是 if 引导的条件从句。注意其中有一个 as...as... 的用法，中间跟的是形容词 desirable，比较的是科学家对 regularity and conformity 的希望和他们论文所反映的要求。这样的构成使主句的主语和谓语 is 发生了倒装，介词 for 后面跟的动名词短语是 blamed 的理由。注意 against 和 in favor of 后面各跟了一种不同类型的 researchers。最后需要注意的是 thinkers 后面跟的是 who 引导的定语从句，起修饰作用。

【译文】如果像他们的论文所反映的那样，科学家也想看到规律性和与某种标准模式的一致性，那么如果管理人员歧视研究人员中的"标新立异者"，而赞赏"善于合作"的具有传统思维模式的人，那也是无可指责的。

答案及解析

86. 【问题】作者举牛顿的例子是为了证明_____。
    A. 爱追根究底的想法远比科学实验更重要
    B. 当富有成效的研究在进行时，科学就进步了
    C. 科学家们很少忘记科学研究的本质
    D. 在科学研究中，未知因素大多是可预测的

    【答案】A

    【解析】细节题的例证题。相关原文信息在第 1 段：Science, in practice, depends far less on the experiments it prepares than on the preparedness of the minds of the men who watch the experiments. 此句意为：在实践中，科学更多依赖

于实验观察者的心理准备状况，而很少依赖于科学所设置的实验。在四个选项中，A 项突出作者的观点，就是牛顿对于苹果为什么会掉下来等事情的好奇心促使他在科学上取得巨大成就。

87.【问题】作者认为科学家_____。

　　A．不应用想象力代替"科学方法"

　　B．不应该忽视对不可预测事情的推测

　　C．应该为科学杂志写更多精炼的文章

　　D．应该对自己的研究发现有信心

【答案】B

【解析】细节题。解题信息在第 2 段：Unpredictability is part of the essential nature of research. If you don't have unpredictable things, you don't have research. 此句意为：不可预知性是研究的重要本质，如果没有不可预测的事情，就不会有研究。根据作者这一观点，B 为正确答案。另外，在第一段作者有关牛顿的事例也是在证明这一观点。

88.【问题】第 2 段中的画线词组"cut and dried"与_____意思最为接近。

【答案】A

【解析】猜词题。画线词组含义为"呆板的，事先准备好的"；A．平庸的，普通的；B．杰出的；C．可以采用的；D．一字不差的。

89.【问题】似乎一些年轻科学家_____。

　　A．对预测十分感兴趣　　　　　　B．经常揣测未来

　　C．对有创造力的思维大加赞赏　　D．坚持"科学的方法"

【答案】D

【解析】细节题。此题目有关年轻科学家的内容。原文相关信息在第 3 段，年轻科学家给人们的印象是：他们认为 the "scientific method" a substitute for imaginative thought，即科学方法可以替代想象思维。

90.【问题】作者暗示科学研究的成果_____。

　　A．可能没有预期的那样有利润　　B．可以用美元衡量

　　C．有赖于遵循一个标准模式　　　D．大多数情况下被管理阶层低估了

【答案】A

【解析】推断题。谈到研究结果的原文信息在最后一段：If experiments are planned and carried out according to plan as faithfully as the reports in the science journals indicate, then it is perfectly logical for management to expect research to produce results measurable in dollars and cents. 此句意为：如果按照科学杂志上的报告所指出的那样进行实验，按照计划去实施，那么对于管理者来说，期望研究产生可以用钱来衡量的结果就是完全合乎逻辑的。作者的言外之意表示科学实验不可能如此。故答案为 A。

经过前面系统的复习和 18 篇专项训练，您一定已经有所收获。下面是最近几年的阅读真题，每一套都请在限定的时间内做完，以更准确地检验你的复习效果。

2018 年医学博士统考阅读理解部分真题

Passage One

When Tony Wagner, the Harvard education specialist, describes his job today, he says he's "a translator between two hostile tribes"— the education world and the business world, the people who teach our kids and the people who give them jobs. Wagner's argument in his book "Creating *Innovators: The Making of Young People Who Will Change the World*" is that our K-12 and college tracks are not consistently "adding the value and teaching the skills that matter most in the marketplace".

This is dangerous at a time when there is increasingly no such things as a high-wage, middle-skilled job — the thing that sustained the middle class in the last generation. Now, there is only a high-wage, high-skilled job. Every middle-class job today is being pulled up, out or down faster than ever. That is, it either requires more skill or can be done by more people around the world or is being buried — made obsolete — faster than ever. Which is why the goal of education today, argues Wagner, should not be to make every child "college ready" but "innovation ready" — ready to add value to whatever they do.

That is a tall task. I tracked Wagner down and asked him to elaborate ."Today," he said via e-mail, "because knowledge is available on every Internet-connected device, what you know matters far less than what you can do with what you know. The capacity to innovate — the ability to solve problems creatively or bring new possibilities to life — and skills like critical thinking, communication and collaboration are far more important than academic knowledge. As one executive told me, 'We can teach new hires the content. And we will have to because it continues to change, but we can't teach them how to think — to ask the right questions — and to take initiative.'"

My generation had it easy. We got to "find" a job. But, more than ever, our kids will have to "invent" a job. Sure, the lucky ones will find their first job, but, given the pace of change today, even they will have to reinvent, re-engineer and reimagine that job much often than their parents if they want to advance in it.

"Finland is one of the most innovative economies in the world," Wagner said,"and it is the only country where students leave high school 'innovation-ready'. They learn concepts and creativity more than facts, and have a choice of many electives — all with a shorter school day, little homework, and almost no testing. There are a growing number of 'reinvented' colleges like the Olin College of Engineering, the M.I.T. Media Lab and the 'D-school' Stanford where students learn to innovate."

61. In his book, Wagner argues that _____.

    A. the education world are hostile to our kids

    B. the business world are hostile to those seeking jobs

    C. the business world are too demanding on the education world

    D. the education world should teach what the marketplace demands

62. What does the "tall task" refer to in the third paragraph?

    A. Sustaining the middle class.

    B. Saving high-wage, middle-skilled jobs.

    C. Shifting from "college ready" to "innovation ready".

    D. Preventing middle-class jobs from becoming obsolete fast.

63. What is mainly expressed in Wagner's e-mail?

    A. New hires should be taught the content rather than the ways of thinking.

    B. Knowledge is more readily available on Internet-connected devices.

    C. Academic knowledge is still the most important to teach.

    D. Creativity and skills matter more than knowledge.

64. What is implied in the fourth paragraph?

    A. Jobs favor the lucky ones in every generation.

    B. Jobs changed slowly in the author's generation.

    C. The author's generation led an easier life than their kids.

    D. It was easy for the author's generation to find their first job.

65. What is the purpose of the last paragraph?

    A. To orient future education.

    B. To exemplify the necessary shift in education.

    C. To draw a conclusion about the shift in education.

    D. To criticize some colleges for their practices in education.

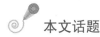 本文话题

如今的就业市场是需要创造工作的地方。作者认为，教育领域，尤其是高等教育应该随其革新，不能再故步自封，与世界变化隔绝。

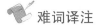 难词译注

consistently [kənˈsɪstəntlɪ] *ad.*   一贯地，坚持地

obsolete 英 [ˈɒbsəliːt] *a.*   废弃的；老式的，已过时的

 难句译注

1. This is dangerous at a time when there is increasingly no such things as a high-wage, middle-skilled job — the thing that sustained the middle class in the last

generation.

【分析】at a time when... 是常见的先行词 + 定语从句的结构，when 引导的定语从句中主干结构为 there be 句型。破折号后为名词 + 定语从句结构，作为 job 的同位语来进行解释说明。

【译文】这是很危险的，因为现在高工资、中等技能之类的工作越来越见不着了，而这些工作曾维持了上一代的中产阶级。

2. Which is why the goal of education today, argues Wagner, should not be to make every child "college ready" but "innovation ready"—ready to add value to whatever they do.

【分析】该句的主谓结构为 Wagner argues，倒装后插入到表语从句中的主谓之间。表语从句中有 not...but... 的并列结构。

【译文】瓦格纳认为，这就是为什么今天的教育目标不应该让每个孩子都"准备好上大学"，而是"准备好创新"，准备为他们所做的任何事情增加价值。

答案及解析

61. 【问题】瓦格纳在他的书中认为_____。

A. 教育领域对孩子们充满了敌意

B. 商业世界对求职者充满敌意

C. 商业世界对教育领域过于苛刻

D. 教育领域应该教授市场所需要的技能

【答案】D

【解析】细节题。由题干中的 book 定位到第一段：Wagner's argument in his book … is that our K-12 and college tracks are not consistently "adding the value and teaching the skills that matter most in the marketplace". 即他认为教育应该教给孩子市场最需要的技术。因此本题正确答案为 D。

62. 【问题】第三段中的 tall task 指的什么？

A. 维持中产阶级

B. 保留高工资、中等技能的工作

C. 从"准备好上大学"向"准备好创新"转移

D. 防止中产阶级的工作太快地废弃

【答案】C

【解析】指代题。定位到第三段首句"That is a tall task."，这里的 that 指代的是上一段的末尾，不难判断 C 为本题的正确答案。

63. 【问题】瓦格纳的邮件主要表达了什么？

A. 新的求职者应该被教授内容，而不是思维方式。

B. 知识在连接互联网的设备上更容易获得。

C. 学术知识仍然是教学的最重要的内容。

D. 创造性和技巧比知识更重要。

【答案】D

【解析】细节题。通过 email 可定位到文中第三段 "… what you know matters far less than what you can do with what you know … and collaboration are far more important than academic knowledge.",即学术知识远没有创造性解决问题的能力和在生活中创造新可能性重要,因此本题正确答案为 D。

64. 【问题】第四段隐含了什么意义?

    A. 工作垂青于每一代人中的幸运者。

    B. 工作在作者这一代改变很慢。

    C. 作者这一代比其子女生活更为容易。

    D. 作者这一代人更容易找到自己的第一份工作。

【答案】D

【解析】推理题。从第四段中得知,作者说他们这一代很容易。他们必须"找到"一份工作。但是,他们的孩子比以往任何时候都需要"发明"一份工作。当然,幸运儿们会找到他们的第一份工作,但是,考虑到今天的变化速度,若他们想要进步,他们也不得不重新设计和重新构思这项工作。从这里不难看出,作者这一代的压力比下一代要小多了。因此本题正确答案为 D。

65. 【问题】最后一段的目的是什么?

    A. 引导教育的方向。

    B. 举例说明教育转型的必要性。

    C. 对教育转型的总结。

    D. 谴责某些大学的教育实践。

【答案】B

【解析】写作目的题。最后一段作者讲到了芬兰、奥林工程学院,M.I.T. 媒体实验室和"D 学校"斯坦福大学的教学模式,也是举例说明现有的教学模式改革。因此 B 选项是作者的写作目的。

2017 年医学博士统考阅读理解部分真题

This issue of *Science* contains announcements for more than 100 different Gordon Research Conferences, on topics that range from atomic physics to developmental biology. The brainchild(某人的主意) of Neil Gordon of Johns Hopkins University, these week-long meetings are designed to promote intimate, informal discussions of frontier science. Often confined to fewer than 125 attendees, they have traditionally been held in remote places with minimal distractions. Beginning in the early 1960s, I attended the summer Nucleic Acids Gordon Conference in rural New Hampshire, sharing austere(简朴的)dorm facilities in a private boy's school with randomly assigned roommates. As a beginning scientist, I found the question period after each talk especially fascinating, providing valuable insights into the personalities and ways of thinking of many senior scientists whom I had not encountered previously. Back then, there were no cellphones and no Internet, and all of the speakers seemed to stay for the entire week. During the long, session-free afternoons, graduate students mingled freely with professors. Many lifelong friendships were begun, and—as Gordon intended—new scientific collaborations began. Leap forward to today, and every scientist can gain immediate access to a vast store of scientific thought and to millions of other scientists via the Internet. Why, nevertheless, do in-person scientific meetings remain so valuable for a life in science?

Part of the answer is that science works best when there is a deep mutual trust and understanding between the collaborators, which is hard to develop from a distance. But most important is the critical role that face-to-face scientific meetings play in stimulating a random collision of ideas and approaches. The best science occurs when someone combines the Knowledge gained by other scientists in non-obvious ways to create a new understanding of how the world works. A successful scientist needs to deeply believe, whatever the problem being tackled, that there is always a better way to approach that problem than the path currently being taken. The scientist is then constantly on the alert for new paths to take in his or her work, which is essential for making breakthroughs. Thus, as much as possible, scientific meetings should be designed to expose the attendees to ways of thinking and techniques that are different from the ones that they already know.

66. Assembled at Gordon Research Conference are those who _____.

　　A. are physicists and biologists

　　B. just start doing their sciences

　　C. stay in the forefront of science

　　D. are accomplished senior scientists

67. Speaking of the summer Nucleic Acids Gordon Conference, the author thinks highly of _____.

　　A. the personalities of senior scientists

　　B. the question period after each talk

　　C. the austere facilities around

　　D. the week-long duration

68. It can be inferred from the author that the value of the in-person scientific conference _____.

　　A. does not change with times

　　B. can be explored online exclusively

　　C. lies in exchanging the advances in life science

　　D. is questioned in establishing a vast store of ideas

69. The author believes that the face-to-face scientific conferences can help the attendees better _____.

　　A. understand what making a breakthrough means to them

B. expose themselves to novel ideas and new approaches

C. foster the passion for doing science

D. tackle the same problem in science

70. What would the author most probably talk about in the following paragraphs?

A. How to explore scientific collaborations.

B. How to make scientific breakthroughs.

C. How to design scientific meetings.

D. How to think like a genius.

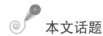 本文话题

现场科学会议的重要意义。

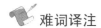 难词译注

frontier science	前沿科学
randomly ['rændəmli] v.	随便地，未加计划地
mingle [miŋgl] v.	混合，混淆

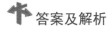 答案及解析

66. 【问题】聚集在戈登研究会议的是那些_____.

    A. 物理学家和生物学家

    B. 刚在科学研究上起步的人

    C. 科学前沿的人

    D. 功成名就的资深科学家

【答案】C

【解析】推理题。从首段中 designed to promote intimate, informal discussions of frontier science 可知，与会者都是前沿科学的参与人。C 为正确答案。

67. 【问题】说到夏季核酸戈登会议，作者高度赞扬了_____。

    A. 资深科学家们的性格

    B. 每个发言后的提问时间

    C. 周围简朴的设备

    D. 长达一周的时间

【答案】B

【解析】细节题。首段中讲到 I found the question period after each talk especially fascinating，他发现提问环节非常棒，因为他可以充分了解未曾谋面的科学家们的思想和个性。因此 B 为正确答案。

68. 【问题】可推理得知，作者认为现场科学会议的价值_____。

    A. 不会随着时间改变而改变

B．只能在线开发

C．存在于生命科学进步成果的交流中

D．在树立一系列观点时被质疑

【答案】A

【解析】推理题。从第一段中的最后一句"Why, nevertheless, do in-person scientific meetings remain so valuable for a life in science"可知，无论在过去还是在互联网时代，现场会议的价值是保持不变的。因此正确答案为 A。

69.【问题】作者认为面对面的科学会议能帮助参会者更好地_____。

A．理解突破性进展的含义

B．接触新颖的观点和方法

C．培养科研热情

D．处理科学中相通的问题

【答案】B

【解析】细节题。从第二段中"But most important is the critical role that face-to-face scientific meetings play in stimulating a random collision of ideas and approaches"可知，面对面的科学会议在刺激思想和方法的随机碰撞方面发挥关键作用，B 选项符合文意。

70.【问题】下一段作者最可能谈到什么？

A．如何开发科研协作。

B．如何进行科技创新。

C．如何设计科研会议。

D．如何像天才一样思考。

【答案】C

【解析】推理题。第二段末尾讲到科学会议的设计应该尽最大可能让与会者充分接触不同的思维方式和技巧，由此可推断，作者极有可能在第三段讲述如何安排一场好的现场科学会议。故本题正确答案为 C。

2016 年医学博士统考阅读理解部分真题

Passage One

Parents are on a journey of discovery with each child whose temperament, biology, and sleep habits result in a unique sleep-wake pattern. It can be frustrating when children's sleep habits do not conform to the household schedule. Helping the child develop good sleep habits in childhood takes time and parental attention, but it will have beneficial results throughout life. An understanding of the changing patterns of the typical sleep-wake cycle in children will help alleviate any unfounded concerns. Maintaining a sleep diary for each child will provide the parents with baseline information in assessing the nature and severity of childhood sleep problems. Observant patents will come to recognize unusual sleep disruptions or those that persist or intensify.

Developmental changes throughout childhood bring differences in the sleep-wake cycle and in the type and frequency of parasomnias that may interrupt sleep. Medical consultation to rule out illness, infection or injury is prudent if the child's sleep problems prevent adequate sleep and result in an ongoing sleep deficit. As reported by *News-Medical* in Child Health News, children's sleep problems should be taken seriously as they may be a "marker" for predicting later risk of early adolescent substance use . In the same article. University of Michigan psychiatry professor Kirk Brower, who has studied "the interplay of alcohol and sleep in adults", stressed that " The finding does not mean there's a cause-and-effect relationship."

Consultation with a child psychologist may be helpful if frightening dreams intensity and become more frequent as this may indicate a particular problem or life circumstance that needs to be changed or one that the child may need extra help working through.

Most childhood sleep disturbance will diminish over time as the brain matures and a regular sleep-wake cycle is established. Parental guidance is crucial to development of healthy sleep habits in children.

61. To have journey of discovery with each child, according to the passage, is_____.
   A. to discover their unique sleep-wake cycles
   B. to follow their behavioral preferences
   C. to alleviate their sleeping problems
   D. to explore their asset

62. In the first paragraph, the author suggests that parents_____.
   A. seek professional consultation for their child's sleep problem
   B. adjust their household schedule to the child's sleeping habit
   C. take their child's unfounded concerns into consideration
   D. keep a diary on sleep pattern for their child

63. Where there exists a "marker" in the child, according to the passage_____.
   A. it might lead to his or her early substance use
   B. he or she will carry it all his or her life
   C. it might interrupt his or her sleep pattern
   D. he or she is destined to be an alcoholic

64. What is the author trying to tell us in the third paragraph?
   A. It takes time to combat sleeping problem in children.
   B. Sometimes parents need to seek professional assistance.
   C. Parents cannot afford to neglect their child's sleeping problem.
   D. Much importance should be attached to the child's life circumstance.

65. What is the main idea of the passage?

    A. Child sleep disturbance and its future impact.

    B. Child sleep disturbance and its family history.

    C. Parent's role in building their child's healthy sleeping habit.

    D. A psychological perspective on sleep disturbance in children.

Passage Two

The United States and England each has a major — and unique — health-care challenge, according to a study comparing the health of senior citizens in the two countries. The study, conducted by researchers from RAND Corporation in the United States and Institute for Fiscal Studies in the United Kingdom, found that disease and health disorder incidence was higher among U.S. senior citizens, but mortality rates were higher among English senior citizens.

Americans aged 65 and older have almost twice the rate of diabetes found among their English counterparts and more than double the rate of cancer. Nevertheless, death rate among Americans 65 and older is lower.

"Americans are a sicker group of people who tend to live longer," says James Smith, a study co-author. He attributes the U.S. health problems to lifestyle factors, including poor eating habits and inadequate exercise. Americans tend to eat much larger servings of food, for example, "There is what I call an <u>American plate.</u> When we go to a restaurant, it's a plate I can't even eat any more. It's a plate with so much food on if it's not even appealing to me."

Smith also says that English adults are generally much more physically active than Americans. Biking and walking are much common in everyday life in England. He observes that "there is a lot of walking in London, and there is a lot of bicycle riding. I don't see people in downtown Los Angeles on their bicycles".

On the other hand, England's problem is that doctors fail to diagnose serious conditions each enough. American doctors tend to screen patients for cancer, diabetes, and other illnesses more frequently. Smith notes, "American medicine is much more aggressive. It leads to high costs, but it has benefits, too. "

66. The study's results indicated _____.

    A. an urgent call for health promotion among English and American senior citizens

    B. health disparities between English and American senior citizens

    C. a close relation between disease incidence and mortality rate

    D. a significant rise in mortality rates among senior citizens

67. Which of the following is a unique health care challenge for English senior citizens when compared with their American counterparts?

    A. A higher death rate.   B. A higher rate of cancer.

    C. A higher incidence of disease.   D. A lower tendency to have diabetes.

68. What does James Smith imply by "an American plate"?

    A. A sedentary American lifestyles.

    B. American junk foods on the table.

    C. A large portion of food consumed by Americans.

    D. Severe malnutrition among American senior citizens.

69. The Americans' unique health-care challenge according to James Smith, is derived from _____.

    A. their unusual forms of physical activities
    B. their different geographic location
    C. their genetic likelihood of obesity
    D. their unhealthy lifestyle factors

70. Even though it is much more aggressive, the American medicine _____.

    A. better improves the quality of life among its senior citizens

    B. benefits more seniors who need medical care

    C. facilitates its senior citizens to live longer

    D. helps its senior citizens live healthier

Passage One

本文话题

孩子睡眠状况以及父母的作用。

难词译注

temperament ['temprəmənt] *n.*	性格
parasomnia ['pærəsɔmniə] *n.*	深眠状态
prudent ['pru:dnt] *a.*	小心谨慎的

答案及解析

61. 【问题】根据文章，探索发现每一个孩子的过程是_____。

    A. 发现他们独特的睡眠—觉醒周期　　B. 跟随他们的喜好

    C. 缓解他们的睡眠问题　　　　　　　D. 挖掘他们的潜力

    【答案】A

    【解析】此题为细节理解题。根据题干可以定位到文章第一段第一句。此句提到家长正在探索发现孩子的过程中，孩子的性格和睡眠习惯都会产生独特的睡眠觉醒周期。因而我们可以得知父母探索孩子是为了了解他们的睡眠—觉醒周期。所以答案为 A

62. 【问题】在第一段，作者建议父母_____。

    A. 孩子睡眠问题寻求专业咨询

    B. 根据孩子睡眠习惯调整家庭作息

    C. 重视孩子未被发现的问题

    D. 记录孩子的睡眠模式

【答案】D

【解析】此题为细节理解题。第一段提到帮助孩子在童年时期建立很好的睡眠习惯虽然费时费力，但终身受益。对孩子睡眠习惯的了解也能缓解他们的睡眠问题。随后作者建议父母记录孩子的睡眠情况就能识别睡眠问题以及严重程度。因而答案为D。

63.【问题】根据文章，当孩子出现"标记物"时_____。

  A．这可能导致孩子过早吸毒   B．孩子终身携带

  C．可能影响孩子睡眠模式   D．孩子注定要酗酒

【答案】A

【解析】此题为细节理解题。文章第二段第三句出现题干关键词 marker，这句话也提到marker 的出现，预示着孩子在青少年时期开始吸毒的危险性。因而答案为 A。

64.【问题】第三段作者想告诉我们什么？

  A．解决孩子的睡眠问题是需要时间的。

  B．有时父母需要寻求专业帮助。

  C．父母绝不能忽视孩子的睡眠问题。

  D．孩子的生活环境至关重要。

【答案】C

【解析】此题为推断题。本段提到如果父母发现孩子噩梦情况严重或者频繁发生，有必要咨询医生，因为这些变化可能预示着一个病症，或者生活环境需要改变，也或者表示孩子的问题需要更多帮助。这些都说明作为父母一定要密切关注孩子的睡眠状况，出现情况要及时寻求专业人士的帮助，因而答案为 C。

65.【问题】全文主要内容是什么？

  A．孩子的睡眠问题及对今后的影响。

  B．孩子的睡眠问题及家族史。

  C．在建立孩子正确睡眠习惯中父母的作用。

  D．从心理学视角看孩子的睡眠问题。

【答案】C

【解析】此题为主旨题，解题可结合段落含义或者综合前几道细节题的答案。文章最后一段也提到大多数孩子的睡眠问题随着年龄增长而逐渐消失，但在这一过程中父母的指导作用至关重要。因而答案为 C。

Passage Two

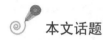

本文话题

英美两国各自老年人健康问题及对比。

66.【问题】研究结果表明_____。

  A．提高英美两国老年人健康水平迫在眉睫

  B．英美两国老年人健康水平相差悬殊

C. 发病率与死亡率之间紧密相关

D. 老年人死亡率显著上升

【答案】A

【解析】第一段第一句提到英美两国各有各的主要医疗问题。随后对两国老年人的健康状况进行研究，结果表明在美国老年人的患病率偏高，而在英国老年人的死亡率偏高。这说明两国老年人的健康状况均不乐观，因而答案为 A。尽管对比两国老年人健康状况，但都不乐观，因而选项 B 错。选项 C 和 D 文章没有提到。

67. 【问题】与美国老年人相比，下列哪一项是英国老年人特有的健康问题？

A. 较高死亡率。

B. 较高的患癌率。

C. 较高的发病率。

D. 患糖尿病的可能性较低。

【答案】A

【解析】此题为细节定位题。根据题干，可以定位到第一段第一句。具体到英国老年人的健康问题是在第一段最后一句话提到该国老年人死亡率偏高。因而答案为 A。

68. 【问题】通过 "An American Plate"，James Smith 暗示什么？

A. 美国人不爱运动的生活方式。

B. 美国人餐桌上的垃圾食品。

C. 美国人食量大。

D. 美国老人严重营养不良。

【答案】C

【解析】根据题干关键词，定位到文章第三段。研究者 James Smith 将美国人的健康问题归因为不健康的生活方式，例如不良的饮食习惯和不爱运动。作者随后谈到美国人食量很大，用 an American plate 作为实例。因而答案为 C。

69. 【问题】根据 James Smith 的看法，美国人特有的健康问题来源于_____。

A. 不寻常的体育锻炼形式   B. 不同的地理位置

C. 基因肥胖概率   D. 不健康的生活方式

【答案】D

【解析】此题为细节定位题。此题定位在第三段。第二句提到他认为美国人的健康问题来源于生活方式，因而答案为 D。

70. 【问题】尽管过于激进，但是美国医学_____。

A. 能更好地提高美国老年人的生活质量

B. 惠及更多有需要的老年人

C. 帮助老年人延年益寿

D. 帮助老年人活得更健康

【答案】C

【解析】此题根据题干定位到文章最后一段。本段提到英国的问题在于疾病的早期筛查，而在这方面美国做得好多了。文章最后提到虽然美国医学激进，成本高，但也有好处。这里的益处指的就是疾病的早期筛查。因而答案为 C。

2015 年医学博士统考阅读理解部分真题

Passage One

The American Society of Clinical Oncology wrapped its annual conference this week, going through the usual motions of presenting a lot of drugs that offer some added quality or extension of life to those suffering from a variety of as-yet incurable diseases. But buried deep in an AP story are a couple of promising headlines that seems worthy of more thorough review, including one treatment study where 100 percent of patients saw their cancer diminish by half.

First of all, it seems pharmaceutical companies are moving away from the main cost-effective one-size-fits-all approach to drug development and embracing the long cancer treatments, engineering drugs that only work for a small percentage of patients but work very effectively within that group.

Pfizer announced that one such drug it's pushing into late-stage testing is targeted for 4% of lung cancer patients. But more than 90% of that tiny cohort responded to the drug initial tests, and 9 out of ten is getting pretty close to the ideal ten out of ten. By gearing toward more boutique treatments rather than broad umbrella pharmaceuticals that try to fit for everyone it seems cancer researchers are making some headway. But how can we close the gap on that remaining ten percent?

Ask Takeda Pharmaceutical and Celgene, two drug makers who put aside competitive interests to test a novel combination of their treatments. In a test of 66 patients with the blood disease multiple myeloma, a full 100 percent of the subjects saw their cancer reduced by half. Needless to say, a 100 percent response to a cancer drug (or in this case a drug cocktail) is more or less unheard of. Moreover, this combination never would've been tried if two competing companies hadn't sat down and put their heads together.

Are there more potentially effective drug combos out there separated by competitive interest and proprietary information? Who's to say, but it seems like with the amount of money and research being pumped into cancer drug development, the outcome is pretty good. And if researchers can start pushing more of their response numbers toward 100 percent, we can more easily start talking about oncology's favorite four-letter word: cure.

61. Which of the following can be the best title for the passage?
    A. Competition and Cooperation.
    B. Two Competing Pharmaceutical Companies.
    C. The Promising Future of Pharmaceuticals.
    D. Encouraging News: a 100% Response to a Cancer Drug.

62. In cancer drug development, according to the passage, the pharmaceuticals now＿＿＿＿＿.
    A. are adopting the cost-effective one-size-fits-all approach

    B. are moving towards individualized and targeted treatments

    C. are investing the lion's shares of their money

    D. care only about their profits

63. From the encouraging advance by the two companies, we can infer that _____.

    A. the development can be ascribed to their joint efforts and collaboration

    B. it was their competition that resulted in the accomplishment

    C. other pharmaceutical companies will join them in the research

    D. the future cancer treatment can be nothing but cocktail therapy

64. From the last paragraph it can be inferred that the answer to the question _____.

    A. is nowhere to be found

    B. can drive one crazy

    C. can be multiple

    D. is conditional

65. The tone of the author of this passage seems to be _____.

    A. neutral   B. critical   C. negative   D. optimistic

Passage Two

Liver disease is the 12th-leading cause of death in the U.S., chiefly because once it's determined that a patient needs a new liver it's very difficult to get one. Even in case where a suitable donor match is found, there's no guarantee a transplant will be successful. But researchers at Massachusetts General Hospital have taken a huge step toward building functioning livers in the lab, successfully transplanting culture-grown livers into rats.

The livers aren't grown from scratch, but rather within the infrastructure of a donor liver. The liver cells in the donor organ are washed out with a detergent that gently strips away the liver cells, leaving behind a biological scaffold of proteins and extracellular architecture that is very hard to duplicate synthetically.

With all of that complicated infrastructure already in place, the researchers then seeded the scaffold（支架）with liver cells isolated from healthy livers, as well as some special endothelial cells to line the bold vessels. Once repopulated with healthy cells, these livers lived in culture for 10 days.

The team also transplanted some two-day-old recellularized livers back into rats, where they continued to thrive for eight hours while connected into the rats' vascular systems. However, the current method isn't perfect and cannot seem to repopulate the blood vessels quite densely enough and the transplanted livers can't keep functioning for more than about 24 hours (hence the eight-hour maximum for the rat transplant).

But the initial successes are promising, and the team thinks they can overcome the blood vessel problem and get fully functioning livers into rats within two years. It still might be a decade before the tech hits the clinic, but if nothing goes horribly wrong — and especially if stem-cell research establishes a reliable way to create health liver cells from the very patients who need transplants — lab-generated livers that are perfect matches for their recipients could become a reality.

66. It can be inferred from the passage that the animal model was mainly intended to _____ .
    A. investigate the possibility of growing blood vessels in the lab
    B. explore the unknown functions of the human liver
    C. reduce the incidence of liver disease in the U.S.
    D. address the source of liver transplants

67. What does the author mean when he says that the livers aren't grown from scratch?
    A. The making of a biological scaffold of proteins and extracellular architecture.
    B. A huge step toward building functioning livers in the lab.
    C. The building of the infrastructure of a donor liver.
    D. Growing liver cells in the donor organ.

68. The biological scaffold was not put into the culture in the lab until _____ .
    A. duplicated synthetically
    B. isolated from the healthy liver
    C. repopulated with the healthy cells
    D. the addition of some man-made blood vessels

69. What seems to be the problem in the planted liver?
    A. The rats as wrong recipients.
    B. The time point of the transplantation.
    C. The short period of the recellularization.
    D. The insufficient repopulation of the blood vessels.

70. The research team holds high hopes of _____ .
    A. creating lab-generated livers for patients within two years
    B. the timetable for generating human livers in the lab
    C. stem-cell research as the future of medicine
    D. building a fully functioning liver into rats

Passage One

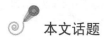 本文话题

制药公司在治疗癌症药物研发方面取得的成就。

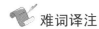 难词译注

cost-effective [kɔst i'fektiv] *a.*   划算的

one-size-fits-all   一刀切，万全之策

headway [hedwei] *n.*   进展，前进

proprietary [prə'praiətri] *a.*   专有的，专利的

答案及解析

61. 【问题】下列哪一个是文章最好的标题？

        A．竞争与合作。

        B．两家竞争的制药公司。

        C．制药业的光明前景。

        D．令人兴奋的消息：某种抗癌药物的 100% 回应。

【答案】C

【解析】主旨题。本文的中心思想是制药公司在治疗癌症的问题上的努力以及取得的成就。因此，C 选项（制药业的光明前景）是正确答案。

62. 【问题】在抗癌药物的开发中，制药公司现在 _____。

        A．正在采用有成本效益的一刀切方式

        B．正朝个性化和针对性的治疗方式发展

        C．正在进行巨大的投资

        D．只在乎他们的利益

【答案】B

【解析】通过 cancer drug development 回到原文定位到第二段，一些制药公司正由成本效益高的"一刀切"的发展模式向注重药物发展方面转变，并且接受长期癌症治疗，以及研发适用于特定患者群的高效药物。由此可知，制药公司正向治疗个体化和目标特定化前进。individualized and targeted 与原文中的 work for a small percentage of patients 对应。

63. 【问题】从两大公司令人鼓舞的进步中，我们可推理得知 _____。

        A．所取得的进展是共同努力和合作的结果

        B．正是他们的竞争才有后来的成绩

        C．其他制药公司会加入研究

        D．将来癌症的治疗方案只不过是鸡尾酒疗法

【答案】A

【解析】细节题。用 two companies 回到原文定位到倒数第二段，从最后一句可知，如果两家公司不坐下来商榷，就不会有这项研究。故本题答案为 A（归因于两家公司的共同努力和协作）。

64. 【问题】从最后一段可推理得知，对该问题的答案 _____。

        A．无处可寻   B．能使人疯狂

C．可以多元化　　　　　　　　　D．是有条件的

【答案】A

【解析】细节题。最后一段中讲到，（对这个问题）谁都说不准，因为两家竞争公司之间存在竞争效益和信息专有的问题。由此可知，没人能告知答案。

65．【问题】本文作者的语气是 _____。

A．中立的　　　　B．批判的　　　　C．负面的　　　　D．积极的

【答案】D

【解析】细节题。从末段最后一句可知，如果研究人员开始把药物效率向百分之百推进，那我们也能更加容易地开始探讨肿瘤界最令人神往的一个词：治愈。即作者很乐观，充满了希望。故本题答案为D。

Passage Two

 本文话题

人工培植肝脏可能成为肝脏疾病的治疗方法。

 难词译注

culture ['kʌltʃə] *n.*	养殖；（微生物等的）培养
detergent [di'tə:dʒənt] *n.*	洗涤剂
endothelial [,endə'θi:liəl] *n.*	内皮的
recipient [ri'sipiənt] *n.*	接受者，容器

答案及解析

66．【问题】从文中可推理得知，动物模型的主要目的是 _____。

A．检验实验室中血管生长的可能性

B．研究人类肝脏未知的功能

C．减少美国肝脏疾病的发生概率

D．解决肝脏移植的肝源问题

【答案】D

【解析】推理题。从文中首段可知，目前美国第十二大致命杀手便是肝脏疾病，主要是因为一旦患上这种疾病，患者需要移植一颗新的肝脏，但是要找到完全匹配的肝脏非常困难。因此动物模型主要是为了解决肝脏来源的问题。故本题答案为D。

67．【问题】作者说肝脏无法"无中生有"的意思是什么？

A．蛋白质的生物支架和细胞外结构的形成。

B．在实验室中培养功能性肝脏的巨大一步。

C. 捐赠者肝脏的基本框架。

D. 捐赠者器官生长的肝脏细胞。

【答案】C

【解析】细节题。通过 grow from scratch 回到原文定位到第二段首句，大意是这些肝脏不是无中生有，而是在供体肝的框架里培养出来的。因此首先要搭建这样一个 infrastructure。故本题答案为 C。

68. 【问题】生物支架先要 _____，然后才会放进实验室的培养液中。

A. 合成复制　　　　　　　　B. 从健康的干细胞中分离

C. 植入健康的肝脏细胞　　　D. 增加一些人造血管

【答案】C

【解析】细节题。用 culture 回到原文定位到第三段，可知这些复杂的基础框架准备好后，研究者将从健康肝脏里分离出来的肝脏细胞和粗血管上的内皮细胞植入蛋白质支架之中。健康的肝脏细胞植入之后，肝脏便能够在培养基中存活 10 天。因此正确答案应该是"植入健康的肝脏细胞"。故本题答案为 C。

69. 【问题】移植肝脏的问题是什么？

A. 白鼠是不合适的受体。　　B. 移植的时间点。

C. 再细胞化的时间短。　　　D. 血管的密度不够。

【答案】D

【解析】细节题。答案在第四段：目前采用的这种肝脏移植的方法并不尽善尽美，因为血管再生密度不够。另外，移植肝脏发挥正常功能的时间不超过 24 小时。因此本题正确答案为 D。

70. 【问题】研究团队对 _____ 报以很大希望。

A. 两年内为病人创造实验室培育的肝脏

B. 实验室培育人类肝脏的时间表

C. 医学未来的干细胞研究

D. 将正常功能的肝脏移植到白鼠体内

【答案】D

【解析】细节题。文章最后一段首句讲到，研究团队认为他们能在两年之内解决肝脏移植过程中遇到的血管问题，从而培养出功能完全正常的肝脏，并移植入老鼠体内。因此正确答案为 D。

2014 年医学博士统考阅读理解部分真题

Passage One

I have just returned from Mexico, where I visited a factory making medical masks. Faced with fierce competition, the owner has cut his costs by outsourcing some of his production. Scores of people work for him in their homes, threading elastic into masks by hand. They are paid below the minimum wage, with no job security and no healthcare provision.

Users of medical masks and other laboratory gear probably give little thought to where their equipment comes from. That needs to change. A significant proportion of these products are made in the developing world by low-paid people with inadequate labor rights. This leads to human misery on a tremendous scale.

Take lab coats. Many are made in India, where most cotton farmers are paid an unfair price for their crops and factory employees work illegal hours for poor pay.

One-fifth of the world's surgical instruments are made in northern Pakistan. When I visited a couple of a years ago I found most workers toiling 12 hours a day, seven days a week, for less than a dollar a day, exposed to noise, metal dust and toxic chemicals. Thousands of children, some as young as 7, work in the industry.

To win international contracts, factory owners must offer rock-bottom prices, and consequently drive down wages and labor conditions as far as they can. We laboratory scientists in the developed world may unwittingly be encouraging this: we ask how much our equipment will cost, but which of us asks who made it and how much they were paid?

This is no small matter. Science is supposed to benefit humanity, but because of the conditions under which their tools are made, many scientists may actually be causing harm.

What can be done? A knee-jerk boycott of unethical goods is not the answer; it would just make things worse for workers in those manufacturing zones. What we need is to start asking suppliers to be transparent about where and how their products are manufactured and urge them to improve their manufacturing practices.

It can be done. Many universities are committed to fair trade in the form of ethically sourced tea, coffee or bananas. That model should be extended to laboratory goods.

There are signs that things are moving. Over the past few years I have worked with health services in the IK and in Sweden. Both have recently instituted ethical procurement practices. If science is truly going to help humanity, it needs to follow suit.

1. From the medical masks to the lab coats, the author is trying to tell us _____.
   A. the practice of occupational protection in the developing world
   B. the developing countries plagued by poverty and disease
   C. the cheapest labor in the developing countries
   D. the human misery behind them

2. The concerning phenomenon the author had observed, according to the passage _____.
   A. is nothing but the repetition of the miserable history
   B. could have been even exaggerated
   C. is unfamiliar to the wealthy west
   D. is prevailing across the world

3. The author argues that when researchers in the wealthy west buy tools, they should
   _____.
   A. have the same concern with the developing countries
   B. be blind to their sources for the sake of humanity
   C. pursue good bargains in the international market
   D. spare a thought for how they were made

4. A proper course of action suggested by the author is _____.
   A. to refuse to import the unethical goods from the developing world
   B. to ask scientists to tell the truth as the prime value of their work
   C. to urge the manufacturers to address the immoral issues
   D. to improve the transparency of international contracts

5. By saying at the end of the passage that if science is truly going to help humanity, it
   needs to follow suit, the author means that _____.
   A. the scientific community should stand up for all humanity
   B. the prime value of scientists' work is to tell the truth
   C. laboratory goods also need to be ethically sourced
   D. because of science, there is hope for humanity

Passage Two

A little information is a dangerous thing. A lot of information, if it's inaccurate or confusing, even more so. This is a problem for anyone trying to spend or invest in an environmentally sustainable way. Investors are barraged with indexes purporting to describe companies eco-credentials, some of dubious quality Green labels on consumer products are ubiquitous, but their claims are hard to verify. **The confusion** is evident from the *New Scientists*' analysis of whether public perception of companies' green credentials reflect reality. It shows that many companies considered "green" have done little to earn that reputation, while others do not get sufficient credit for their efforts to reduce their environmental impact. Obtaining better information is crucial, because decisions by consumers and big investors will help propel us towards a green economy.

At present, it is too easy to make unverified claims. Take disclosure of greenhouse gas emission, for example. There are voluntary schemes such as a Carbon Disclosure Project, but little scrutiny of the figures companies submit, which means investors may be misled.

Measurements can be difficult to interpret, too, like those for water use. In this case, context is crucial: a little from rain-soaked Ireland is not the same as a little drawn from the Arizona desert.

Similar problems bedevil "green" labels attached to individual products. Here, the computer equipment rating system developed by the Green Electronics Council show the way forward.

Its criteria come from the IEEE, the world's leading, professional association for technology.

Other schemes, such as the "sustainability index" planned by US retail giant Walmart, are broader. Devising rigorous standard for a large number of different types of product will be tough, placing a huge burden on the academic-led consortium that is doing the underlying scientific work.

Our investigation also reveals that many companies choose not to disclose data. Some will want to keep it that way. This is why we need legal requirements for full disclosure of environmental information, with the clear message that the polluter will eventually be required to pay. They market forces will drive companies to lean up their acts.

Let's hope we can rise to this challenge. Before we can have a green economy we need a green information economy — and it's the quality of information, as well as its quality, that will count.

6. "The confusion" in the first paragraph refers to _____.
   A. where to spend or invest in a sustainable way
   B. an array of consumer products to choose
   C. a fog of unreliable green information
   D. little information on eco-credibility

7. From the *New Scientists* analysis it can be inferred that in many cases _____.
   A. eco-credibility is abused
   B. a green economy is crucial
   C. an environment impact is lessened
   D. green credentials promote green economy

8. From unverified claims to difficult measurements and then to individual products, the author suggests that _____.
   A. eco-credibility is a game between scientists and manufactures
   B. neither scientists nor manufactures are honest
   C. it is vital to build a green economy
   D. better information is critical

9. To address the issue, the author is crying for _____.
   A. transparent corporate management　　B. establishing sustainability indexes
   C. tough academic-led management　　D. strict legal weapon

10. Which of the following can be the best inference from the last paragraph?
    A. The toughest challenge is the best opportunity.
    B. It is time for another green revolution.
    C. Information should be free at all.
    D. No quantity, no quality.

Passage One

 本文话题

医用物品的生产环境堪忧。

 难词译注

outsource ['əutsɔ:s] *v.*	将……外包
gear [giə] *n.*	装备
toil [tɔil] *v.*	辛苦工作
unwittingly [ʌn'witiŋli] *ad.*	不知不觉地，不经意地
knee-jerk	膝反射

答案及解析

1. 【问题】从医用口罩到实验服，作者想要告诉我们 _____。
   A. 发展中国家对职业保护的做法
   B. 发展中国家饱受贫穷和疾病的困扰
   C. 发展中国家最廉价的劳动力
   D. 背后的人类疾苦

   【答案】D

   【解析】此题为信息理解题。本文第一段作者在工厂观察到医用器具生产的恶劣环境，由此作者产生忧虑，因而答案是 D。

2. 【问题】根据文章，作者过去所观察到的令人关注的现象 _____。
   A. 只是悲惨历史的重现
   B. 可能被夸大了
   C. 在富有的西方不常见
   D. 在全世界都普遍存在

   【答案】C

   【解析】此题为细节信息题。根据第一至第四段我们得知，西方国家的医疗用品都是来源于发展中国家，因而答案为 C。

3. 【问题】作者认为当西方富国的研究者购买工具时，他们应该 _____。
   A. 与发展中国家有同样的担心
   B. 出于人道考虑，对他们的材料源头视而不见
   C. 在国际市场追求赚钱的买卖
   D. 想想这些器具是如何制成的

   【答案】D

   【解析】此题为细节信息题。原文出处是在第五段最后一句话，这一问句说明我们关心的是产品价格，但很少关心产品的出产地和生产状况，这一问题应该引起我们

的关注。因而答案为 D。

4. 【问题】作者建议的恰当做法是 _____。

    A．禁止进口来自发展中国家的不道德的产品

    B．作为他们工作的首要价值，科学家要告知真相

    C．敦促生产商解决不道德的问题

    D．提高国际合同的透明度

【答案】C

【解析】此题为细节信息题。原文信息在文章第七段最后一句话：我们需要做的是让货品提供商在产品产地和制作方法上更加透明，敦促他们改善生产做法。因而答案为 C。

5. 【问题】在文章结尾，作者提到：如果科学是真的要造福人类，它就应该照着做。作者的意思是 _____。

    A．科学界应该支持所有人类

    B．科学家工作的首要价值就是告知真相

    C．实验室用品也需要有公德

    D．科学给人类带来了希望

【答案】C

【解析】此题为信息理解题。文章最后一段提到在英国和瑞典，他们已经开始了更为符合道德的采购做法，作为造福人类的科学也应如此，即关注实验室用品的来源，因而答案为 C。

Passage Two

本文话题

为了环保绿色经济，信息的数量和准确性事关重要。

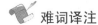

难词译注

barrage ['bærɑ:ʒ] n.	密集轰炸
dubious ['dju:biəs] a.	可疑的
ubiquitous [ju:'bikwitəs] a.	普遍存在的
propel [prə'pel] v.	激励，促使
thorny ['θɔ:ni] a.	苦恼的，多刺的
bedevil [bi'devl] v.	使痛苦，使苦恼
consortium [kən'sɔ:tiəm] n.	财团，合伙

答案及解析

6. 【问题】第一段中的 "The confusion" 指的是 _____。

    A．在哪里以可持续的方式进行投资消费

B．大量的产品供选择

C．不可靠的环保信息

D．环保资质信息很少

【答案】C

【解析】此题为指代题。confusion 指代的应该是前句中提到的"dubious quality green labels"，再根据文章首句告诉我们信息量虽然很大，但不准确或者迷惑人可能更加危险。因而答案为 C。

7. 【问题】从《新科学人》的分析可以推断出在很多情况下 _____。

A．环保信誉被滥用

B．绿色环保经济很重要

C．环境影响弱化了

D．环保资质促进绿色环保经济

【答案】A

【解析】此题为细节信息题。根据题干定位到文章第一段第五句。第六句话告诉我们该分析表明大多数企业被认为是环保型的，但名不副实，因而答案为 A。

8. 【问题】从未经证实的说法到测量的困难，再到个人产品，作者想说 _____。

A．环保信誉是科学家和生产商之间的较量

B．科学家和生产商都不诚实

C．建立绿色环保经济很重要

D．更完善的信息很重要

【答案】D

【解析】根据题干提到的三个方面，可以定位到文章的第二、三、四段。这三个方面都是举例说明，为的是证明文章第一段最后一句话：获取更完善的信息很重要。因而答案为 D。

9. 【问题】为了解决问题，作者呼吁 _____。

A．透明的企业管理　　　　B．确立可持续性指标

C．严格的以学术为先导的管理　　D．严格的法律武器

【答案】D

【解析】文章第五段提到为各种产品制定严格的标准很难，而且也会给学术机构造成很大负担，所以可以排除选项 B 和 C。答案的原文出处在最后一段，作者提到对企业环保信息公开提出法律要求很必要，因而答案为 D。

10. 【问题】下面哪一个是对最后一段最好的推测？

A．难度最大的挑战是最好的机会。

B．是开始另一场绿色革命的时候了。

C．信息应该完全免费。

D．没数量，就没质量。

【答案】B

【解析】本题的解题要结合文章的主题，文章开头就提到不准确且迷惑人的信息尽管数量很大，但造成的结果更危险。因而为了实现绿色环保经济，首当其冲要确保信息的正确性，因而答案为 B。

2013 年医学博士统考阅读理解部分真题

Passage One

There is plenty we don't know about criminal behavior. Most crime goes unreported so it is hard to pick out trends from the data, and even reliable sets of statistics can be difficult to compare. But here is one thing we do know: those with a biological predisposition to violent behavior who are brought up in abusive homes are very likely to become lifelong criminals.

Antisocial and criminal behavior tends to run in families, but no one was sure whether this was due mostly to social-environmental factors or biological ones. It turns out both are important, but the effect is most dramatic when they act together. This has been illustrated in several studies over the past six years which found that male victims of child abuse are several times as likely to become criminals and abusers themselves if they were born with a less-active version of a gene for the enzyme monoamine oxidase A (MAO-A), which breaks down neurotransmitters crucial to the regulation of aggression.

Researchers recently made another key observation: kids with this "double whammy" of predisposition and an unfortunate upbringing are likely to show signs of what's to come at a very early age. The risk factors for long-term criminality — attention deficit hyperactivity disorder, low IQ, language difficulties — can be spotted in kindergarten. So given what we now know, shouldn't we be doing everything to protect the children most at risk?

No one is suggesting testing all boys to see which variant of the MAO-A gene they have, but what the science is telling us is that we should redouble efforts to tackle abusive upbringings, and even simple neglect. This will help any child, but especially those whose biology makes them vulnerable. Thankfully there is already considerable enthusiasm in both the US and the UK for converting the latest in behavioral science into parenting and social skills: both governments have schemes in place to improve parenting in families where children are at risk of receiving poor care.

Some people are uncomfortable with the idea of early intervention because it implies our behavior becomes "set" as we grow up, compromising the idea of free will. That view is understandable, but it would be negligent to ignore what the studies are telling us. Indeed, the cost to society of failing to intervene — in terms of criminal damage, dealing with offenders and helping victims of crime — is bound to be greater than the cost of improving parenting. The value to the children is immeasurable.

1. Researchers have come to a consensus: to explain violent behavior _____.
    A. in terms of physical environment   B. from a biological perspective
    C. based on the empirical data   D. in a statistical way

2. When we say that antisocial and criminal behavior tends to run in families, as indicated by the recent findings, we can probably mean that _____.
    A. a particular gene is passed on in families
    B. child abuse will lead to domestic violence
    C. the male victims of child abuse will pass on the tendency
    D. the violent predisposition is exclusively born of child abuse

3. The recent observation implicated that to check the development of antisocial and criminal behavior _____.
    A. boys are to be screened for the biological predisposition
    B. high-risk kids should be brought up in kindergarten
    C. it is important to spot the genes for the risk factors
    D. active measures ought to be taken at an early age

4. To defend the argument against the unfavorable idea, the author makes it a point to consider _____.
    A. the immeasurable value of the genetic research on behavior
    B. the consequences of compromising democracy
    C. the huge cost of improving parenting skills
    D. the greater cost of failing to intervene

5. Which of the following can be the best title for the passage?
    A. Parenting Strategies for Kids.   B. The Making of a Criminal.
    C. Parental Education.   D. Abusive Parenting.

Passage Two

After 25 years battling the mother of all viruses, have we finally got the measure of HIV? Three developments featured in this issue collectively give grounds for optimism that would have been scarcely believable a year ago in the wake of another failed vaccine and continuing problems supplying drugs to all who need them.

Perhaps the most compelling hope lies in the apparent "cure" of a man with HIV who had also developed leukemia. Doctors treated his leukemia with a bone marrow transplant that also vanquished the virus. Now US Company Sangamo Biosciences is hoping to emulate the effect using gene therapy. If it works, and that is still a big if, it would open up the possibility of patients being cured with a single shot of gene therapy, instead of taking antiretroviral drugs for life.

Antiretroviral therapy (ART) is itself another reason for optimism. Researchers at the World Health Organization have calculated that HIV could be effectively eradicated in Africa and other hard-hit places using existing drugs. The trick is to test everyone often, and give those who test positive ART as soon as possible. Because the drugs rapidly reduce circulating levels of the virus to almost zero, it would stop people passing it on through sex. By blocking the cycle of infection in this way, the virus could be virtually eradicated by 2050.

Bankrolling such a long-term program would cost serious money — initially around $3.5 billion a year in South Africa alone, rising to $85 billion in total. Huge as it sounds, however, it is peanuts compared with the estimated $1.9 trillion cost of the Iraq war, or the $700 billion spent in one go propping up the US banking sector. It also looks small beer compared with the costs of carrying on as usual, which the WHO says can only lead to spiraling cases and costs.

The final bit of good news is that the cost of ART could keep on falling. Last Friday, GlaxoSmithKline chairman Andrew Witty said that his company would offer all its medicines to the poorest countries for at least 25 percent less than the typical price in rich countries. GSK has already been doing this for ART, but the hope is that the company may now offer it cheaper still and that other firms will follow their lead.

No one doubts the devastation caused by AIDS. In 2007，2 million people died and 2.7 million more contracted the virus. Those dismal numbers are not going to turn around soon — and they won't turn around at all without huge effort and investment. But at least there is renewed belief that, given the time and money, we can finally start riddling the world of this most fearsome of viruses.

6. Which of the following can be most probably perceived beyond the first paragraph?
   A. The end of the world.
   B. A candle of hope.
   C. A Nobel prize.
   D. A Quick Fix.

7. According to the passage, the apparent "cure" of the HIV patient who had also developed leukemia would _____.
   A. make a promising transition from antiretroviral medication to gene therapy
   B. facilitate the development of effective vaccines for the infection
   C. compel people to draw an analogy between AIDS and leukemia
   D. change the way we look at those with AIDS

8. As another bit of good news, _____.
   A. HIV will be virtually wiped out first in Africa
   B. the cycle of HIV infection can be broken with ART
   C. the circulating levels of HIV have been limited to almost zero
   D. the existing HIV drugs will be enhanced to be more effective in 25 years

9. The last reason for optimism is that _____.
    A. governments will invest more in improving ART
    B. the cost of antiretroviral therapy is on the decline
    C. everybody can afford antiretroviral therapy in the world
    D. the financial support of ART is coming to be no problem

10. The whole passage carries a tone of _____.
    A. idealism   B. activism   C. criticism   D. optimism

Passage Three

Archaeology can tell us plenty about how humans looked and the way they lived tens of thousands of years ago. But what about the deeper questions? Could early humans speak? Were they capable of self-conscious reflection? Did they believe in anything?

Such questions might seem to be beyond the scope of science. Not so. Answering them is the focus of a burgeoning field that brings together archaeology and neuroscience. It aims to chart the development of human cognitive powers. This is not easy to do. A skull gives no indication of whether its owner was capable of speech, for example. The task then is to find proxies（替代物）for key traits and behaviors that have stayed intact over millennia.

Perhaps the most intriguing aspect of this endeavor is teasing out the role of culture as a force in the evolution of our mental skills. For decades, development of the brain has been seen as exclusively biological. But increasingly, that is being challenged.

Take what the Cambridge archaeologist Colin Renfrew calls "the sapient（智人的）paradox（矛盾）". Evidence suggests that the human genome, and hence the brain, has changed little in the past 60,000 years. Yet it wasn't until about 10,000 years ago that profound changes took place in human behavior: people settled in villages and built shrines. Renfrew's paradox is why, if the hardware was in place, did it take so long for humans to start changing the world?

His answer is that the software — the culture — took a long time to develop. In particular, the intervening time saw humans vest（赋予）meaning in objects and symbols. Those meanings were developed by social interaction over successive generations, passed on through teaching, and stored in the neuronal connections of children.

Culture also changes biology by modifying natural selection, sometimes in surprising ways. How is it, for example, that a human gene for making essential vitamin C became blocked by junk DNA? One answer is that our ancestors started eating fruit, so the pressure to make vitamin C "relaxed" and the gene became unnecessary. By this reasoning, early humans then became addicted to fruit, and any gene that helped them to find it was selected for.

Evidence suggests that the brain is so plastic that, like genes, it can be changed by relaxing selection pressure. Our understanding of human cognitive development is still fragmented and confused, however. We have lots of proposed causes and effects, and hypotheses to explain them. Yet the potential pay-off makes answers worth searching for. If we know where the human mind came from and what changed it, perhaps we can gauge where it is going. Finding those answers will take all the ingenuity the modern human mind can muster.

11. The questions presented in the first paragraph _____.
    A. seem to have no answers whatever
    B. are intended to dig for ancient human minds
    C. are not scientific enough to be answered here
    D. are raised to explore the evolution of human appearance

12. The scientists find the proxy to be _____.
    A. the role of culture   B. the passage of time
    C. the structure of a skull   D. the biological makeup of the brain

13. According to Renfrew's paradox, the transition from 60,000 to 10,000 years ago suggests that _____.
    A. human civilization came too late
    B. the hardware retained biologically static
    C. it took so long for the software to evolve
    D. there existed an interaction between gene and environment

14. From the example illustrating the relation between culture and biology, we might conclude that _____.
    A. the mental development has not been exclusively biological
    B. the brain and culture have not developed at the same pace
    C. the theory of natural selection applies to human evolution
    D. vitamin C contributes to the development of the brain

15. Speaking of the human mind, the author would say that _____.
    A. its cognitive development is extremely slow
    B. to know its past is to understand its future
    C. its biological evolution is hard to predict
    D. as the brain develops, so as the mind

Passage One

本文话题

犯罪行为的原因。

难词译注

predisposition [ˌpriːdispəˈziʃn] *n.*	倾向
double whammy [ˈdʌbl] [ˈwæmi]	祸不单行
neurotransmitter [ˌnjuərətrænzˈmitə] *n.*	神经递质

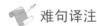 难句译注

This has been illustrated in several studies over the past six years which found that male victims of child abuse are several times as likely to become criminals and abusers themselves if they were born with a less-active version of a gene for the enzyme monoamine oxidase A (MAO-A), which breaks down neurotransmitters crucial to the regulation of aggression.

【分析】此句为复合句，句中有多个定语从句。主句为：This has been illustrated in several studies over the past six years. 后面 which 引导定语从句（which found…oxidase A）修饰 studies。在定语从句中有一个 if 引导的条件状语从句。最后 which 引导的非限制性定语从句（which break down…）修饰 MAO-A。

【译文】过去的六年间多个研究已经阐述了这个观点。研究发现，如果虐待儿童案件中受害的男孩出生时就带有相对不活跃的单胺氧化酶基因，（那么）他们将来成为罪犯和施暴者的可能性多达几倍。而这种酶可以分解为对控制人的进攻行为至关重要的神经传递素。

答案及解析

1. 【问题】研究者已经达成共识：从 _____ （方面）解释犯罪行为。
　　　A. 自然环境　　　　　　　B. 生物角度
　　　C. 经验数据　　　　　　　D. 统计方法

　　【答案】B

　　【解析】此题为细节定位题。根据第一段得知，对于犯罪行为，由于多数未报道，因而采集数据或者用可靠的统计方法都很困难, 故排除选项B和D, 选项A也没提到。第一段最后一句话是此题的有效信息。

2. 【问题】当说到"正如最近的研究结果指出，反社会和犯罪行为通常发生在家族中"，我们的意思可能是 _____ 。
　　　A. 由家族中一个特殊的基因遗传下来
　　　B. 虐待儿童会导致家庭暴力
　　　C. 虐待儿童案件中受害的男孩将会继续这种倾向
　　　D. 暴力倾向仅仅出现在虐待儿童的家庭

　　【答案】A

　　【解析】此题为细节理解题。根据题干信息，可以定位到文章的第二段，最后一句话是解题的有效信息，句义理解详见难句译注。

3. 【问题】最近的观察暗示，为了探究反社会和犯罪行为的发展，_____。

    A．要筛查男孩的生理倾向性　　B．高危孩子应该在幼儿园养育

    C．发现危险因素基因很重要　　D．在早期应采取积极措施

【答案】D

【解析】此题为细节定位题。根据题干信息，可以定位到第三段。解题有效信息为最后一句。根据本段主题句可以得知有暴力倾向的孩子在早期会出现迹象。而最后一句用反问的方式提出，我们是否应该就我们目前了解的知识，采取措施保护那些处于危险中的孩子们。因而答案为 D。

4. 【问题】为了支持反对不利观点的论点，作者认为要考虑_____。

    A．行为基因研究的无限价值。　　B．妥协民主的后果。

    C．提高父母教育的技巧。　　D．干涉失败成本更大。

【答案】D

【解析】此题为细节理解题。根据题干信息，可以定位到文章最后一段。解题有效信息是第三句，句意为：事实上，社会干预失败所付出的成本必定大于提高父母教育能力的成本。考虑到成本的差异，作者指出，尽管不利观点可以理解，但对于孩子来说家庭教育提升这一早期介入意义重大。因而答案为 D。

5. 【问题】文章最恰当的题目是什么？

    A．父母对子女教育的策略。　　B．罪犯的形成。

    C．父母教育。　　D．虐待型的父母教育。

【答案】B

【解析】此题为主旨题。根据文章第一段的主题句以及每段的主题句可以得知，文章围绕犯罪行为的形成因素展开讨论，因而选项 B 为答案。

Passage Two

 本文话题

HIV 的治疗进展。

 难词译注

leukemia [luːˈkiːmiə] n.	白血病
vanquish [ˈvæŋkwiʃ] v.	征服，抑制
emulate [ˈemjuːleit] v.	仿效
antiretroviral drug [ænti,retrəuˈvairəl] [drʌg]	抗逆转录病毒药
bankroll [ˈbæŋkrəul] n./v.	资助
spiral [ˈspaiərəl] n./v.	螺旋，盘旋
devastation [,devəˈsteiʃən] n.	毁坏

🖋 难句译注

　　Three developments featured in this issue collectively give grounds for optimism that would have been scarcely believable a year ago in the wake of another failed vaccine and continuing problems supplying drugs to all who need them.

【分析】主句为：Three developments give grounds for optimism。featured 做定语修饰 development。"that would have been…" 是定语从句，修饰 optimism。in the wake of 的意思是"随着……而来"。

【译文】以这个问题为主的三个进展共同为这个问题的乐观态度提供理由，这在一年前随着另一个疫苗的失败和给予人们的药物不断出现问题的情况下是几乎不可想象的。

🔩 答案及解析

6. 【问题】下列哪一个是通过第一段可以得知的？

    A. 世界的灭亡。   B. 希望之光。

    C. 诺贝尔奖。   D. 快速修复。

【答案】B

【解析】此题为细节定位题。根据第一段最后一句话可以得知，针对 HIV 病毒，研究进展又带给我们希望，因而答案为 B。

7. 【问题】根据文章，对已经患上白血病的 HIV 病毒病人表面上的治愈将 _____。

    A. 有望从抗逆转录病毒治疗转向基因疗法

    B. 有助于有效的抗感染疫苗的研制

    C. 迫使人们将艾滋病与白血病进行类比

    D. 改变我们看待艾滋病患者的方式

【答案】A

【解析】此题为细节定位题。根据题干信息可定位到第二段，解题有效信息为最后一句，意思是希望仿效那些仅采用单一基因疗法患者的疗效，取代终身服用抗逆转录病毒的药物。因而答案为 A。

8. 【问题】另一个好消息是 _____。

    A. HIV 病毒将在非洲首先被消灭

    B. HIV 病毒感染的循环可以被 ART 打破

    C. HIV 病毒的流行程度已经几乎降为零

    D. 现有的 HIV 病毒药物将在 25 年后效力更强

【答案】B

【解析】此题为细节理解题。根据题干和第三段首句信息可以得知，解题有效信息就在第三段。首先，根据第三段第二句话可以排除选项 A，原文信息中没有提到 HIV 病毒首先将在非洲被消灭；另外，根据第四句可排除选项 C，原文信息是"因为药物能快速将病毒流行程度降到零，这就防止人们通过性传播病毒"。选项 D 在文章中没有相应信息。

9.【问题】乐观的最后一个原因是 _____。
　　　　A．政府将为提高 ART 给予更多投资
　　　　B．ART 的成本在下降
　　　　C．世界上的每个人都能承受 ART（费用）
　　　　D．对 ART 的资金支持将不成问题

【答案】B

【解析】此题为细节定位题。根据题干信息，可定位至第五段。本段首句为有效信息，其含义与选项 B 吻合。

10.【问题】全篇的语气是 _____。
　　　　A．理想化　　　　　B．行动性　　　　　C．批评　　　　　D．乐观

【答案】D

【解析】此题为态度推断题，根据每段的主题句内容以及上述细节题可以得出，全篇语气态度为乐观积极的，因而答案为 D。

Passage Three

 本文话题

人类大脑思维的形成与进化。

 难词译注

archaeology [ˌɑːkiˈɔlədʒi] *n.*	考古学
burgeoning [ˈbəːdʒəniŋ] *a.*	增长迅速的，生机勃勃的
intact [inˈtækt] *a.*	完整的，原封不动的
millennia [miˈleniə] *n.*	千年
intriguing [inˈtriːgiŋ] *a.*	有趣的，迷人的
endeavor [enˈdevə] *n./v.*	努力，尽力
gauge [geidʒ] *n./v.*	测量
ingenuity [ˌindʒiˈnjuiti] *n.*	心灵手巧，独创性
muster [ˈmʌstə] *n./v.*	召集，集合

答案及解析

11.【问题】第一段提出的问题 _____。
　　　　A．似乎没有答案　　　　　B．想要挖掘古人类的思维
　　　　C．不够科学，无法回答　　　D．为探究人类相貌进化而提出

【答案】B

【解析】此题为细节定位题，解题有效信息在第一段最后一句话。

12. 【问题】科学家们寻找的替代物是 _____。
    A. 文化的作用   B. 时间推移
    C. 头颅的结构   D. 大脑的生理结构
    【答案】A
    【解析】此题为细节定位题。根据题干可以定位到第二段最后一句话，而解题有效信息是第三段的第一句话，因而答案为 A。

13. 【问题】根据 Renfrew 的悖论，从 6 万年前到 1 万年前的转变说明 _____。
    A. 人类文明来得太晚了   B. 硬件仍旧在生理上没有变化
    C. 软件的进化经历了太长时间   D. 基因和环境间存在着联系
    【答案】C
    【解析】此题为推断题，根据题干定位到第四段。段落大意是：证据表明，人类基因组及大脑在过去的 6 万年间几乎没有变化，然而直到 1 万年前人类行为才发生深远的变化……如果硬件保持不变，人类为什么要花费如此长的时间开始改变世界呢？因而答案为 C。

14. 【问题】从文化和生理关系的实例中我们可以得出的结论是 _____。
    A. 心智发展已不仅仅是生理上的
    B. 大脑和文化不是同步发展的
    C. 自然选择理论应用于人类进化
    D. 维生素 C 有助于大脑发育
    【答案】C
    【解析】此题为推论题。解题有效信息在第六段，这两段主要论述文化与人类生理变化的关系。本段首句指出：文化也通过修改自然选择而改变生理。因而选项 C 为答案。

15. 【问题】提到人类思维，作者想要说 _____。
    A. 认知发展十分地缓慢   B. 知晓过去就是了解未来
    C. 生理进化很难预测   D. 随着大脑的发育，心智也随之发育
    【答案】B
    【解析】此题为推断题，解题有效信息在最后一段。解题有效信息是最后三句：可能的回报使得探寻答案是有意义的，如果我们知道人类的思维从何而来并且如何改变，也许我们就可以测算它今后的发展方向……选项 B 与此句含义吻合。

2012 年医学博士统考阅读理解部分真题

Passage One

As the defining epidemic of a modern age notable for overconsumption and excess, obesity is hard to beat. The increased availability of high-fat, high-sugar foods, along with more sedentary lifestyles, has helped push the number of obese people worldwide to beyond 400 million, and the number of overweight to more than 1.6 billion. By 2015, those figures are likely to grow to 700 million and 2.3 billion respectively, according to the World Health Organization. Given the health implications — increased risk of heart disease, stroke, diabetes and some cancers — anything that helps people avoid piling on the pounds must be a good thing, right?

Those who agree will no doubt welcome the growing success of researchers striving to develop "diet pills" that provide a technical fix for those incapable of losing weight any other way. Last week a study published in *The Lancet* showed that tesofensine, which works by inducing a sense of fullness, is twice as effective as any other drug at enabling patients to lose weight.

There is no question that advances such as this are good news for those with a strong genetic predisposition to obesity. But for the rest of us it is dangerous to see treatment as a more effective solution than prevention. There are several reasons for this. For a start, the traditional ways of maintaining a safe weight, such as limiting what you eat, increasing consumption of fruit and vegetables and taking more exercise, are beneficial for our health in many ways.

Second, overindulgence in fatty foods has implications for the entire planet. Consider the deleterious environmental effects of the rising demand for meat. As demonstrated in our special issue on economic growth, technological fixes will not compensate for excessive consumption. Third, interfering with the brain circuits that control the desire for food can have an impact on other aspects of a person's personality and their mental and physical health.

We need two approaches: more research into the genetics of obesity to understand why some people are more susceptible, and greater efforts to help people avoid eating their way to an early death. Cynics will say we've tried education and it hasn't worked. That is defeatist: getting people to change their behavior takes time and effort, held back as we are by our biological tendency to eat more than we need, and by the food industry's ruthless opportunism in exploiting that.

Drugs will be the saving of a few — as a last resort. But the global obesity problem is one of lifestyle, and the solution must be too.

1. In the first paragraph all the figures surrounding obesity reflect_____.
    A. a close link between growing obese and developing disease
    B. the inevitable diseases of modern civilization
    C. the war against the epidemic we have lost
    D. the urgency of the global phenomenon

2. When it comes to the recently reported diet pills, the author would say that_____.
    A. drugs are no replacement of prevention
    B. the technical advance is not necessarily good news
    C. the technical fix does help reverse the obesity epidemic
    D. the mechanism of tesofensine still remains to be verified

3. Which of the following can be referred to as the environmental perspective of the author's argument?
    A. Belittling good health behavior.

B. Imposing a heavy burden on our planet.

C. Making trouble for our social environment.

D. Having implications for mental and physical health.

4. The author argues that we make greater efforts to help people fight against _____.

A. their biological overeating tendency and aggressively marketed foods

B. the development of diet pills as a technical fix for obesity

C. their excuses for their genetic susceptibility to obesity

D. the defeatism prevailing in the general populations

5. Which of the following can be the best title for the passage?

A. No Quick Fix.   B. Disease of Civilization.

C. Pursuing a Technical Fix.   D. A War on Global Obesity.

Passage Two

An abandoned airfield near a former Nazi concentration camp may soon feature pagodas and Tai Chi parks. A $700 million project aims to give Germany its own Chinatown 22 miles north of Berlin in the town of Oranienburg, housing 2,000 residents by 2010.

The investor group behind the scheme hopes the new Chinatown will attract tourists and business to rival the famed Chinatowns of San Francisco and New York by delivering an "authentic Chinese experience". "You'll be able to experience China, go out for a Chinese meal, and buy Chinese goods," says Stefan Kunigam, managing director of Bandenburg-China-Project-Management GmbH.

The project has attracted investors in both Germany and China, reports Christoph Lang of Berlin's Trade and Industry promotion Office. "Chinese investors have already asked if we have a Chinatown here." He says. "The cultural environment is very important for them. You cannot build a synthetic Chinatown."

Germany is home to about 72,000 Chinese migrants (2002 Federal Statistical Office figures), but the country has not had a Chinatown since the early 1930s in Hamburg, when most of the city's 2,000 Chinese residents fled or were arrested by the Nazis.

German's more-recent history with anti-foreigner extremism remains a problem even within the government, reports Deutsche Welle (DW), Germany's international broadcaster. DW notes that National Democratic Party lawmaker Holger Apfel's xenophobic（恐外的）comments about "state-subsidized Oriental mega-families" at first went largely uncriticized.

"Every fourth German harbors anti-foreigner sentiments," DW quotes Miriam Gruss, a Free Democratic Party parliamentarian. "Right-wing extremism is clearly rooted in the middle of society. It's not a minor phenomenon." The German government initiated a special youth for Democracy and Tolerance program in January 2007 as part of its tolerance-building efforts.

While it is not clear how many Chinese migrants will ultimately settle in the new

German Chinatown, developers hope the project will increase Germans' understanding for China and Chinese culture.

6. If set up, according to the passage, the new German Chinatown will probably be _____.
   A. a rival to the Chinatowns of San Francisco and New York
   B. mainly made of pagodas and Tai Chi parks
   C. located in the north suburbs of Berlin
   D. the biggest one in Germany

7. When he says that you cannot build a synthetic Chinatown, Lang means _____.
   A. the real imported goods made in China
   B. the authoritative permission for the project
   C. the importance of the location for a Chinatown
   D. the authentic environment to experience Chinese culture

8. By mentioning the population of Chinese migrants in Germany, the author most probably means that _____.
   A. it is too late to build a Chinatown
   B. it is their desire to save a Chinatown
   C. it is important to create jobs for them
   D. it is necessary to have a Chinatown there

9. According to the passage, German anti-foreigner extremism _____.
   A. can seed the new community with hatred
   B. could be an obstacle to the project
   C. will absolutely kill the plan
   D. is growing for the scheme

10. The message from the plan is clear _____.
    A. to build a new community
    B. to fight against right-wing extremism
    C. to promote more cultural understanding
    D. to increase Chinese's understanding of Germany

Passage One

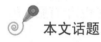

本文话题

减肥药的危害以及如何应对肥胖的方式。

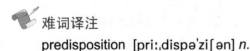

难词译注

predisposition [priːˌdɪspəˈzɪʃən] *n.*   倾向，易染病的体质

deleterious [ˌdeliˈtiəriəs] *a.*   有毒的，有害的

答案与解析

1. 【问题】第一段中有关肥胖的所有数据反映出 _____。

    A. 越来越胖与患病的密切关系   B. 现代文明不可避免的疾病

    C. 我们已经输掉了抗争流行病的战役   D. 这一全球现象的紧迫性

    【答案】D

    【解析】此题为总结概括题。第一段的数据清楚地表明肥胖已经成为全球性的趋势，解决该问题刻不容缓，因而答案为 D。

2. 【问题】当谈到最近报道的减肥药时，作者认为 _____。

    A. 药物无法取代预防

    B. 科技进步不一定是好消息

    C. 技术手段确实有助于逆转肥胖的流行趋势

    D. tesofensine 的原理仍需证实

    【答案】B

    【解析】此题为转折处命题。根据减肥药的专有名词定位到第二段，第二段主要讲述该药的作用。第三段第二句话转折后说，对于其他人（没有明显的遗传肥胖基因的人）来说，将治疗看作比预防更有效的手段是很危险的。因而答案为 B。对于有遗传肥胖基因的人来说这种药确实有效，因而 A 过于绝对。

3. 【问题】下列哪一个指的是作者对环境方面的观点？

    A. 轻视有利于健康的行为。   B. 对我们的星球添加过重的负担。

    C. 给我们的社会环境增添麻烦。   D. 对身心健康有意义。

    【答案】B

    【解析】此题参看文章第四段。

4. 【问题】作者认为我们要更努力帮助人类抵抗 _____。

    A. 生理上饮食过度的趋势和被过度营销的食品

    B. 减肥药这一技术手段的发展

    C. 以遗传导致肥胖为借口

    D. 大众中流行的挫败心理

    【答案】C

    【解析】根据题干定位到第五段的第一句话：…greater efforts to help people avoid eating their way to an early death. 这句话说明更多的人将自己的肥胖归因于有肥胖的遗传基因，而忽视了生活方式的影响。因而选项 C 正确。

5. 【问题】下列哪一个是文章最好的标题？

    A. 没有快速的办法。   B. 文明病。

    C. 寻求技术上的办法。   D. 针对全球肥胖的斗争。

    【答案】D

【解析】此题为主旨题。本文利用众多数据表明肥胖问题刻不容缓，随后阐述了减肥药的作用。但作者对于这一药物的弊端进行了分析，最后指出两种应对措施：一是研究肥胖基因，二是努力避免人们消极对待这一问题而坐以待胖。文章最后作者提到减肥药可以救助一些人，但全球肥胖的问题是生活方式问题，因而其解决方法也应由此入手。选项 D 为答案。

Passage Two

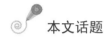

本文话题

德国准备建造唐人街。

答案与解析

6. 【问题】根据文章，如果建立，新的德国唐人街将可能 _____。
   A．是旧金山和纽约唐人街的劲敌　　B．主要由古塔和太极公园组成
   C．位于柏林的北部郊区　　　　　　D．是德国最大的一个

   【答案】A

   【解析】此题为细节定位题，原文信息参考第二段的第一句话。文章第一段提到这个唐人街将以古塔和太极公园为特征，所以选项 B 错误；同时第一段提到新建的唐人街位于柏林以北 22 英里的 Oranienburg，因而选项 C 错误；选项 D 没提到。

7. 【问题】当 Lang 说你不能建造一个综合性的唐人街时，他的意思是 _____。
   A．真正进口中国制造的物品　　　　B．该项目的官方准许
   C．唐人街位置的重要性　　　　　　D．感受中国文化的真实环境

   【答案】D

   【解析】此题参见文章第三段。倒数第二句提到文化环境很关键，因而我们可以推断出 Lang 的意思是指的是文化氛围，故选项 D 正确。

8. 【问题】通过提及德国的中国移民者，作者最可能的意思是 _____。
   A．建造唐人街太晚了　　　　　　　B．拯救唐人街是他们的愿望
   C．为他们创造工作机会很重要　　　D．在那里有个唐人街很必要

   【答案】D

   【解析】此题参见文章第四段，德国有很多中国移民者，但没有一个唐人街，因而作者的意思是 D 项。

9. 【问题】根据文章，德国排外极端主义 _____。
   A．可能充满仇恨地建造这个新社区　　B．可能阻碍这个项目
   C．一定会扼杀这个计划　　　　　　　D．正为这个计划发展壮大

   【答案】B

   【解析】文章倒数第二段提到德国的右翼极端排外主义扎根于社会中，并且不是一个小问题。因此我们可以推断德国排外极端主义可能会阻碍建唐人街的计划。

10.【问题】这个计划传递出的信息很清楚：_____。

    A. 建立一个新的社区   B. 对抗右翼极端主义

    C. 更好地促进文化上的理解   D. 增进德国人对中国的了解

【答案】C

【解析】此题参见文章最后一句：建造者们希望这个建造唐人街的计划能增进两国之间的文化了解，所以选项 C 正确。

2011 年医学博士统考阅读理解部分真题

Passage One

Patients can recall what they hear while under general anesthetic even if they don't wake up, concludes a new study.

Several studies over the past three decades have reported that people can retain conscious or subconscious memories of thinks that happened while they were being operated on. But failure by other researchers to confirm such findings has led skeptics to speculate that the patients who remembered these events might briefly have regained consciousness in the course of operations.

Gitta Lubke，Peter Sebel and colleagues at Emory University in Atlanta measured the depth of anesthesia using bispectral analysis, a technique which measures changes in brainwave pattern in the frontal lobes moment by moment during surgery. Before this study researchers only took an average measurement over the whole operation, says Lubke.

Lubke studied 96 traurna patients undergoing emergency surgery, many of whom were too severely injured to tolerate full anesthesia. During surgery, each patient wore headphones through which a series of 16 words was repeated for 3 minutes each. At the same time bispectral analysis recorded the depth of anesthesia.

After the operation Lubke tested the patients by showing them the first three letters of a word such as "limit"，and asking them to complete it. Patients who had had a word starting with these letters played during surgery — "limit"，for example — chose that word an average of 11 per cent more often than patients who had been played a different word list. None of the patients had any conscious memory of hearing the word lists.

Unconscious priming was strongest for words played when patients were most lightly anaesthetized. But it was statistically significant even when patients were fully anaesthetized when the word was played.

This finding which will be published in the journal *Anesthesiology* could mean that operating theatre staff should be more discreet. What they say during surgery may distress patient afterwards, says Philip Merikle，a psychologist at the University of Waterloo，Ontario.

1.   Scientists have found that deep anesthesia _____.

    A. is likely to affect hearing

B．cannot block surgeons' words

C．can cause serious damages to memory

D．helps retain conscious or subconscious memories

2. By the new study the technique of bispectral analysis helps the scientists _____．

A．acquire an average measurement of brainwave changes over the whole surgery

B．decide whether the patient would retain conscious or subconscious memories

C．relate their measurements and recordings to the verbal sounds during surgery

D．assure the depth of anesthesia during surgery

3. To test the patients the scientists _____．

A．prepared two lists of words

B．used 96 headphones for listening

C．conducted the whole experiment for three minutes

D．voiced only the first three letters of 16 words during surgery

4. The results from the new study indicate that it was possible for the patients _____．

A．to regain consciousness under the knife

B．to tell one word from another after surgery

C．to recall what had been heard during surgery

D．to overreact to deep anesthesia in the course of operations

5. What can we infer from the finding?

A．How surgery mispractice can be prevented.

B．Why a surgeon cannot be too careful.

C．Why surgeons should hold their tongues during surgery.

D．How the postoperative patients can retain subconscious memories.

Passage Two

Scientists used to believe adult brains did not grow any new neurons, but it has emerged that new neurons can sprout in the brains of adult rats, birds and even humans. Understanding the process could be important, for finding ways to treat diseases such as Alzheimer's in which neurons are destroyed.

Most neurons sprouting in adulthood seem to be in the hippocampus, a structure involved in learning and memory. But they rarely survive more than a few weeks. "We thought they were possibly dying because they were deprived of some sort of input," says Elizaberh Gould, a neuroscientist at Princeton. Because of the location, Gould and her colleagues suspect that learning itself might bolster the new neurons' survival, and that only tasks involving the hippocampus would do the trick.

To test this, they injected adult male rats with a substance that labeled newborn neurons so that they could be tracked. Later, they gave some of the rats standard tasks. One involved using visual and spatial cues, such as posters on a well, to learn to find a platform hidden under murky water. In another, the rats learnt to associate a noise with a tiny shock half a second later. Both these tasks use the hippocampus — if this structure is damaged, rats can't do them.

Meanwhile, the researchers gave other rats similar tasks that did not require the hippocampus finding a platform that was easily visible in water, for instance. Other members of the control group simply paddled in a tub of water or listened to noises.

The team reported in *Nature Neuroscience* that the animals given the tasks that activate the hippocampus kept twice as many of their new neurons alive as the others. "Learning opportunities increase the number of neurons," says Gould.

But Fred Gage and his colleagues at the Salk Institute for Biological Studies in La Jolla, California, dispute this. In the same issue of *Nature Neuroscience*, they reported that similar water maze experiments on mice did not help new neurons survive.

Gould thinks the difference arose because the groups labeled new neurons at different times. She gave the animals tasks two weeks after the neurons were labeled. When the new cells would normally be dying, she thinks the Salk group put their mice to work too early for new neurons to benefit. "By the time the cells were degenerating, the animals were not learning anything," she says.

6. Not until recently did scientists find out that _____.
   A. new neurons could grow in adult brains
   B. neurons could be man-made in the laboratory
   C. neurons were destroyed in Alzheimer's disease
   D. humans could produce new neurons as animals

7. Gould's notion was that the short-lived neurons _____.
   A. did survive longer than expected
   B. would die much sooner than expected
   C. could actually better learning and memory
   D. could be kept alive by stimulating the hippocampus

8. Which of the following can clearly tell the two groups of rats from each other in the test?
   A. The water used.   B. The noises played.
   C. The neurons newly born.   D. The hippocampus involved.

9. Gould theorizes that the Salk group's failure to report the same results was due to _____.
   A. the timing of labeling new neurons   B. the frequency of stimulation
   C. the wrongly labeled neurons   D. the types of learning tasks

10. Which of the following can be the best title for the passage?

　　A. Use It or Lose It.　　　　　　　B. Learn to Survive.

　　C. To Be or Not to Be.　　　　　　D. Stay Mentally Healthy.

Passage Three

Here's yet another reason to lose weight. Heavier people are more likely to be killed or seriously injured in car accidents than lighter people.

That could mean car designers will have to build in new safety features to compensate for the extra hazards facing overweight passengers. In the US, car manufacturers have already had to redesign air bags so they inflate to lower pressures making them less of a danger to smaller women and children. But no one yet knows what it is that puts overweight passengers at extra risk.

A study carried out in Seattle, Washington, looked at more than 26,000 people who had been involved in car crashes, and found that heavier people were at far more risk. People weighing between 100 and 119 kilograms are almost two-and-a-half times as likely to die in a crash as people weighing less than 60 kilograms.

And importantly: the same trend held up when the researchers looked at body mass index (BMI) — a measure that takes height as well as weight into account. Someone 1.8 meters tall weighing 126 kilograms would have a BMI of 39, but so would a person 1.5 meters tall weighing 88 kilograms. People are said to be obese if their BMI is 30 or over.

The study found that people with a BMI of 35 to 39 are over twice as likely to die in a crash compared with people with BMIs of about 20. It's not just total weight, but obesity that's dangerous.

While they do not yet know why this is the case, the evidence is worth pursuing, says Charles Mock, a surgeon and epidemiologist at the Harborview Injury Prevention and Research Center in Seattle, who led the research team. He thinks one answer may be for safety authorities to use heavier crash-test dummies when certifying cars as safe to drive.

Crash tests normally use dummies that represent standard-sized males weighing about 78 kilograms. Recently, smaller crash-test dummies have also been used to represent children inside crashing cars. But larger and heavier dummies aren't used, the US National Highway Traffic Safety Administration in Washington, D.C. told *New Scientist*.

The reasons for the higher injury and death rates are far from clear. Mock speculates that car interiors might not be suitably designed for heavy people. Or obese people, with health problems such as high blood pressure or diabetes, could be finding it tougher to recover from injury.

11. When they redesigned air bags to hold less pressure, the American car manufacturers _____.

　　A. found it hard to set standards without the definition of obesity

B. incidentally brought about extra risks to obese passengers

C. based their job on the information of car accidents

D. actually neglected smaller women and children

12. When they categorized the obese people, the researchers _____.

A. showed a preference for BMI in measurements

B. achieved almost the same results as previously

C. found the units of kilogram more applicable than BMI

D. were shocked to know the number of obese people killed in car crashes

13. To address the problem, Mock _____.

A. suggested that the safety authorities use heavier crash-test dummies

B. cried for the standardization of crash-test dummies

C. reduced the weights of crash-test dummies

D. encouraged obese people to lose weight

14. While exploring the reason for the higher injury and death rates, Mock would most probably say that _____.

A. cars can be made safer to avoid crashes

B. it is wise for obese people not to drive drunk

C. it is not just total weight, but obesity itself that is dangerous

D. the main reason behind the problem is drinkers of heavy weight

15. Which of the following questions is closely related to the passage?

A. Are air bags really necessary to be built in cars?

B. Are cars certified as safe to drive?

C. Are crash-test dummies too thin?

D. Are car accidents preventable?

Passage One

本文话题

麻醉状态下人们仍有记忆。

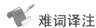

难词译注

anesthetic [ˌænisˈθetik] *n. / a.*	麻醉剂；麻醉的
anesthesia [ˌænisˈθiːzjə] *n.*	麻醉
skeptic [ˈskeptik] *n.*	怀疑者
bispectral analysis	双谱分析
frontal lobe	大脑额叶

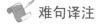 难句译注

But failure by other researchers to confirm such findings has led skeptics to speculate that the patients who remembered these events might briefly have regained consciousness in the course of operations. (Paragraph 2)

【分析】 主句的主语为 failure, by other researchers… such findings 作为定语修饰 failure；主句谓语为 has led；不定式 to speculate 后面接一个宾语从句。宾语从句的主语为 the patients，谓语动词结构为 might briefly have regained，宾语从句主语 the patients 由定语从句 who remembered these events 修饰。

【译文】 然而其他研究者没能证实上述结果，这导致怀疑者推测，回忆起这些事情的病人在手术过程中可能暂时恢复了意识。

答案及解析

1. 【问题】科学家们已经发现深度麻醉_____。

   A. 可能影响听力
   B. 不能阻碍医生的言语
   C. 可造成记忆的严重损伤
   D. 可保留有意识或潜意识的记忆

   【答案】D

   【解析】此题考点为细节定位题，原文有效信息是第二段第一句。

2. 【问题】新研究中，双谱分析有助于科学家_____。

   A. 在手术过程中获取脑波变化的平均测量数据
   B. 决定病人是否保持有意识的或潜意识的记忆
   C. 把测量数据和记录与手术中的语言发音联系起来
   D. 确保手术中的麻醉程度

   【答案】B

   【解析】根据题干中的关键词"bispectral analysis"定位到文章的第三段。本段第一句中出现该技术，并且同位结构解释说明这一技术的作用，即测量手术大脑额叶脑波形式的时时刻刻的变化。本段最后一句提到在这项研究前，研究者们仅对整个手术进行平均测量。A 项错在这一作用不是双谱分析的作用；C 项没提到；D 项错在 assure。

3. 【问题】为了测试病人，科学家们_____。

   A. 准备了两套词汇
   B. 使用 96 个耳机
   C. 使整个试验持续 3 分钟
   D. 手术中仅念出 16 个单词的前 3 个字母

   【答案】B

   【解析】此题可通过定位选项中的数字进行判断。第五段第二句提到使用不同的单词表，

但没有提到两套，故 A 项排除；第四段第二句话提到 16 个单词，每个单词重复 3 分钟，因而可判断选项 C 错误；第五段第一句话提到手术后测试病人，每个单词仅展示前 3 个字母，因而 D 项错误。B 项信息在第四段，整个研究的受试者为 96 人，每个病人都戴上耳机，所以 B 项为答案。

4. 【问题】新研究的结果表明病人可能 _____。

    A. 在手术中恢复意识   B. 会在术后区分词汇

    C. 回忆起手术中听到的内容   D. 在手术中对深度麻醉反应过激

【答案】C

【解析】此题为细节定位题，原文第一段开门见山地提到新研究的结果。

5. 【问题】从研究结果中我们可以推断出什么？

    A. 手术误操作如何避免。

    B. 为什么外科大夫多小心都不为过。

    C. 为什么外科大夫应该在手术中保持沉默。

    D. 术后病人如何能保持潜意识的记忆。

【答案】C

【解析】此题为推断题。文章最后一段提到研究结果可能意味着手术医务人员应该更加谨慎，手术中他们交谈的内容可能影响到病人，病人术后可能回忆起手术中听到的内容，因而外科大夫应该在手术中保持沉默，以免影响到病人。故答案为 C。

Passage Two

 本文话题

成人大脑中也可以产生新的神经元，这一新发现为老年痴呆症的治疗提供了新的方法。

 难词译注

hippocampus [ˌhipəˈkæmpəs] *n.*   海马状突起（脑组织）

bolster [ˈbəulstə] *v.*   支持，支撑

murky [ˈmə:ki] *a.*   朦胧的

答案及解析

6. 【问题】直到最近科学家才发现 _____。

    A. 成人大脑可以生长出新的神经元

    B. 在实验室中神经元可以人为制造

    C. 老年痴呆症患者的神经元被损

    D. 人类同动物一样可以生产出新神经元

【答案】A

【解析】此题为细节定位题，文章第一段直接说明新研究的研究结果。

7. 【问题】Gould 的观点是：短命的神经元 _____。

  A．比预期存活的时间更长   B．比预期死亡得更快

  C．实际上更有助于学习和记忆力   D．通过刺激海马状突起而存活

【答案】D

【解析】此题根据人名定位到文章的第二段最后一句话。第二段的第一句提到海马状突起涉及学习和记忆力。而最后一句提到学习本身有助于新神经元的存活。因而答案为 D。

8. 【问题】下列哪一个可以清楚地分清试验中的两组小鼠？

  A．使用的水。   B．播放的声音。

  C．新生的神经元。   D．海马状突起。

【答案】D

【解析】此题为细节定位题，由原文中的第四段第一句话可以得出答案。

9. 【问题】Gould 认为 Salk 小组没能得出相同的结果是因为 _____。

  A．标记新神经元的时间   B．刺激的频率

  C．误标的神经元   D．学习任务的类型

【答案】A

【解析】此题为细节定位题，参考最后一段的第一句话。

10. 【问题】下列哪一个是文章最好的标题？

  A．使用它，或失去它。   B．学会生存。

  C．是活还是不活。   D．保持精神健康。

【答案】A

【解析】此题为主旨题。通过第二段可知，学习（learning）可以促使新的神经元生长，而缺乏输入（input）则会使其死亡（dying），故 A 为正确的题目。

Passage Three

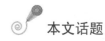 本文话题

本文讨论体重较大者可能在车祸中更危险。

答案及解析

11. 【问题】当重新设计安全气囊以承受较少压力的时候，美国汽车制造商 _____。

  A．发现若没有肥胖的定义则很难制定标准

  B．意外地给肥胖乘客带来了额外的危险

  C．根据车祸的相关信息进行工作

  D．实际上忽略了娇小女性和儿童

【答案】B

【解析】此题考点为细节信息定位。文章第二段第二句话提到美国汽车制造商重新设计气囊，因为他们减少气囊的压力，从而降低娇小女性和儿童面临的危险。因而D项错误。最后一句话转折结构揭示这样的做法可能给超重乘客带来更多的危险，答案为B项。

12. 【问题】当对肥胖人群进行分类时，研究者们 _____。

    A. 对BMI测量情有独钟

    B. 几乎得出和先前一样的结果

    C. 发现公斤单位比BMI更实用

    D. 震惊地获知车祸中肥胖人致死的人数

【答案】B

【解析】此题解题关键在文章第四段第一句话。这句话的意思是：当研究者们看BMI测量值时，得出同样的结论。这句话中的hold up的含义是"证明属实，经得起检验"。因而答案为B。

13. 【问题】为了解决这个问题，Mock _____。

    A. 建议安全权威部门使用更重的碰撞测试假人

    B. 迫切呼吁碰撞测试假人的标准化

    C. 减少碰撞测试假人的重量

    D. 鼓励肥胖者减肥

【答案】A

【解析】此题为细节信息定位题，根据人名定位到文章第六段。本段最后一句提到，他认为问题答案可能就在于要检验汽车行驶安全时，权威部门应该使用更重的碰撞测试假人。

14. 【问题】当探究重伤和致死率的原因时，Mock最可能的观点是 _____。

    A. 汽车要更安全，以避免车祸

    B. 肥胖者最好不要饮酒驾车

    C. 不仅是总重量的问题，而是肥胖本身很危险

    D. 问题背后的主要原因是饮酒者的过重体重

【答案】C

【解析】此题为推断题。文章最后一段提到Mock推断汽车内部设计不太适合体重较大的人，或者有高血压、糖尿病等疾病的肥胖者很难从事故受伤中康复。因此我们可以推断Mock的观点在于肥胖本身可能是该问题的原因。

15. 【问题】下面哪一个问题与文章紧密联系？

    A. 车内确实有必要安装气囊吗？   B. 汽车真的能保证安全驾驶了吗？

    C. 碰撞测试假人重量不够？   D. 车祸可以避免吗？

【答案】C

【解析】此题参考文章主旨：文章第一段。并且可以参考第73题。

2010 年医学博士统考阅读理解真题

Passage One

Children should avoid using mobile phones for all but essential calls because of possible health effects on young brains. This is one of the expected conclusions of an official government report to be published this week. The report is expected to call for the mobile phone industry to refrain from promoting phone use by children, and to start labeling phones with data on the amount of radiation they emit.

The Independent Expert Group on Mobile Phones, chaired by former government chief scientist William Stewart, has spent eight months reviewing existing scientific evidence on all aspects of the health effects of using mobile phones. Its report is believed to conclude that because we don't fully understand the nonthermal effects of radiation on human tissue, the government should adopt a precautionary approach, particularly in relation to children.

There is currently no evidence that mobile phones harm users or people living near transmitter masts. But some studies show that cell-phones operating at radiation levels within current safety limits do have some sort of biological effect on the brain.

John Tattersall, a researcher on the health effects of radiation at the Defense Evaluation and Research Agency's site at Porton Down, agrees that it might be wise to limit phone use by children. "If you have a developing nervous system, it's known to be more susceptible to environmental insults," he says. "So if phones did prove to be hazardous—which they haven't yet—it would be sensible."

In 1998, Tattersall showed that radiation levels similar to those emitted by mobile phones could alter signals from brain cells in slices of rat brain. "What we've found is an effect, but we don't know if it's hazardous," he says.

Alan Preece of the University of Bristol, who found last year that microwaves increase reaction times in test subjects, agreed that children's exposure would be greater. "There's a lot less tissue in the way, and the skull is thinner, so children's heads are considerably closer," he says.

Stewart's report is likely to recommend that the current British safety standards on energy emissions from cell-phones should be cut to the level recommended by the International Commission on Non-Ionizing Radiation Protection, which is one-fifth of the current British limit. "The extra safety factor of five is somewhat arbitrary," says Michael Clark of the National Radiological Protection Board. "But we accept that it's difficult for the UK to have different standards from an international body."

1. Just because it has not been confirmed yet whether mobile phone emissions can harm human tissue, according to the government report, does not mean that _____.
    A. the government should prohibit children from using cell phones
    B. we should put down the phone for the sake of safety

C. the industry can have a right to promote phone use

D. children are safe using cell phones

2. Tattersall argues that it is wise to refrain mobile phone use by children in terms of _____.

A. their neural development

B. their ill-designed cell-phones

C. the frequency of their irrational use

D. their ignorance of its possible health effects

3. On the issue in question, Preece _____.

A. does not agree with Tattersall

B. tries to remove the obstacles in the way

C. asks for further investigation

D. would stand by Stewart

4. What is worrisome at present is that the UK _____.

A. is going to turn deaf ears to the voice of Stewart's plan

B. finds it difficult to cut the current safety standards on phone use

C. maintains different standards on safety limit from the international ones

D. does not even impose safety limit on the mobile phones' energy emissions

5. Which of the following can be the best candidate for the title of the passage?

A. Brain Wave.

B. For Adults Only.

C. Catch Them Young.

D. The Answer in the Air.

Passage Two

Advances in cosmetic dentistry and plastic surgery have made it possible to correct facial birth defects, repair damaged teeth and tissue, and prevent or greatly delay the onset of tooth decay and gum disease. As a result, more people smile more often and more openly today than ever in the past, and we can expect more smiles in the future.

Evidence of the smile's ascent may be seen in famous paintings in museums and galleries throughout the world. The vast majority of prosperous bigwigs（要人）, voluptuous nudes, or middle-class family members in formal portraits and domestic scenes appear to have their mouths firmly closed. Soldiers in battle, children at play, beggars, old people, and especially villains may have their mouths open; but their smiles are seldom attractive, and more often suggest strain or violence than joy.

Smiles convey a wide range of meanings in different eras and cultures, says art historian Angus Trumble, currently curator（馆长）of Yale University's Center for British Art, in his book *A Brief History of the Smile*. Compare, for instance, the varying impressions made by the shy dimples（酒窝）of Leonardo's Mona Lisa; the rosy-cheeked, mustachioed Laughing Cavalier of Frans Hals; and the "Smiley Face" logo perfected (though not invented) in 1963 by American graphic artist Harvey R. Ball.

In some non-Western cultures, Trumble notes, even a warm, open smile does not necessarily indicate pleasure or agreement. It can simply be a polite mask to cover emotions considered too rude or shocking to be openly displayed.

Subtle differences in muscle movement can convey enormous differences in emotion, from the tranquility of bronze Buddhas, to the erotic bliss of couples entwined in stone on Hindu temples, to the fierce smirk（假笑）of a guardian demon at the entrance to a Chinese tomb.

Trumble expects the impact of Western medicine and mass media to further increase the pressure on people to grin broadly and laugh openly in public. "Faint smiles are increasingly thought of in scientific and psychological circles as something that falls short of the true smile," and therefore suggest insincerity or lack of enthusiasm, he says.

With tattooing, body piercing, and permanent cosmetics already well established as fashion trends, one can imagine tomorrow's beauty shops adding plastic surgeons and dentists to their staffs. These comer-store cosmeticians would offer style makeovers to reshape our lips, teeth, and jawlines to mimic the signature smile of one's favorite celebrity.

What can you say to that except "Have a nice day"？

6. Had it not been for cosmetic advances, as inferred from the passage, _____.
    A. people would not have been as happy as they are today
    B. the rate of facial birth defect would not have declined
    C. there would not have been many more open smiles
    D. we would not have seen smiling faces in public

7. According to the passage, it seems that whether there is a smile or not in the portraits or pictures is decided by _____.
    A. one's internal sense of the external world
    B. one's identity or social position
    C. one's times of existence
    D. All of the above

8. Trumble's study on smiles shows that _____.
    A. an open smile can serve as a cover-up
    B. the famous portraits radiate varying smiles
    C. even the human muscles can arouse varying emotions
    D. smiles can represent misinterpretations of different eras and cultures

9. What Trumble expects to see is _____.
    A. the increasing tendency of broad grins and open smiles in public
    B. further impact of Western medicine upon non-Western cultures
    C. a wider range of meanings to be conveyed by smiles
    D. more of sincerity and enthusiasm in public

10. At the end of the passage, the author implicates _____.
   A. a fortune to come with cosmetic advances
   B. an identical smile for everybody
   C. future changes in lifestyle
   D. the future of smiles

Passage *Three*

Adolf Hitler survived an assassination attempt in 1944 with the lamp of penicillin made by the Allies, a microbiologist in the UK claims. If the Nazi leader had died from bacterial infection of his many wounds, the Second World War might have been over a year earlier, saving millions of lives, says Milton Wainwright of the University of Sheffield, a noted historian of microbiology.

In a paper to be published soon in *Perspectives in Biology and Medicine*, Wainwright reveals first-hand evidence that Hitler was treated with penicillin by his personal doctor, Theo Morrell, following an assassination attempt in which a bomb in a suitcase exploded next to Hitler's desk. Hitler was badly hurt, fleeing the scene with his hair and trousers on fire, a badly bleeding arm and countless wooden splinter wounds from the oak table that probably saved his life.

Wainwright found confirmation that Morrell gave Hitler antibiotics as a precaution in a recent translation of Morrell's own diary. "I happened to be reading it for interest when the word penicillin jumped out at me," he says. He then set about trying to establish where Morrell might have got the drug.

At the time, penicillin was available only to the Allies. German and Czechoslovakian teams had tried without much success to make it, Wainwright says, but the small quantities that were available were weak and impure. "It's generally accepted that it was no good," says Wainwright.

He reasons that Morrell would only have risked giving Hitler penicillin to prevent infections if he were confident that the antibiotic would cure, not kill the German premier. "My research shows that Morrell, in a very dodgy（危险的）position as Hitler's doctor, would only have used pure stuff." And the only reliable penicillin was that made by the Allies. So where did Morrell get it?

Wainwright's investigations revealed that Allied airmen carried penicillin, so the Germans may have confiscated some from prisoners of war. The other more likely source is from neutral countries such as Spain, which received penicillin from Allied countries for humanitarian purposes, perhaps for treating sick children.

"I have proof that the Allies were sending it to these countries," says Wainwright. "I'm saying this would have got through in diplomatic bags, reaching Hitler's doctor and the higher echelons（阶层）of the Nazi party. So this was almost certainly pure, Allied penicillin."

"We can never be certain it saved Hitler's life," says Wainwright. But he notes that one of Hitler's henchmen（死党）, Reinhard Heydrich, died from blood poisoning after surviving a car-bomb assassination attempt. "Hair from his seat went into his wounds and gave him septicaemia," says Wainwright. Morrell may have been anxious to ensure that Hitler avoided the same fate.

11. According to Wainwright, Adolf Hitler _____.
    A. might have used biological weapons in the war
    B. could not have committed suicide as confirmed
    C. could have died of bacterial infection
    D. might have survived a bacterial plague

12. Following his assassination in 1944, Adolf Hitler _____.
    A. began to exercise precautions against his personal attacks
    B. was anxious to have penicillin developed in his country
    C. received an injection of penicillin for blood poisoning
    D. was suspected of being likely to get infected

13. As Wainwright reasons, Hitler's personal doctor _____.
    A. cannot have dared to prescribe German-made penicillin to him
    B. need not have used pure antibiotic for his suspect infection
    C. would have had every reason to assassinate him
    D. must have tried to produce penicillin

14. Wainwright implies that the Third Reich _____.
    A. met the fate of collapse as expected
    B. butchered millions of lives on the earth
    C. was severely struck by bacterial plagues
    D. did have channels to obtain pure penicillin

15. Which of the following can be the best title for the passage?
    A. How Hitler Managed to Survive Assassination Attempts.
    B. Morrell Loyal to His German Premier.
    C. Hitler Saved by Allied Drugs.
    D. Penicillin Abused in German.

Passage Four

Get ready for a new kind of machine at your local gym: one that doesn't involve huffing and puffing as you burn off calories. Instead, all you have to do is stand still for 30 seconds while the machine measures your body fat. It could then tell you exactly where you could do with losing a few pounds and even advise you on exercises for your problem areas. If the body fat scanner turns out to be accurate enough, its makers hope it could one day help doctors spot disease.

The scanner works by simultaneously building up an accurate 3D image of the body, while measuring the body's effect on an electromagnetic field. Combining the two measurements allows the researchers to work out the distribution of fat and water within. Neither method is new on its own, says Henri Tapp, at the Institute of Food Research in Norwich in the UK. "The smart thing is that we've put them in one machine."

And it's not just for gym users. The body fat scanner could be used to study fat deposition as children develop, while patients recover from injury, or during pregnancy. And since it uses radio waves rather than X-rays, Tapp's device is safe to use repeatedly.

Body shape is known to be a risk indicator for heart disease and diabetes. So accurately quantifying fat distribution could help doctors suggest preventive measures to patients before problems arise. At the moment, doctors estimate fat content from knowing body volume and water content. To a good approximation, says Tapp, anything that isn't fat is water. The amount of water in the body is often measured by giving the subject a drink of water that contains a radioactive tracer. The level of tracer in the patient's urine after three hours reveals the total water volume.

To find out a body's volume, subjects are weighed while totally submerged in water, and this is subtracted from their normal weight to give the weight of water displaced, and hence the subject's volume. But it is scarcely practical for seriously ill people.

There are other ways to directly measure body fat, such as passing a minuscule current between the wrists and feet. The overall fat content can then be estimated from the body's resistance. But this method doesn't take body shape into account — so a subject with particularly skinny legs might register a higher fat content than the true value. That's because skinny legs — with a lower cross-sectional area — will present higher resistance to current. So the machine thinks the water content of the body is lower — rating the subject as fatter. Also, the system can only give an overall measurement of fat.

Tapp's method uses similar calculations, but is more sophisticated because it tells you where you are piling on the pounds.

16. The new machine is designed _____.
    A. to picture the body's hidden fat
    B. to identify those at risk for obesity
    C. to help clinically treat specific cases
    D. to measure accurately risky obesity-related effects

17. The beauty of the device, according to Tapp, is that _____.
    A. it performs a dual function
    B. it is of great accuracy in measurement

C. it has significant implications in clinical practice

D. it contributes to the evolution of human anatomy

18. Which of the following, according to the passage, does the machine have the potential to spare?

   A. A minuscule current.   B. A radioactive tracer.

   C. A water tank.   D. All of the above.

19. In comparison with the techniques mentioned in the passage, the body fat scanner _____.

   A. quickens the pace of the patient's rehabilitation

   B. is highly appreciated for its safety

   C. features its measuring precision

   D. is easy to operate in the clinic

20. For scanning, all the subject has to do is to _____.

   A. take up a form of workout in the gym

   B. turn round the body fat scanner

   C. lie on the electromagnetic field

   D. stand in the system

Passage *Five*

There is currently abroad a new wave of appreciation for breadth of knowledge. Curricula at universities and colleges and programs in federal agencies extol（赞扬）the virtues of a broad education. For scientists who work in specialized jobs, it is a pleasure to escape in our spare time to read broadly in fields distant from our own. Some of us have made interdisciplinary study our occupation, which is no surprise, because much of the intellectual action in our society today lies at the interfaces between traditional disciplines. Environmental science is a good example, because it frequently requires us to be conversant in several different sciences and even some unscientific fields.

Experiencing this breadth of knowledge is stimulating, but so is delving deeply into a subject. Both are wonderful experiences that are complementary practical and aesthetic（美学的）ways. They are like viewing the marvelous sculpture of knowledge in two different ways. Look at the sculpture from one perspective and you see the piece in its entirety, how its components connect to give it form, balance, and symmetry. From another viewpoint you see its detail, depth, and mass. There is no need to choose between these two perspectives in art. To do so would subtract from the totality of the figure.

So it is with science. Sometimes we gaze through a subject and are reluctant to stop for too much detail. As chemists, we are fascinated by computer sciences or molecular genetics, but not enough to become an expert. Or we may be interested in an analytical technique but not enough to stay at its cutting edge. At other times, we become immersed in the detail of a subject and see its beauty in an entirely different way than when we browse. It is as if we penetrate the surface of the sculpture and pass through the crystal structure to the molecular level where the code for the entire structure is revealed.

Unfortunately, in our zeal for breadth or depth, we often feel that it is necessary to diminish the value of the other. Specialists are sometimes ridiculed with names such as "nerd" or "technocrats", generalists are often criticized for being too "soft" or knowing too little about any one thing. Both are ludicrous（可笑的）accusations that deny a part of the reality of environmental science. Let us not be divided by our passion for depth or breadth. The beauty that awaits us on either route is too precious to stifle, too wonderful to diminish by bickering（争吵）.

21. From a broad education to interdisciplinary study, we can see _____.
    A. the integration of theory with practice
    B. the enthusiasm for breadth of knowledge
    C. the rapid division of traditional disciplines
    D. the confrontation between specialists and generalists

22. The commentator would say that the totality of the sculpture of knowledge _____.
    A. is mainly composed of two elements
    B. presents two different points of view
    C. cannot be perceived from one perspective
    D. is a whole made up of complementary elements

23. Just because we become engrossed in the detail of a subject, according to the comment, does not mean that we _____.
    A. can have an understanding of it
    B. will develop into an expert
    C. will perceive its entirety
    D. are interested in it

24. It is commentator's contention that neither specialists nor generalists _____.
    A. have zeal for the totality of the knowledge for sculpture
    B. represent the depth and breadth of knowledge
    C. are necessarily supposed to belittle the other
    D. can be qualified as environmental scientists

25. Which of the following can be the best title for the comment?
    A. Interdisciplinary Study as Our Occupation.
    B. Breadth and Depth of Knowledge.
    C. The Ways of Doing Science.
    D. The Beauty of Science.

Passage Six

That shabby unknown bundle of neglect and despair that was dropped off by the police six weeks ago — later to be identified by his mother, who turns up occasionally — is now a driving force on the infants' ward. Once he was bathed a few times and his rashes were treated, he turned out to be a 14-month-old boy named Vergil, still recovering from premature birth — birth weight, 2.5 pounds. It came obvious that he had never received any real attention, and practically no solid food, and it was never very clear who assumed responsibility for him in his family, if anyone. Miraculously he survived, with almost no outside help.

At first he just lay there, withdrawn, sucking on an empty bottle as he had been used to doing at home. After a few days it became clear that he was ravenously hungry and he downed bottle after bottle of milk. Slowly he began to respond to the ward staff around him who hung over the side of his crib, tempting him back to life.

He started by cautiously "chewing" on people, sniffing and tasting them warily like a little wild creature. Gradually he climbed to a standing position, pulling himself up on the bars of his crib. Then he began to discover noise — that came from himself. When he learned that it was acceptable, in this place, to scream when enraged, he filled his corner of the room with garbled speech-like sounds, and loud baby-bellows of demand. If nobody responded he would fix each passerby with a coy look that evolved into a seductive grin, revealing four widely space little teeth. Someone always stopped, grinning back at this adorable creature, then picking him up and cuddling him. We all the staff took personal pride and delight in his steady progress.

During the day we moved his crib from the infants' ward to the playroom where there are people coming and going. He loved it, standing and cruising in his crib, commenting happily on the scene, crowing and babbling. One afternoon, when his crib was moved adjacent to the wall, he became unusually quiet, deep in concentration. With the stealth of a cat, using his little fingers like tiny screwdrivers, he had taken apart the wall oxygen unit. Our delight in his progress turned to real respect. Perhaps we could steer him toward the right path before it was too late.

Vergil definitely had a future.

26. In the infants' ward, Vergil _____.

    A. was treated as an orphan   B. was born prematurely

    C. had himself renamed   D. drove the staff busy

27. The ward staff must have been marveled at Vergil's _____.

    A. vitality   B. shabbiness

    C. premature birth   D. physical well-being

28. How did Vergil begin to respond to people?

    A. By making loud baby-bellows of demand.

    B. By fixing each passerby with a coy look.

    C. By sniffing and tasting them.

    D. By yelling at them.

29. From the observation made by the physician in the clinic, we can say that Vergal _____.

    A. was appreciative of the ward staff

    B. was growing in a favorable environment

    C. was growing faster in mind than in body

    D. was proud of his physical and mental growth

30. Through the mention of Vergil's improper act, the writer is trying to imply _____.

    A. the existence of dangers in the infants' ward

    B. the importance of guidance on babies' growth

    C. the acceptance of inborn mischief

    D. the existence of a future for him

2010 年真题阅读理解答案与解析

Passage One

 本文话题

出于健康考虑，儿童应避免使用手机。

 难词译注

refrain [riˈfrein] v.	克制，节制
nonthermal effects [ˌnɔnˈθəːməl]	无热量效应
precautionary [priˈkɔːʃənəri] a.	预防的
mast [mɑːst] n.	天线杆

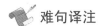 难句译注

    Stewart's report is likely to recommend that the current British safety standards on energy emissions from cell phones should be cut to the level recommended by the International Commission on Non-Ionizing Radiation Protection, which is one-fifth of the current British limit.

【分析】that the current British safety standards 是 recommend 的宾语从句，which 引

导非限制性定语从句修饰 the level recommended by ICNIRP。

【译文】 Stewart 的报告可能是在建议，目前英国有关手机能量释放的安全标准应该降低，降到国际非电离辐射保护委员会所建议的级别，这一标准是目前英国限制标准的五分之一。

答案与解析

1. 【问题】根据政府报告，虽然还不能证实手机辐射对人体细胞的伤害，但这并不意味着_____。
   - A．政府应该禁止儿童使用手机
   - B．我们应该为了安全放下手机
   - C．该产业有权利促进手机使用
   - D．儿童使用手机是安全的

   【答案】D

   【解析】此题根据题干可以定位在文章第 2 段最后一句话：因为我们不能完全理解辐射对人体细胞非热能效应，政府应该采取预防措施，尤其是和儿童相关的措施。可知这句话的含义与选项 D 吻合。

2. 【问题】Tattersall 认为限制儿童使用手机是考虑到_____。
   - A．他们神经系统的发育
   - B．他们的手机有设计缺陷
   - C．他们非理性使用的频率
   - D．他们忽视可能的健康影响

   【答案】A

   【解析】根据题干中的人名，可以定位在第 4 段第一句，Tattersall 认为限制儿童使用手机是明智之举，这句话与题干吻合。此题解题关键信息在这句话的后面，他说："如果你有一个正在发育的神经系统，那么它会更加容易受环境的侵扰。所以如果手机被证明确实是危险的，当然现在还没得到证实，那么限制儿童使用手机就是明智的。"故选项 A 正确。

3. 【问题】就讨论中的这个问题，Preece_____。
   - A．不同意 Tattersall 的观点
   - B．试图移除障碍
   - C．要求进一步的调查
   - D．会支持 Stewart

   【答案】D

   【解析】此题解题较为麻烦。首先根据题干中的人名可以定位到文章的第 6 段，寻找 Preece 对限制手机使用的观点态度，即第 6 段第 2 句话，其大概含义是：他认为孩子接触得会更多。有许多较小的组织堵在那里，并且头颅骨更小，所以儿童的头就会离手机更近。这说明 Preece 也认为应限制儿童使用手机，据此可以排除 A。选项 B 和 C 没提到，也被排除。根据第 7 段可知，Stewart 建议英国政府提高对儿童手机能量发射的限制，与国际通用一个标准，故选项 D 正确。

4. 【问题】目前令人担心的是英国_____。
   - A．会对 Stewart 计划的呼声充耳不闻
   - B．觉得降低手机使用时能量辐射的安全标准值会很难
   - C．继续保持和国际标准不同的安全限制标准
   - D．甚至不就手机能量辐射做任何限制

【答案】C

【解析】此题根据题干关键词可以定位到文章最后一段。

5. 【问题】下面哪一个是这篇文章最好的标题？

  A．脑电波。   B．仅限成年人。

  C．抓住年轻人。   D．答案仍旧悬而未决。

【答案】B

【解析】文章第1段开门见山提出文章的主题，即儿童应该避免使用手机。故选项B正确。

Passage Two

 本文话题

本文通过对不同文化以及社会地位的人的笑的研究，希望人们能多开口笑。

 难词译注

cosmetic dentistry [ˈdentistri] *n.*	牙科整形，牙科
plastic surgery [ˈsɜːdʒəri] *n.*	整形外科
ascent [əˈsent] *n.*	进步，登高，坡路
voluptuous nude	体态丰满的裸体人像
villain [ˈvilən] *n.*	恶棍
tranquility [trænˈkwiliti] *n.*	宁静
erotic bliss	性爱欢愉，鱼水之欢
entwine [inˈtwain] *v.*	编织，盘绕
demon [ˈdiːmən] *n.*	魔鬼
mimic [ˈmimik] *v.*	模仿

答案与解析

6. 【问题】按照文章所暗示的，假设没有美容方面的进步_____。

  A．人们就不会像现在这样快乐 B．出生面部缺陷率就不可能下降

  C．就不会有更多的开口笑   D．在公众场合我们就不会看见笑容

【答案】C

【解析】此题解题信息在文章第1段。这个段落开门见山点出文章的主题。因为整形牙科和整形外科使得人们比以往更能开口大笑，而且我们希望未来可以有更多的笑容。所以如果没有这些进步，人们就不可能像现在这样开口大笑，选项C为正确答案。

7. 【问题】根据文章所述，似乎人像画或照片上是否有笑容取决于_____。

  A．一个人对于外部世界的内心感受 B．一个人的身份或社会地位

  C．一个人所处的时代   D．以上都是

【答案】B

【解析】根据题干中的 portraits 可以定位到文章第 2 段。这一段作者给出很多实例，大多数人像或照片上富有的要人，体态丰满的裸体人像，或是中产阶级家庭成员看上去都是紧闭着嘴。而战争中的士兵、玩耍的孩子、乞丐、老人，尤其是坏蛋可能都张着嘴，但他们的笑却鲜有魅力，更多情况下让人感觉僵硬或者暴力多于快乐。根据这些具体信息可以得知，一个人的身份地位决定了画像上是否有笑容，故选项 B 正确。

8. 【问题】Trumble 有关笑容的研究表明_____。

    A．开口笑是一种掩饰　　　　　　B．名人画像呈现不同的笑

    C．甚至人类肌肉也可以产生不同的笑　D．笑可以体现不同时代和文化的误解

【答案】A

【解析】细节题。本题题意是：Trumble 有关微笑的研究表明开朗的笑容可以作为一种掩饰。根据第 4 段 "Trumble 指出，在一些非西方文化中，即使是温和、开朗的笑容也并不一定代表愉快或者同意。它可能仅仅是礼貌的面具来遮盖那些被认为是太粗鲁或太吃惊也不应明显表示出来的情绪。" 故选 A。

9. 【问题】Trumble 希望看到的是_____。

    A．公开场合开怀大笑的增长趋势　　B．西药对非西方文化的进一步影响

    C．笑传递更加广泛的含义　　　　　D．公开场合多一些真诚和热情

【答案】D

【解析】细节题。A 项内容是实现期望的方式，D 项内容是最终的期望。所以选 D。

10. 【问题】文章最后，作者暗指_____。

    A．美容进步所带来的财富　　　　　B．每个人的笑都一样

    C．未来生活方式的变化　　　　　　D．笑的未来

【答案】D

【解析】根据文章最后一段可以推断出，由于整形技术和专业人士进入美容院，他们能有助于人们重塑完美的面容。

Passage Three

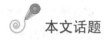

本文话题

有科学家发现，二战期间，希特勒在被暗杀后活了下来是因为他的私人医生给他用了青霉素，本文就此展开讨论。

难词译注

splinter ['splintə] *n.*	碎片
confiscate ['kɔnfiskeit] *v.*	查抄，没收，扣押
humanitarian [hju(:),mæni'teəriən] *a.*	人道主义的
septicaemia [,septi'si:miə] *n.*	败血症

答案与解析

11. 【问题】根据 Wainwright 的观点，阿道夫·希特勒_____。

    A．在战争中可能使用了生化武器   B．不可能像人们证实的那样自杀

    C．可能死于细菌感染   D．可能在细菌感染中活了下来

    【答案】D

    【解析】此题定位在第 1 段：由于盟军生产的青霉素，希特勒在 1944 年的暗杀中活了下来。如果这个纳粹头子死于多处伤口的细菌感染，那么第二次世界大战就可能提早一年结束，可能拯救了百万人的生命。故选项 D 正确。

12. 【问题】1944 年遭到一次暗杀后，阿道夫·希特勒_____。

    A．开始采取针对他个人遇袭的预防措施

    B．急切希望在他的国家研制青霉素

    C．因为败血症接受青霉素注射

    D．被怀疑可能感染了

    【答案】C

    【解析】细节题。利用题干关键词 following an assassination in 1944 可以定位到文章的第二段：在一期名为《生物学和医学展望》的杂志上，温莱特披露了一手资料，证明在经历过一次暗杀后，希特勒的私人医生 Theo Morrel 用青霉素对其进行了治疗。由此可知答案为 C "接受青霉素的注射来防止血液中毒"。而下一段说道 "Wainwright 在研究中发现 Morrell 在他的日记中写道，他给希特勒用了抗生素作为预防"，可知这只是一种预防措施，并不确定一定会感染，所以 D 项与原文表述不一致。

13. 【问题】正如 Wainwright 所推论的，希特勒的私人医生_____。

    A．不可能敢给希特勒开德国产的青霉素

    B．不需要使用纯的抗生素来预防可能的感染

    C．有充分理由要暗杀希特勒

    D．一定在试图制造青霉素

    【答案】A

    【解析】此题定位在文章第 4 和第 5 段。第 4 段提到当时只有盟军有青霉素，德国试图生产但没成功，他们只有少量青霉素，但不够纯，一般认为这不会有效。第 5 段提到：作为希特勒的私人医生他处于很危险的境地，因而他只可能使用纯的青霉素。这说明为了自己的性命，他的私人医生不会给希特勒使用不纯的青霉素，故选项 A 正确。

14. 【问题】Wainwright 暗指第三帝国_____。

    A．正如预料的那样，免不了崩溃的命运

    B．屠杀了地球上数以百万计的生命

    C．遭受细菌灾害的重创

    D．确实有渠道可以获得纯青霉素

    【答案】D

【解析】第 5 段最后一句话是这道题关键的定位，意味着后面段落将谈论 Morrell 如何获得纯的青霉素。第 6 段和第 7 段提到了可能获得青霉素的途径，故选项 D 正确。

15. 【问题】下面哪一个是这篇文章最合适的标题？

    A. 希特勒如何从暗杀中活下来。

    B. Morrel 对他的德国总理忠诚吗？

    C. 希特勒是盟军的药救活的吗？

    D. 青霉素在德国被滥用了吗？

【答案】C

【解析】如文中所述，Wainwright 揭示希特勒可能因为有盟军的青霉素而在一次暗杀后活了下来，这就是文章的主题，故选项 C 正确。

Passage Four

 本文话题

介绍一款新型的测量体内脂肪的仪器。

 难词译注

huff and puff	沉重的呼吸
fat deposition	脂肪堆积
radioactive tracer	放射性指示剂
minuscule current	微电流

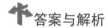 答案与解析

16. 【问题】设计这个新机器是为了_____。

    A. 显示人体隐藏的脂肪

    B. 识别那些存在肥胖隐患的人

    C. 有助于在临床上治疗特定病例

    D. 精准测量和肥胖有关的危险影响

【答案】A

【解析】参见第一段第二句，你只需要在机器上站 30 秒，它就会测出你身体中的脂肪。故选 A。

17. 【问题】根据 Tapp 的观点，这个装置的魅力在于_____。

    A. 它运行双重功能

    B. 在测量方面有极高的准确性

    C. 对临床工作有着重要意义

    D. 对人类解剖学的发展做出贡献

【答案】A

【解析】根据题干中的人名和问题可以定位到文章第 2 段的最后一句话：这款机器最聪

明的设计在于我们把两个测量方式放在一台机器上，故选项 A 正确。

18. 【问题】根据文章所述，下面哪一个不是这台机器所具有的潜质？

    A. 微电流。   B. 放射性指示剂。   C. 一个水箱。D. 以上都不是。

【答案】D

【解析】根据第 1 段可知这台仪器只需让受试者站在上面保持不动 30 秒，即可知道受试者体内的脂肪含量。故这三个东西都是这台仪器不需要的。

19. 【问题】和文章中提到的技术相比，身体脂肪扫描仪＿＿＿＿＿＿。

    A. 加速病人康复的进程   B. 因为它的安全性而备受赞扬

    C. 以测量的精准性为特征   D. 在诊所易于操作

【答案】C

【解析】参见最后一段，Tapp 的方法也使用了相似的计算方法，但是却更准确（sophisti-cated），因为它会告诉你哪里超重了。故选 C。

20. 【问题】为了扫描，所有受试者都必须＿＿＿＿＿＿。

    A. 在健身房参加一种锻炼   B. 转动身体脂肪扫描仪

    C. 躺在电子磁场中   D. 站在系统上

【答案】D

【解析】此题参见文章第 1 段第 2 句话：所有你必须做的就是站在上面保持 30 秒不动，这台机器就可以测量出你的体内脂肪，故选项 D 正确。

Passage Five

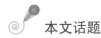 本文话题

现在有一个新的潮流：崇尚知识的广度。作者就知识的广度和深度谈了自己的看法。

难词译注

interface ['intə(:),feis] *n.*	界面，分界处
conversant [kən'və:sənt] *a.*	熟悉的，熟知的
delve [delv] *v.*	探究，探索
complementary [kɔmplə'mentəri] *a.*	互补的
analytical [ˌænə'litikəl] *a.*	分析的
at the cutting edge	前沿
diminish [di'miniʃ] *v.*	轻视，贬低
accusation [ækju(:)'zeiʃən] *n.*	谴责，控告

答案与解析

21. 【问题】从广义教育到跨学科研究，我们可以看到＿＿＿＿＿＿。

    A. 理论与实际的融合   B. 追求知识广度的热情

C．传统学科的迅速解体　　　　　D．专家和全才的对抗

【答案】B

【解析】根据题干可以定位到文章的第 1 段。题干提到的广义教育和跨学科研究均作为实例出现在第 1 段。因此解答本题的关键在于理解本段的主要论点，也即本段的第一句话，其大概含义是：目前在国外有一个新的潮流，崇尚知识的广度。全段的实例都在说明各个领域注重知识的广度，故选项 B 符合题意。

22．【问题】评论家会说雕塑知识的全部_____。

A．主要由两个元素组成　　　　　B．呈现两种不同的观点

C．不能从一个视角去理解　　　　D．是由互补元素构成的一个整体

【答案】D

【解析】根据题干的关键词 "the totality of the sculpture of knowledge" 可以定位在文章第 2 段。本段第 3 句话提到：这就如同用两种不同的方法观察伟大的雕塑。这说明例证关系的"证"应该在前面，即本段的前两句话，其大意是：体验知识的广度很刺激，但是深度探索一个物体同样刺激。这两种美妙的体验是实际和美学两种方式的互补。故选项 D 正确。

23．【问题】根据评论，虽然我们专心于一个物体的细节，但不意味着我们_____。

A．对它有了解　　　　　　　　　B．将成为专家

C．将理解全部　　　　　　　　　D．对此感兴趣

【答案】C

【解析】此题根据题干，可以定位到文章第 3 段。由第 3 段第 1 句话可知，本段主要围绕专注细节进行论述。本段提到专注细节，例如作为化学家，痴迷于计算机科学或者分子遗传学，不意味着会成为这方面的专家。这些论述揭示，仅仅深究一个细节不意味着能够理解全部。故选项 C 正确。选项 B 和 D 均在例子中，是错误答案。

24．【问题】评论家的论点是专家和全才_____。

A．都没有对雕塑知识的整体充满热情

B．都不代表知识的深度和广度

C．都没必要轻视彼此

D．都没有资格成为环境科学家

【答案】C

【解析】根据题干中的关键词 "specialist" 和 "generalist" 可以定位在文章的最后一段。这段的主题句就是第 1 句话，其大意是：不幸的是，在我们很热情地追求知识的广度或深度时，总是贬低另一方的价值，故选项 C 正确。

25．【问题】下面哪一个是文章最好的标题？

A．跨学科研究，我们的职业。　　B．知识的广度和深度。

C．做科学研究的方式。　　　　　D．科学的魅力。

【答案】B

【解析】全文都是在就知识的广度和深度进行探讨，故选项 B 正确。

Passage Six

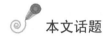 本文话题

本文作者介绍病房里的一个早产儿，作者观察他的一举一动，以及作者个人的感受。

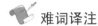 难词译注

miraculously [miˈrækjuləsli] *ad.*	奇迹般地，不可思议地
withdrawn [wiðˈdrɔːn] *a.*	内向的，沉默寡言的
ravenously [ˈrævinəsli] *ad.*	饿极地，渴望地
warily [ˈweərili] *ad.*	谨慎地
enrage [inˈreidʒ] *v.*	激怒
garbled [ˈɡɑːbld] *a.*	含糊不清的
baby-bellow	婴儿的大叫
seductive [siˈdʌktiv] *a.*	有魅力的
cuddle [ˈkʌdl] *v.*	搂抱
crib [krib] *n.*	有围栏的童床
babble [ˈbæbl] *v.*	含糊不清的喃语，儿语
adjacent [əˈdʒeisənt] *a.*	临近的
stealth [stelθ] *n.*	秘密行动
screwdriver [ˈskruːdraivə] *n.*	螺丝刀，改锥
steer [stiə] *v.*	引导，指导

答案与解析

26. 【问题】在婴儿病房，Vergil_____。

　　　　A. 被当作孤儿对待　　　　　　　　　B. 早产

　　　　C. 改了名字　　　　　　　　　　　　D. 让医护人员很忙碌

【答案】D

【解析】细节题。这里的关键信息是 "In the infants' ward"（在婴儿房里），找到了母亲所以不是（孤儿）A，B（早产）不是发生在婴儿房里的事，C（更名）在文章中未提及，所以答案为D，也就是孩子在婴儿房里得到了很好的照顾和治疗。

27. 【问题】病房的医护人员一定对 Vergil 的_____感到惊讶。

　　　　A. 生命力　　　　B. 衣衫褴褛　　　　C. 早产　　　　D. 身体健康

【答案】A

【解析】此题定位在第 1 段最后一句话，大意是：几乎没有外界的帮助，他奇迹般地活了下来。故选项 A 正确。

28. 【问题】Vergil 开始怎样回应人们？

　　　　A. 通过有需求时的大声哭闹。

B. 用羞答答的表情看着每一个经过的人。

C. 闻和尝。

D. 朝他们大叫。

【答案】C

【解析】第2段最后一句话说："渐渐地，他开始对站在他婴儿床边逗他的医护人员做出了反应。"而第三段第一句话告诉我们："他首先谨慎地研究人们，像个小野兽一样小心地用鼻子闻闻、用小嘴尝尝。"

29. 【问题】从医院里医生的观察，我们可以说 Vergil _____ 。

A. 很感谢病房医护人员　　　　　B. 在一个很有利的环境下成长

C. 心理要比身体成长得快　　　　D. 很自豪他的身心健康

【答案】C

【解析】此题需要概括文章大意。本文描述了他所观察的这个早产儿在医院里的一举一动，可以看出虽然他是早产儿，但其生命力极其顽强，而且通过描述他在医院里与人交流的一举一动以及他在活动室里的表情、神态，可以说都是在对小孩的心智方面进行描述，而对于小孩身体方面的进展着墨偏少。所以我们可知这个孩子在心智方面确实恢复或者说发展更快一些。另外题目是问通过医护人员的观察说明这个孩子如何，所以选项 B 不符合逻辑结构。

30. 【问题】通过提及 Vergil 不恰当的举动，作者试图暗示：_____ 。

A. 在婴儿病房存在危险　　　　　B. 婴儿成长过程中指导的重要性

C. 接受孩子先天的淘气　　　　　D. 对他而言的未来

【答案】B

【解析】此题可以先排除选项 A 和 C。对于选项 D，能够对应的原文信息是文章最后一句话，选项 D 是最后一句话的近义改写，故不是答案。选项 B 的解题信息是文章第 4 段的最后一句话，大意是：也许我们可以趁现在还不晚将他带到正确的道路上来。故选项 B 正确。此题注意：推断题的解不是原文信息的近义改写。

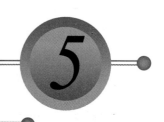

第五章 CHAPTER 5 写 作

一、考试大纲的要求

考试大纲要求书面表达测试考生使用英语书面表达自己思想的能力。此部分共计 20 分，考试时间约为 50 分钟。测试题型共有以下两种：

1. **文章摘要。**要求考生阅读一篇 800 ~ 1000 字中文文章，然后用英文写出一篇约 200 词的文章摘要。所概括的内容应简洁、全面、准确。在行文上，要求文字通顺，基本符合英语表达习惯，无重大语法错误。近几年文章摘要为主要测试题型，而且中文文章的篇幅也在逐年递增，平均字数约为 1200 字左右。

2. **翻译与写作。**这种测试题型包括两个部分，即段落翻译和段落写作。翻译要求忠实原文；段落写作要求切题且意思连贯。在行文上，要求与摘要写作相同。

从近几年的真题来看，一直使用的测试题型就是摘要写作，因而考生应该在此测试题型上多加练习，掌握摘要写作的要领。对于段落翻译和段落写作在平时备考其他测试题型时可以作为基本功，加以训练。

二、摘要写作基本流程

在备考阶段，考生一定要注意：摘要写作绝对不是将千字中文文章翻译成英文文章。摘要写作依然是写作，因而摘要写作要注意以下基本写作流程：

第一步：浏览中文篇章。

第二步：在中文篇章中画出各段主题句及关键的细节内容。

第三步：根据各段主题句及关键内容组织英文摘要的各主要部分及内容。

第四步：根据中文摘要的内容写相应的英文摘要。

第五步：检查有无拼写、语法、用词等错误，查看有无逻辑关系不明确、语句不通顺等。

↗ 例题解析（2017 年真题解析）

环境污染与肺癌

近几十年来，许多国家的流行病学调查资料都表明，不少传染病的发病率和死亡率在不断下降，而癌症的发病率和死亡率却在不断上升。大量的调查研究表明，癌症等疾病的发病率的上升与环境污染有关。由于环境污染对人体的作用一般具有剂量小、作用时间长等特点，所以容易被人们所忽视。往往病发之日，尚不知谁是元凶。

环境污染就像邪恶的阴影，悄悄吞噬着人体的健康。肺及呼吸道是一个开放器官，与外界直接接触，外界很多致癌因素都可以导致肺癌。环境污染就是导致肺癌的一个重要原因。环境污染中最为重要的就是大气污染。大气污染的许多学者惊奇地发现，近50年来，随着工业和经济的发展，人们生活水平的提高，肺癌的发病率也显著提高，特别是世界经济发达地区的患者成倍地增加。例如，美国的病人在50年中，男性增加了18倍，女性增加了6倍。每4名癌症死亡病例中，就有1名是肺癌患者；每100名死亡病人中，有5名死于肺癌。就我国情况看，也有明显增加的趋势。从全国恶性肿瘤排列顺序来看，肺癌占第5位；每100名癌症病人中，大约有8名是患的肺癌。

肺癌是最常见的恶性肿瘤之一，据WHO统计，每年全球估计有120万以上新发肺癌病例，死亡约110万人，平均每隔30秒就有人死于肺癌。近年来，我国肺癌发病率及死亡率亦不断上升。国内外流行病学研究报告指出，大气污染易诱发肺癌而使死亡率增高。

在公认的大气污染物中，颗粒物对健康的危害最大，可增加患肺癌的危险。随着交通的发展、机动车辆的增加、环境的日益破坏，PM2.5污染越来越严重。研究发现，大气中PM2.5在总悬浮颗粒物中的比率逐年增加，沉积在下呼吸道的96%的颗粒物是PM2.5。对肺癌死亡率进行分析表明市区大气总悬浮颗粒物与肺癌死亡率增高有一定的相关性。这在世界上许多国家都被证实。美国癌症协会收集的16年资料，涉及50万名美国人的死亡原因数据，发现空气中的PM2.5与总死亡率和肺癌死亡相关。在日本进行的PM2.5与疾病关系研究也发现，PM2.5水平与女性肺癌呈正相关。

↗ 写作解析

1. 分析中文原文

本文共有四段。第一段开门见山点明文章主旨：癌症等疾病的发病率的上升与环境污染有关。第二段主要讲环境污染与肺癌的直接关系。第三段讲肺癌在全球范围内的严重情况。第四段着重讲大气中颗粒物对健康的影响。

2. 摘要的中文大纲

写作的中文提纲大致如下：

第一段：大量的调查研究表明，癌症等疾病的发病率的上升与环境污染有关。

第二段：环境污染是导致肺癌的一个重要原因。环境污染中最为重要的就是大气污染。近50年来，随着工业和经济的发展，人们生活水平的提高，肺癌的发病率也显著提高，特别是世界经济发达地区的患者成倍地增加。大气污染易诱发肺癌而使死亡率增高。

第三段：大气污染物中的颗粒物对健康的危害最大，可增加患肺癌的危险。对肺癌死亡率进行分析表明市区大气总悬浮颗粒物与肺癌死亡率增高有一定的相关性。

3. 参考的表达

流行病学	epidemiology
传染病	infectious disease

发病率	incidence rate
死亡率	mortality rate
环境污染	environmental pollution
大气污染	air pollution
肺癌	lung cancer
恶性肿瘤	malignant tumor
公认的	widely accepted
悬浮	suspension，suspend
颗粒物	particulate
相关性	relevance
正相关	positive relevance

4. 参考范文

Environmental Pollution and Lung Cancer

According to some epidemiological data, a number of malignant tumors have been caused by the deteriorated environmental conditions, and their incidence rate and mortality rate are increasing.

Environmental pollution is one of the essential factors leading to lung cancer. From some statistics, in recently 50 years, with the industrial and economic development as well as the improvement of people's living standard, the incidence of lung cancer is increasing significantly, especially in the advanced areas where lung cancer patients are doubled. Air pollution leads to higher mortality of lung cancer.

PM2.5 may be the crucial factor in air pollution. According to a new research from the USA, the pm2.5 are abundant in the fog and haze because of overusing cars and destroy of air condition could increase the morbidity of lung cancer. Another research says that the total particle suspending has been found in respiratory system, and there is a positive relevance between the pm2.5 and lung cancer. The above analysis has been approved by scientists in Japan. We have to make efforts to improve the air condition. Not only will it reduce the risk to the lethal disease, but it also can give us a better environment and living quality. The way to the destination, however, is not easy and smooth.

↗ 例题解析（2016 年真题解析）

全科医生培养及发展思路

随着医疗卫生事业的不断发展，人们对社区卫生服务的要求也越来越高。目前我国社区卫生服务发展还不平衡。高素质的全科医生（general practitioner）缺乏成为滞后社区卫生发展的主要原因。规范全科医生培养，大力发展全科医生培训工作势在必行。全科医生在社区卫生服务中的功能包括治疗、保健、预防、护理、健康调查、咨询及健康教育等。虽然我国全科医学（general family medicine）已经得到了普及和发展，但其教育与培训还存在一些问题。本文就全科医生的培养和今后的发展做一浅析。

全科医生需具备的基本素质

全科医生需要较全面的知识。某些严重疾病的早期症状可能比较轻微，与一些常见病、多发病表现并无太大区别。这就要求全科医生从众多的疾病中筛选可能的情况，因此要求全科医生临床学科知识面要广。社区卫生工作中，一名合格的全科医生，也应是一名出色的社会工作者。全科医生服务的对象是社区内的居民，而且有可能需要长期面对，因此要求全科医生要有良好的人际关系、协调能力和高度的工作热情，并与患者建立一种亲密而长期的友情，成为病人家庭的良师益友，要具有良好的职业道德。

目前全科医生存在的问题

全科医生工作热情不高。一方面与专业医生相比，收入与社会地位存在差距；另一方面工作环境较艰苦，医疗设备落后，导致全科医生的工作热情和人员稳定性不高。合格的全科医生人员不多。由于全科医学专业在我国发展历史较短，很多医学院校近年刚开设全科医学的专业。全科医生实际工作能力与居民的要求还有距离，同时社区工作也是在逐渐摸索、完善过程中，因此社区卫生服务的工作开展仍不太理想。

解决的方法与思考

制定全科医学相关领域的政策和规划、社区卫生服务发展策略和相关人力资源政策，特别是推动全科医学毕业生致力于社区群众服务的激励机制等，促使全科医疗得到健康持续的发展。以全科医生岗位培训为重点，低年资的全科医生要进行专科轮转，至少3年，掌握专科学校的基本理论和基本技能；高年资的全科医生可通过远程教育，参加各省、市中心培训机构组织的临床技能培训，逐步提高技术水平。各省、市可以根据实际需要，增加一些社区工作急需的培训内容。对部分基础较好的医生进行重点培养，然后由这些合格的全科医生再去培养更多的全科医生，促进全科医生的全面提高，进而提高防治社区常见疾病解决社区健康问题的能力，达到全科医生的岗位要求。

↗ 写作解析

1. 分析中文原文

本文共有4段，话题突出，并有小标题，这对于考生梳理中文内容、提炼文章结构大有益处。本文话题围绕社区卫生服务中全科医生的培养以及发展思路展开，第一段为背景介绍，谈到社区卫生服务的主要功能、重要性以及全科医学、全科医生教育培养存在不足。第二段主要介绍全科医生的基本素质：知识全面、高度的工作热情以及良好的协调沟通能力。第三段阐述目前全科医生存在的问题及原因。第四段阐述解决方法与思考，既有政策调整又有岗位培训重点及方法。

2. 摘要的中文大纲

通过提炼、总结画线部分的内容，写作的中文提纲大致如下：

第一段：随着医疗卫生事业的不断发展，社区卫生服务日益重要，其主要功能包括医疗、保健、预防、护理、健康调查、咨询及健康教育等。然而我国全科医学教育培训还存在一些问题，缺乏高素质的全科医生，这些都制约着社区卫生服务的发展。因而规范全科医生培养、大力发展全科医生培训的工作势在必行。

第二段：谈到基本素质，全科医生首先需要知识全面。一些严重疾病的早期症状可能较为轻微，与一些常见多发疾病并无太大区别，这就要求全科医生能筛选出可能的情况。其次，作为社会工作者，全科医生需要与社区内居民长期接触，因而饱满的工作热情以及良好的协调沟通能力很必要。

第三段：然而，目前全科医生还存在诸多问题。收入与社会地位相对较低，工作环境艰苦，医疗设备较为落后，这导致全科医生工作热情不高。全科医学专业开展时间不长，全科医生实际能力还很欠缺。

第四段：为了使全科医疗健康持续发展，首先相关政策、规划的制定以及激励机制很必要。其次全科医学教育应以岗位培训为重点，低年资全科医生要进行至少 3 年的专科轮转，以掌握基本理论及技能；高年资全科医生可通过多种渠道（例如远程教育或培训班）进一步提高技术水平。对于部分基础较好的医生进行重点培养，再由他们培养更多的全科医生。

3. 供参考的表达

全科医生	general practitioner
全科医学	general family medicine
社区卫生服务	community health service
保健	healthcare
护理	nursing
健康调查	health survey
咨询	consultation
规范（培养）	standardized training
势在必行	imperative
知识全面	well-rounded
（工作）热情	enthusiasm
协调沟通能力	communication and coordination skills
激励机制	incentive mechanism
岗位培训	on-the-job training
低年资的	junior
高年资的	senior
专科轮转	rotation and training
远程教育	distance education

4. 参考范文

With the continuous development of health care, community health services are increasingly significant, which mainly include health care, prevention, health survey, consultation and health education and so on. However, imperfect general practice education and lack of high-qualified general practitioners inevitably restrict the development of community health services. Thus, standardized training and vigorous devotion to general practice education are very imperative.

When it comes to basic qualities of general practitioners, well-rounded knowledge comes first. Some severe diseases tend to be characterized with mild symptoms, which are similar with some common disorders. Therefore, general practitioners are required to identify possible cases. Moreover, as social workers, general practitioners are bound to constantly contact people in the community, and hence, enthusiasm in work as well as good communication and cooperation skills is crucial.

Unfortunately many problems arise currently. Unsatisfactory income, lower social status and tough working conditions lead to less devotion to the work. Besides, it has not been long since the major of general family medicine was established. General practitioners have not been equipped with adequate practical skills.

In order to enhance the sustainable development of community health care, firstly, related policies, projects and incentive mechanism are indispensable. Secondly, general practice education should put emphasis on on-the-job training. On the one hand, junior general practitioners are required to take rotation and training for three years at least, so as to master basic theories and skills. On the other hand, senior general practitioners improve their skills through distance education or training programs. Some potential talents may be chosen as the very group to be trained, in the hope that they can further cultivate more qualified general practitioners.

↗ 例题解析（2015 年真题解析）

什么是健康

人的健康包括身体健康和心理健康两个方面。一个人的身体和心理都健康才称得上真正的健康。联合国世界卫生组织对健康下的定义是：健康的人不但没有身体疾患，而且有完整的生理、心理状态和社会适应能力。

目前在我们国家，无论在健康人与病人中或者在医务人员中，大都在不同程度上忽略了心理健康。这对提高人的健康水平与提高医疗效果都产生消极的影响。例如在现实生活中，人们往往重视营养，而忽视饮食时的心理因素作用。人们注意身体的锻炼，而不重视心理的锻炼。甚至不知道什么是心理健康以及如何锻炼。在临床实践中，有些医务人员在病因上，重视病毒、感染等因素，忽视疾病的心理因素的作用；在诊断上重视物理诊断等，忽视心理诊断；在治疗上重视药物治疗，忽视心理治疗。其实，身体健康与心理健康是同等重要的。二者是相互联系、相互制约的。身心两方面健康是相辅相成的。

随着 21 世纪的到来，人们更加专注自身的健康。追求长寿、健康生活已成为一种时尚。但是，如何才能健康，怎样才能长寿？健康与长寿的大敌又是什么呢？众多医学保健专家指出，介于疾病与健康之间的"第三状态"是人类健康与长寿的大敌。所谓第三状态，指人们经常感到自己身体难受不适的状态。主要表现为时常感觉身体很累，很疲倦，很想好好睡上一觉。此外，经常出现懒言、少气、食欲欠佳、对什么都不感兴趣，无精打采等症状，也就是人们常说的亚健康状态（sub-health condition）。如果说健康是人的第一状态，疾病是人的第二状态，那么亚健康则为人的第三状态。

有关调查表明，随着经济的高速发展，竞争日趋激烈，生活节奏逐渐加快，亚健康人群的增多已成为一种不可回避的现实。该人群以中年人居多，职业涉及很广。一般来讲，越是有成就，收入越高，亚健康状态的出现频率越高，如经理、秘书、管理人员等都是亚健康状态的高发职业。此外，记者、律师、医生、自由职业者出现亚健康状态的比例也比较高。

目前很"时髦"的"疲劳综合征"（exhaustion syndrome）就是亚健康状态的典型代表。疲劳综合不仅在发达国家有相当高的发病率，在发展中国家也不少见。这类疾病表面看来对人体并无多大妨碍，仅仅表现为生理功能低下，但其潜伏的危险性却不容忽视，因为疲劳综合征往往就是某些慢性病的先兆。比如大家所熟悉的高血压、心脑血管疾病、肿瘤等，很多都继发于疲劳综合征。

对于亚健康状态，目前国内、国外尚无特效治疗方法，而学会自我调节，对于缓解、纠正人体的亚健康状态非常重要。这里提醒您注意以下几点：一是学会以轻松的心态对待学习、工作和生活，尽量不要故意给自己加压；二是要吃好。所谓吃好，不是指大吃大喝、大鱼大肉，而是指根据自己的实际情况选择饮食；三是一定要睡好，早睡早起。睡上一个好觉，精力、体力就容易恢复。

（1098 个字）

↗ 写作解析

1. 分析中文原文

本文主题为亚健康，文章共分 6 段，各段的信息有重合，因而需要考生根据文章的主线重新整理细节信息，使得摘要的内容和结构清晰明了。本文的主线为：健康包括身体健康和心理健康，二者相辅相成，但在我国人们往往忽略心理健康。健康有三种状态，其中第三种状态亚健康是人们健康和长寿的大敌。亚健康的典型代表就是疲劳综合征，然后叙述其表现及危害，最后针对亚健康状态提出建议。

2. 摘要的中文大纲

通过提炼、总结画线部分的内容，写作的中文提纲大致如下：

第一段：人的健康包括身体健康和心理健康两个方面。按照世卫组织的定义，健康的人不但没有身体疾患，而且有完整的生理、心理状态和社会适应能力。然而在我国，无论在健康人与病人中或者在医务人员中，大都在不同程度上忽略心理健康。人们注意锻炼身体，而不重视心理锻炼。在临床实践中，有些医务工作者也忽略了致病的心理因素以及心理治疗。其实，身体健康与心理健康是同等重要的。二者是相互联系、相互制约的。

第二段：人们专注自身的健康，追求长寿，而正如众多医学保健专家指出的，介于疾病与健康之间的"第三状态"是人类健康与长寿的大敌。所谓第三状态也就是人们常说的亚健康状态，目前很"时髦"的"疲劳综合征"（exhaustion syndrome）就是亚健康状态的典型代表，其主要表现为时常感觉身体很疲倦。此外，经常出现懒言、少气、食欲欠佳、对什么都不感兴趣、无精打采等症状。有调查表明，亚健康人群以中年人居多，职业涉及很广，从管理人员、记者到医生。疲劳综合征潜伏的危险性不容忽视，因为疲劳综合征往往就是某些慢性病的先兆，比如高血压、心脑血管疾病、肿瘤等。

第三段：对于亚健康状态，虽然尚无特效治疗方法，但自我调节很重要。一是学会以轻松的心态对待学习、工作和生活，尽量不要故意给自己加压，二是要根据自己的实际情况选择饮食。三是一定要睡好，早睡早起。

3. 供参考的表达式

社会适应能力	social adaptability
心理锻炼	mental exercise
相互联系、制约	interrelated and mutually restricted
介于疾病和健康之间 / 亚健康	subhealth
疲劳综合征	exhaustion syndrome
食欲不佳	poor appetite
无精打采	listlessness
潜伏的危险性	potential risks
慢性病	chronic diseases
高血压	hypertension
心脑血管疾病	cardiovascular and cerebrovascular diseases
肿瘤	tumor
调节情绪	regulate mood
放松心态	relax

4. 参考范文

Health includes people's physical and mental health. WHO defines it as a state of complete physical, mental, and social well-being and not merely the absence of disease or infirmity. People, healthy or not, along with medical staff ignore the mental health to some extent. People tend to attach importance to physical exercise regardless of mental exercise. In clinical practice, some medical staff pay less attention to mental factors and psychological treatments. In fact, physical and mental health are equally significant, which are interrelated and mutually restricted.

People care about their own health and pursue the longevity, however the "third state", being subhealthy, serves as the barrier to people's health. Exhaustion syndrome is the typical representative of such a state, which is characterized by fatigue, listlessness and poor appetite. It is reported that subhealthy people are mainly the middle-aged in a variety of professions ranging from administrators to doctors. Potential risks of exhaustion syndrome should not be ignored, which tend to trigger some chronic diseases, such as hypertension, cardiovascular and cerebrovascular diseases and even cancers.

Although there has not been effective treatments towards subhealth, self-regulation would work. First we should be positive towards our study, work and life and try not to impose much pressure on ourselves. Additionally, we'd better choose proper diet and have a sound sleep. Keeping early hours is recommended.

(222 words)

↗ 例题解析（2012 年真题解析）

电脑、网络与健康

电脑已经成为人们生活和工作不可缺少的工具，它在给人们带来诸多方便的同时，也带来了一些烦恼和忧虑，因为人们长期从事电脑工作对健康的影响是比较直接的。

电脑和网络使用不当危害健康

一是对身体健康的直接影响。电脑显示器是利用电子枪发射电子束来产生图像，并伴有辐射与电磁波，长期使用会伤害人们的眼睛，诱发一些眼病，如青光眼等；键盘上键位密集，键面有一定的弹力和阻力，长期击键会对手指和上肢不利；操作电脑时，体形和全身难得有变化，操作向着高速、单一、重复的特点发展，强迫体位比重越来越大，容易导致肌肉骨骼系统的疾患，其中，计算机操作时所累及的主要部位有腰、颈、肩、肘、腕部等。操作电脑过程中注意力高度集中，眼、手指快速频繁运动，使生理、心理过度重负，从而产生失眠多梦、神经衰弱、头部酸胀、机体免疫力下降，甚至会诱发一些精神方面的疾病。这时人易丧失自信，内心时常紧张、烦躁、焦虑不安，最终导致身心疲惫。

二是导致网络综合征。长时间无节制地花费大量时间和精力在互联网上持续聊天、浏览，会导致各种行为异常、心理障碍、人格障碍、交感神经功能部分失调，严重者发展成为网络综合征，该病症的典型表现为：情绪低落、兴趣丧失、睡眠障碍、生物钟紊乱、食欲下降和体重减轻、精力不足、精神运动性迟缓和激动、自我评价降低、思维迟缓、不愿意参加社会活动、很少关心他人、饮酒和滥用药物等。

三是电脑散发的气体危害呼吸系统。英国过敏症基金会的研究人员最近发表的一份研究报告指出，办公设备会释放有害人体健康的臭氧气体，而主要元凶是电脑、激光打印机等。这些臭氧气体不仅有毒，而且可能造成某些人呼吸困难，对于那些哮喘病和过敏症患者来说，情况就更为严重了。另外，较长时间待在臭氧气体浓度较高的地方，还会导致肺部发生病变。

怎样减少电脑网络的危害

客观地说，电脑对人体生理和心理方面的负面影响已日益受到人们的重视。在电脑普及程度比较高的国家里，"电脑综合征"已成为很普遍的现代病。为此科学使用电脑，减少电脑和网络的危害是十分必要的。

一是要增强自我保健意识。如工作间隙注意适当休息，一般来说，电脑操作人员在连续工作 1 小时后应该休息 10 分钟左右。并且最好到操作室之外活动活动身体。平时要加强体育锻炼，增强体能，要定期进行身体检查和自我心理测定，一旦发现生理、心理上的有关症状，可在一段时间内适当调整上机时间，缓解症状。

二是注意工作环境。电脑室内光线要适宜，不可过亮或过暗，避免光线直接照射在荧光屏上而产生干扰光线，工作室要保持通风干爽，使那些有害气体尽快排出，尽量用非击打式打印机减少噪音等。

三是注意补充营养。电脑操作者在荧光屏前工作时间过长，视网膜上的视紫红质会被消耗掉，而视紫红质主要由维生素 A 合成。因此，电脑操作者应多吃些胡萝卜、白菜、豆芽、豆腐、红枣、橘子以及牛奶、鸡蛋、动物肝脏、瘦肉等食物，以补充人体内维生素 A 和蛋白质。多饮些茶，茶叶中的茶多酚等活性物质会有利于吸收与抵抗放射性物质。

（共 1222 字）

↗ 写作解析

1. 分析中文原文

本文中心意思清晰：标题已表明这篇文章的主题为电脑以及网络对健康的影响。不仅如此，文章中的副标题更是帮助考生掌握文章的要点，因此考生应围绕文章的标题以及副标题的提示构建摘要的写作要点，即电脑和网络使用不当的危害及如何减少其危害。各个要点的重要细节参见中文文章中的划线部分。

2. 摘要的中文大纲

通过提炼、总结画线部分的内容，写作的中文提纲大致如下：

第一段：（第 1～5 段）：电脑成为人们日常生活和工作的重要工具，它带来便利的同时不利于人们的健康。首先对身体健康的直接影响，电脑辐射诱发眼病，长时间操作电脑可导致腰、颈、腕等部位的疾患。操作过程中的注意力高度集中和手眼的频繁快速移动会产生多梦、神经衰弱，甚至诱发精神方面的疾病。其次，长时间且无节制地使用电脑或网络会导致网络综合征，其典型表现为睡眠障碍、情绪低落、食欲下降等。第三，电脑释放出的有害臭氧气体可造成呼吸困难，甚至导致肺部发生病变。

第二段：（第 6～10 段）：科学使用电脑，减少危害十分必要。首先要增强自我保健意识。工作中每 1 小时应休息 10 分钟，到室外活动身体。平时也要注意加强锻炼，定期检查，出现症状适当调整上机时间。其次，工作环境中光线要适宜，保持通风干爽，有助于有害气体的排出。第三，电脑操作者要补充维生素 A 和蛋白质，如胡萝卜、白菜、牛奶、鸡蛋等。多饮茶，有利于抵抗放射性物质。

3. 供参考的表达式

显示器	screen
辐射	radiation
青光眼	glaucoma
键盘	keyboard
肌肉骨骼系统	musculoskeletal system
神经衰弱	neurasthenia
烦躁	irritable
焦虑不安	agitated
网络综合征	Net Synthesis
行为异常	abnormal behavior
心理障碍、人格障碍	mental disorder, personality disorder
食欲下降	loss of appetite
思维迟缓	slow thought; thinking retardation
滥用药物	drug abuse
呼吸系统	respiratory system
臭氧	ozone
呼吸困难	respiratory difficulty

哮喘病	asthma
自我保健意识	self-awareness of health care
通风	air the room
茶多酚	Tea Polyphenols

4. 参考范文

Computer along with the Internet brings much convenience, but it does harm to people's health as well. Firstly improper use affects people's health directly. Computer radiation may induce eye diseases. Using computers for a long time will bring about much discomfort of wrist, neck or waist. Tremendous concentration on the computer use as well as frequent quick movements of hands and eyes may also contribute to dreaminess, neurasthenia, and even mental diseases. Secondly, uncontrolled use of computers or net may lead to Net Synthesis, which is characterized by sleep disorder, depression or loss of appetite. Thirdly, ozone released by computers may cause respiratory difficulty, and even lung diseases.

As Net Synthesis is becoming a common disease, reasonable use of computers and net to reduce its risks is crucial. Computer users should enhance their self-awareness of health care and it is suggested to take a 10-minute break every hour, more exercise and regular physical check. In addition, airing the room is beneficial to the emission of harmful gases. People should eat carrot, cabbage, eggs to supplement vitamin A and protein. Moreover, tea is a good choice because tea polyphenols may help absorb and resist to radioactive substances.

（194 words）

三、评卷人掌握的评分原则

1. 摘要或短文写作的评分原则

总体评分法（global scoring）：通过"内容 + 语言"确定考生作文的基本分数段，再酌情加减分数。

2. 摘要或短文写作的评分标准

20～17分	文章切题，体裁正确，文笔流畅，完全没有或仅有个别语法或用词错误
16～13分	文章基本切题，体裁基本符合要求，文笔较流畅，但有数处一般性语法和用词错误
12～9分	文章大体切题，体裁大体符合要求，文章虽不很流畅但能令人理解其意思，有数处重大语法或用词错误
8～5分	词数达不到要求，文章尚能切题，体裁不符合要求，句子结构较单调和松散，有多处重大语法和用词错误，但文章尚能表达一些意思
4～1分	仅写出若干句子符合题意，语法用词和拼写错误较多，表现缺乏写作能力
0分	仅写几个与题意无关的句子，或虽写几句而错误比比皆是，或根本一句未写，表现无写作能力

3. 解释评分标准

● 词数：要求 200 左右，即左右浮动 20，不可词数太少过于明显（词数偏少体现写作能力不强）。

● 切题：要点要全，否则扣分；不可增加个人看法（摘要）。

● 文笔流畅：体现在用词恰当，句句相扣，段段相扣。

● 错误：重大错误是指句法结构或主谓结构相关的错误，如语序、时态语态等；词性错误、用词错误；拼写错误个别不作扣分主要依据，但多次出现错误就要扣分了。

四、写作中存在的问题及对策

针对历年考生在医学博士英语统考中写作测试部分出现的错误分析，我们将考生常出现的问题归纳如下，希望考生能引起重视：

1. 不是写摘要，而是将中文文章翻译为英文；

2. 错误较多，如拼写、搭配等；

3. 中式英文现象严重；

4. 语法错误频繁出现；

5. 文章结构不紧凑，凌乱不堪；

6. 常用词汇积累不够，导致文章关键词无法体现；

7. 试图使用长难句，但语句结构混乱；

8. 字迹潦草，辨认不清。

针对以上罗列的问题，希望考生在备考阶段在如下方面多加训练和积累：

1. 平时要注意中文篇章大意的凝练，这是医学博士考试摘要写作的第一道坎，每年很多考生不是栽在英文上，而是栽在母语中文上，所以考生如果这个步骤还有较大问题，分不清主次，不能提炼出文章的关键信息，就一定要多下功夫。

2. 一定要用笔纸实际进行写作，切忌用在电脑上完成写作。众所周知，电脑有语法和拼写纠错功能，这样使得考生自己不能意识到错误的存在，而是依赖电脑的提醒。

3. 鉴于医学博士英语统考的作文部分测试题材以大众医学科普知识和社会医学问题，例如健康与生活方式类、常见病类以及医疗体制，考生在备考阶段应加强医学相关文章的阅读以及表达式的积累，以免考试时有想法，但没有相应的表达式支持，最终导致自己随意创造。在练习阶段，写作不是一个根据个人喜好创作的过程，一定要注意模仿别人的写作结构、表达式等，必要的积累必不可少！待自己的"语料库"相当丰满的时候，才能够做到把自己的想法流畅地表达出来，故希望考生更多地关注积累、使用、替换：即积累新的，使用新的，替换旧的！积累的途径可以是阅读的任何英文文章。

4. 在平时写作中，针对文章出现的错误要引起重视，及时查漏补缺，认真改正。

5. 在平时写作训练中，要按照写作流程进行构思和写作，养成良好的写作习惯。

6. 考生要熟悉基本的英文写作结构模式，以利于文章结构一目了然。一般说来，各段的主题句（topic sentence）放在段落之首，用以概括段落大意，使得全段其他文字都围绕它展开。而各段的主题句正是文章结构框架的重要体现，它们要围绕文章的中心思想展开。

7. 写作时间分配建议

1）5～10分钟：认真阅读中文原文，大致把握文章的内容。

2）5分钟：对中文文章进行提炼，划出各段主题句以及关键的细节内容。

3）5～10分钟：根据在各段划出的主题句和关键细节内容，组织英文摘要的各主要部分及内容，符合英文的写作结构，即：

- 文章的中心思想（main idea）
- 每段的主题句（topic sentence）
- 每段的扩展句（support sentences）
- 结论句（conclusion）

4）20分钟：根据确定的英文摘要的大纲写摘要。

5）5分钟：检查要点是否齐全、语法有无错误、意思表达是否清楚、拼写有无错误等。

五、写作常用词语和句子

1. 开头句型

1）As far as...is concerned　就……而言

2）It goes without saying that... 不言而喻

3）It can be said with certainty that... 可以很肯定地说

4）As the proverb says 正如谚语所说

5）It has to be noticed that... 必须注意的是

6）It's generally recognized that... 人们普遍认识到

7）It's likely that 很可能

8）It's hardly too much to say that... 几乎不用说太多的是

9）What calls for special attention is that 需要特别关注的是

10）There's no denying the fact that... 无可否认的是

11）Nothing is more important than the fact that... 没有什么比这个事实更重要

12）What's far more important is that... 更为重要的是

2. 衔接句型

1）A case in point is... 举个恰当的例子

2）As is often the case... ……是常有的事

3）As stated in the previous paragraph 如前段所述

4）But the problem is not so simple. Therefore... 然而问题并非如此简单，所以……

5）But it's a pity that... 但是遗憾的是……

6) For all that…In spite of the fact that… 是因为……尽管事实是……

7) Further, we hold opinion that… 更进一步，我们的观点是……

8) However , the difficulty lies in… 然而，困难在于……

9) Similarly, we should pay attention to… 同样，我们应该注意……

10) not (that) …but (that) … 不是……，而是……

11) In view of the present situation 鉴于目前形势

12) As has been mentioned above… 正如前述

13) In this respect, we many as well (say) 从这个角度上，我们可以说

14) However, we have to look at the other side of the coin, that is… 然而，我们还得看到事物的另一方面，即……

15) equally important 同样重要的是

3. 结尾句型

1) I will conclude by saying… 总结说来

2) Therefore, we have the reason to believe that… 因而，我们有理由相信……

3) All things considered 总而言之

4) It may be safely said that… 可以放心地说

5) Therefore, in my opinion, it's more advisable… 因而，按照我的观点，……更明智

6) It can be concluded from the discussion that… 从中我们可以得出这样的结论……

7) From my point of view, it would be better if… 在我看来……也许更好

8) in the long run 从长远来看

9) consequently; in conclusion; in short; in summary 结果；总结说来；简而言之

10) It's high time that strict measures were taken to stop… 该是采取严格措施制止……的时候了

11) Taking all these into account, we… 考虑到所有这些，我们……

4. 常见病医学词汇

癌症	cancer
肺癌	lung cancer
肝癌	liver cancer
宫颈癌	cervical cancer
皮肤癌	skin cancer
乳腺癌	breast cancer
胃癌	stomach cancer
心血管疾病	cardiovascular diseases
心脏病发作	heart attack
冠心病	coronary disease
骨质疏松症	osteoporosis
关节炎	arthritis

皮肤病	skin diseases
带状疱疹	zoster
疹子	rash
湿疹	eczema
痘	pox
荨麻疹	hives
静脉曲张	varix
天花	variola
中风	stroke
肺结核	tuberculosis
溃疡	ulcer
气管炎	tracheitis
扁桃体炎	tonsillitis
糖尿病	diabetes
糖尿病人	diabetic
狂犬病	rabies
高血压	hypertension; high blood pressure
低血压	hypotension
肝炎	hepatitis
肥胖症	obesity
血管的	vascular
肿瘤	tumor
血栓	thrombus
脑梗死	cerebral infarction
急性的	acute
慢性的	chronic
胰岛素	insulin
脂肪肝	fatty liver

5. 常见症状英语词汇

发痒的	itchy
超重	overweight
症状	symptom
呕吐	vomit; bring up
眩晕的	dizzy (*n.* dizziness)
消化不良	indigestion
体重下降	lose weight
反胃	nausea

失眠症	insomnia
紊乱	disorder
气短	short breath
倦怠	listless
抗生素	antibiotics
胆固醇	cholesterol
流鼻涕	runny noses
嗓子痛	sore throats
头疼	headache
昏昏欲睡	drowsy
心不在焉	absent-minded

6. 常用治疗英语词汇及其他

疫苗	vaccine
移植器官	transplant organs
疗法	therapy
物理治疗	physiotherapy
化疗	chemotherapy
临床的	clinical
流行病学	epidemiology
诊断	diagnosis (*v.* diagnose)
副作用	side effect
缩短寿命	shorten lifespan
夺人生命	claim
蛋白质	protein
止痛药	painkiller
维生素	vitamin
发病	incidence

六、真题解析

2008 年真题

珍爱生命从护心开始
生命第一杀手

这些年来，随着我国经济的发展，在人们解决了温饱之后，伴随而来的是与吸烟、缺乏运动、紧张和过度饮食等不良生活方式相关的慢性疾病，尤其是心血管疾病、肿瘤等已经成为危害健康、危及生命的第一杀手。

近年来，"猝死"事件在各地屡有发生。压力过大，劳累过度，使得不少中青年人长期处于亚健康状态，积重难返而猝死。在众多猝死事件中，多数是由心肌梗死引起的。而半数以上的心肌梗死是没有先兆的，突然起病，致死或致残；在心肌梗死的发病早期死亡者中，半数都死在到达医院之前。

在很多人的印象里，高血压、冠心病、心肌梗死好像是中老年人的"专利"，其实不然，现在每天医院急诊室、监护室里都能看到一些非常年轻的心肌梗死患者，而且越来越多。

无知者"无畏"

多数并不是死于无钱，而是死于无知，即缺乏预防意识，缺乏对健康的忧患意识，这在"白骨精"（白领、骨干、精英）中尤为突出。他们白天忙于工作，晚上忙于应酬，很少有人把自己的健康放在心上。

值得注意的是，不健康生活方式所致的心血管病多是"隐形杀手"，平时无明显症状，但在不知不觉或无先兆的情况下，以突然发病的形式瞬间结束人们的生命。相当多的病人第一次发病或第一次有临床表现就是心肌梗死，甚至猝死进而结束生命。

令人担忧的是，现在很多"白骨精"们根本意识不到自己是心血管疾病的高危人群，甚至幻想患病以后再亡羊补牢。实际上，在长期的超负荷"压迫"下，他们一旦发病就会一发不可收拾，第一次就往往可能猝死，所以一定不能心存侥幸。

管住嘴　迈开腿

血脂的异常和胆固醇升高、吸烟、糖尿病、高血压、中心型肥胖、日常生活缺乏运动、饮食缺乏蔬菜水果，都已经被证明是心血管疾病的重要危险因素，既然我们已经知道心血管疾病是一个多种危险因子的疾病，那么应首先从预防危险因素上做起，而不是等到患了高血压再去吃降压药物，得了高血脂再去降血脂。

心血管疾病是可防、可控、可救的。吸烟是万恶之源，不只是危害心血管，也是引起呼吸系统和多种癌症的"罪犯"。吸烟害己更害人，吸烟不是"嗜好"，而是疾病。肥胖和血脂异常也可以明显增加高血压、心肌梗死等的危险。

心血管防治要注重"治未病"，对每一个人来说，要有一个健康的身体，首先要不吸烟，"管住嘴"，特别要从青少年抓起，引导青少年从小养成健康文明的生活习惯，告别吸烟，告别垃圾食品。

"迈开腿"，除了爬山、游泳等运动以外，要把路走起来。如果大家能坚持每天快步走一万步的话，持之以恒，定将受益匪浅。饭吃八成饱，日行万步路，为最有效的减肥方法。

（1024 字）

↗ 写作解析

1. 分析中文原文

本文一共十三段，而且文章各部分均有副标题，这就对于考生来说很容易抓住文章的主要要点。在阅读中文原文后，我们可以确定每一段的段落大意，并在原文画出相应的关键细节内容。关键细节内容请见原文画线部分。各段的段落大意简要如下：

第一段：副标题1：生命第一杀手

第二段：不良生活方式相关的慢性病，尤其是心血管疾病和肿瘤成为第一杀手

第三段："猝死"屡有发生，多数是由心肌梗死引起的，事先没征兆，突然起病

第四段：现在有越来越多的年轻心肌梗死患者

第五段：副标题 2：无知者"无畏"

第六段：多数人死于无知，既缺乏预防和忧患意识，"白骨精"尤为突出

第七段：不健康生活方式所致的心血管疾病是"隐形杀手"

第八段：很多"白骨精"意识不到自己是高危人群

第九段：副标题 3：管住嘴，迈开腿

第十段：心血管疾病的高危因素，从预防危险因素做起

第十一段：吸烟是万恶之源

第十二段："管住嘴"

第十三段："迈开腿"

在确定每段的段落大意后，我们可以很清楚地看到：文章共三个要点，就是三个副标题，因而英文摘要最好是符合副标题，由三个段落组成。根据各个副标题下的具体细节，可以整合内容，形成英文摘要的中文提纲，但要　　　　注意段落和句句间的逻辑关系连接。

2. 摘要的中文大纲

第一部分（第 1～4 段）：生命第一杀手。近些年来，与不良生活方式相关的慢性病，尤其是心血管疾病和肿瘤成为危害健康的第一杀手。压力过大、劳累过度使得不少中青年人长期处于亚健康状态，"猝死"事件屡有发生。心肌梗死趋于年轻化，而且大多没有先兆。

第二部分（第 5～8 段）：无知者"无畏"。多数人死于无知，即缺乏预防和对健康的忧患意识，这在"白骨精"中尤为突出。值得注意的是，不健康生活方式所致的心血管疾病多是"隐形杀手"，即平时无明显症状，在不知不觉中残害人们的健康。但令人担忧的是，很多"白骨精"们根本意识不到自己是高危人群，心存侥幸。

第三部分（第 9～13 段）：管住嘴，迈开腿。血脂异常、胆固醇升高、吸烟、糖尿病、高血压、中心性肥胖、日常生活缺乏运动、饮食缺乏蔬菜水果、紧张都是心血管疾病的重要危险因素，故应从预防危险因素做起。"管住嘴"首先要不吸烟，吸烟是万恶之源，其次要注意饮食，尤其要从青少年抓起。"迈开腿"是指除了爬山、游泳等之外，坚持每天快步走。

3. 供参考的表达式

第一杀手	top killer
不良生活方式	unhealthy lifestyle
慢性病	chronic diseases
心血管疾病	cardiovascular diseases
肿瘤	tumor
压力过大	excess stress
劳累过度	overwork; overloaded work

中青年人	young and middle-aged individuals
亚健康状态	sub-health
猝死	sudden death
心肌梗死	myocardial infarction
趋于年轻化	younger trend
先兆	sign
死于无知	die of ignorance
意识	consciousness
"白骨精"（白领，骨干，精英）	white-collars; backbones; elite
隐形杀手	invisible killer
高危人群	high-risk group; high-risk population
心存侥幸	count on luck
"管住嘴"	control the diet
"迈开腿"	start a workout or exercise
血脂异常	abnormal blood lipid
胆固醇升高	the increasing cholesterol
糖尿病	diabetes
高血压	high blood pressure; hypertension
中心性肥胖	central obesity

4. 参考范文

Love Your Life, Care Your Heart

In recent years, some chronic diseases related to unhealthy lifestyles, particularly cardiovascular disease and tumors have been becoming the top killer. Excess stress and overwork contribute to sub-health among many young and middle-aged individuals, which causes high occurrence of sudden deaths without any signs, even frequently happening among young people.

It is believed that most people die of ignorance, that is, lack of prevention and health consciousness. Unfortunately those white-collar workers and elites, counting on luck, don't realize at all that they are high-risk groups. It is worth noting that the cardiovascular diseases induced by unhealthy lifestyles are invisible killers, which have no any obvious symptoms.

Controlling your diet and enjoying workouts are the optimal solutions. It is accepted that abnormal blood lipid, smoking, diabetes, hypertension, inactive life, lack of vegetables and fruits as well as stress are the high risks of cardiovascular diseases; thus, prevention of those risks comes first. First of all, please quit smoking, in combination with control your diet, which should be required among young people. Besides, apart from climbing and swimming, walking at fast pace can be beneficial.

（182 words）

2009 年真题

水果是否可吃可不吃

水果含有人体必需而又不能自身合成的矿物质，具有强抗氧化作用、防止细胞衰老的维生素以及可以明显降低血液中胆固醇浓度的可溶性纤维等，对人体健康十分有益。但中国人特别是男性，经常吃水果的比例很低。20 世纪 80 年代我在美国分析了美国 100 万人十年追踪研究的资料，发现不吃或很少吃水果的人群，肺癌死亡率为吃水果人群的 1.75 倍。而且从 45 岁到 74 岁的每个 5 岁年龄组均表现出类似的结果，说明这种因果关系非常可靠。美国有句谚语叫："一天一个苹果，不用看医生。"说明他们很早就总结出了水果对疾病的预防作用。世界卫生组织近年来提出了"天天五蔬果"的口号。其含义是，为保障健康，最好每天吃够五种蔬菜和五种水果。近年来美国哈佛大学的一些研究表明，多进食水果和蔬菜还可降低中风和冠心病的发病危险。

那么，到底水果中的什么成分起到了这样的作用？是不是维生素？服用市售维生素制剂是否可起到相同作用？我又进一步分析了肺癌死亡与服用维生素制剂的关系。结果发现，经常服用维生素并不能起到类似的保护作用。再专门分析重度吸烟者肺癌死亡率与进食水果和服用维生素制剂的关系。发现水果仍然起到保护作用，而维生素却没有。该分析研究的结论是人工合成的维生素不能替代水果对肺癌死亡的预防作用。后来的一些研究也得出了同样的结论。对此，营养免疫学家的解释是：天然植物中的维生素并不是单独起作用，而是与其他维生素和营养素相互联合一起工作。一种维生素补充的过多或不足，均会影响和削弱其他营养素或维生素的作用。由于化学合成的维生素是与其他维生素和营养素分离的，复方的各成分间的比例也与天然的不尽相同，所以他们不能产生与天然物质中所含的维生素一样的功效。有些国外的专家把这种现象戏称为"人造的不如神造的"。另外，蔬菜水果中还可能含有些尚未被人类认识的生理活性物质。目前，天然食物的抗氧化作用已成为一个重要的研究领域，各国营养学家正在进行研究开发。研究已证实，有些蔬菜水果具有强抗氧化作用，如大蒜、胡萝卜、柿子、柑橘、猕猴桃等能提高体内超氧化物歧化酶（SOD）的活性，发挥延缓衰老的作用。

综上所述，在日常生活中，水果应作为每日膳食的重要组成部分，绝不是可有可无的东西。对一般人群来说，维生素制剂绝不能也不应当代替日常对水果、蔬菜的进食。另外，过多地服用维生素制剂还可能引致一些副作用，有些甚至非常严重。如服用过量维生素 D 会导致软组织钙化，对肾脏和心血管系统造成损伤；长期服用维生素 E 易引起血栓等。在病态情况下，由于体内某些维生素的大量消耗或吸收合成转化不良，打破了其正常平衡，则必须适当补给，如，发热、手术、患心肌梗死等疾病时需补充维生素 C；肝肾功能不良时需补充维生素 D 等。但这些均需在医生的指导下使用。

（1110 字）

⤴ 写作解析

1. 分析中文原文

本文一共三段，主要讲述水果对健康的好处，以及维生素制剂对人健康的影响。关键细节内容请见原文画线部分。各段的段落大意简要如下：

第一段：水果中的矿物质、维生素和可溶性纤维对人体健康有益

第二段：维生素制剂不能替代天然维生素

第三段：水果是每日膳食必需品，以及维生素制剂的副作用

在确定每段的段落大意后，我们可以根据选取各段主要具体细节作为论据支持三个段落的主旨。文章中的具体重要细节参见原文中的划线部分。

2. 摘要的中文大纲

第一部分（第1段）：水果含有人体必需而又不能自身合成的矿物质，具有强抗氧化作用、防止细胞衰老的维生素以及可以明显降低血液中胆固醇浓度的可溶性纤维等，对人体健康十分有益。但中国人特别是男性，经常吃水果的比例很低。一项研究表明，不吃或很少吃水果的人群，肺癌死亡率为吃水果人群的 1.75 倍。世界卫生组织近年来提出了"天天五蔬果"的口号。其含义是，为保障健康，最好每天吃够五种蔬菜和五种水果。美国哈佛大学的一些研究也表明，多进食水果和蔬菜还可降低中风和冠心病的发病危险。

第二部分（第2段）：服用市售维生素制剂不能起到水果所起到的作用。一项有关肺癌死亡和维生素制剂的研究发现：人工合成的维生素不能替代水果对肺癌的预防作用。天然植物中的维生素是与其他维生素和营养素共同工作的。但化学合成的维生素是与其他维生素和营养素分离的。另外，蔬菜水果中还可能含有些尚未被人类认识的生理活性物质。研究已证实，有些蔬菜水果具有强抗氧化作用，如大蒜、胡萝卜、柿子、柑橘、猕猴桃等能提高体内超氧化物歧化酶（SOD）的活性，发挥延缓衰老的作用。

第三部分（第3段）：因而在日常生活中，水果应作为每日膳食的重要组成部分。对一般人群来说，维生素制剂不能替代蔬果的进食，过多服用维生素制剂会引起一些副作用。在病态情况下，必须适当补给维生素，但须在医生指导下使用。

3. 供参考的表达式

必需	indispensable
合成	synthesize
矿物质	mineral
抗氧化作用	antioxidant effects
可溶性纤维	soluble fibers
死亡率	death rate
中风	stroke
冠心病	coronary heart disease
发病危险	risk factors for developing a disease
市售	over-the-counter
营养素	nutrient
生理活性物质	physiologically active substance
柿子	persimmon
猕猴桃	kiwi fruit
大蒜	garlic

延缓衰老	delay aging process
膳食	diet
替代	substitute
副作用	side effect

4. 参考范文

Fruits, rich in the minerals that human bodies need but cannot be synthesized by themselves, anti-aging vitamins as well as soluble fibers which considerably decrease cholesterol in the blood, are beneficial to human's health. However, Chinese particularly males eat less fruits. It is indicated by a research that people eating less or no fruit have higher risks of lung cancer. WHO has also advocated that consumption of five kinds of vegetable and fruits can improve human's health. Another study also suggests that the increasing vegetable and fruit consumption can lower the risks of stroke and coronary heart disease.

Over-the-counter vitamin supplement cannot play the role that fruit does, such as prevention of lung cancer. It is believed that natural vitamins work together with other vitamins and nutrients while synthetic vitamins are separated from other vitamins and nutrients. In addition, research has verified that some vegetable and fruit such as garlic, carrot, orange and kiwifruit have antioxidant effects which can help delay aging.

Therefore, fruit should be the significant component in daily diet. For ordinary people, vitamin supplements can't substitute natural vegetable and fruit, and excess intake of supplements can cause side effect. As patients, they should consume vitamin supplements with the help of physician's instruction.

（204 words）

2010 年真题

新兴学科：药物心理学

药物作用于人体的病变部位，而病人的心理作用会或多或少地影响药物的作用。为了使药物治疗达到最佳疗效，人们必须研究药物心理学，讲究服药心理。

现代医药学认为：药物大多能产生两种效应。药物通过其药理作用来达到治病的目的，此为药物的生理作用。药物还可通过其非生理作用，在病人的心理上产生良好的感觉，加速疾病的康复，此为药物的心理效应。药物的心理效应可促使药物取得更好的疗效，为治疗奠定良好的基础。

药物的心理效应是指由医生的威信，病人对药物的信任感，接受药物治疗的体验、评价，治疗时外界的暗示及药物的广告效应等共同作用而产生的综合效应。药物心理学正是建立在药物心理效应基础之上的一门新兴边缘学科。众所周知，用同样的药物，由专家、名医开出的则效果会更好，这就是药物心理学最简单而明显的例子。

有人做了一个形象的比喻：药物是治疗疾病的"种子"，而心理状态是种子赖以生长、开花和结果的"土壤"。药物的药理作用是药物治疗疾病的基础，而药物的心理效应则在疾病治疗过程中起着十分微妙的作用。特别是在治疗心因性疾病和心理精神疾病中，良好的心态显得更为重要。

与服药心理关系最密切的是药物的信誉。原因为：虔诚的信念和愉快的心情能影响人体的生理机能，增加肾上腺皮质激素的分泌；而适量的肾上腺素能耐受200～400倍致死量的细菌内毒素。药物的良好信誉，能树立人对药物治病救人的鉴定信念。

为什么不良心态会降低药物的生理效应呢？人体是一个复杂的有机整体，不良心态会影响内分泌、心脑血管系统等的功能，从而减弱人体的抗病能力，体内细菌就乘机繁衍滋生，药效当然就降低了。积极的服药心理，可激活内分泌和潜在的免疫功能，药物在免疫器官分泌抗体增多时，能发挥最佳疗效。

药物心理学对人体的作用，在某些人中表现尤为明显：特别是有神经质、意志薄弱、心理缺陷和易受暗示的人。药物心理学揭示了安慰剂止痛和心理安慰的奥秘：安慰剂可通过心理暗示作用刺激大脑产生内源性脑啡肽，其结构类似天然吗啡，作用于疼痛部位，从而减轻疼痛。

许多人有以自觉症状为主的慢性病。许多慢性病有明显的自觉症状，如恶心呕吐、头晕目眩、失眠多梦、食欲不振、腹胀和隐痛等，这些症状与心理和精神状态密切相关。而药物的心理作用正是通过心理暗示来调整人的心态，在不知不觉中治愈或缓解了原有的慢性病。

医护人员的语言、举止和行为对病人的用药心理影响很大。目前世界各国对癌症、类风湿性疾病和自身免疫疾病等尚无特效药。但医生绝不可对患者说："此病为绝症，无药可治。"如对症适时选用安慰剂，有时会收到真正特效药所没有的神奇作用，至少可解除病人精神上的痛苦，在心灵上得到安慰和鼓励，从而增强战胜疾病的信心。

药物心理学的重要组成部分是暗示疗法和安慰剂。安慰剂通过心理暗示作用而影响病人的心理状态，进而影响机体的生理功能，从而起到积极的治疗作用。现代医学证明：药物心理效应不但具有心理上的安慰作用，而且还有改变器官功能活动和躯体症状的多种作用，故可用于治疗某类躯体疾病及多种心理疾病。

（1228字）

➚ 写作解析

1. 分析中文原文

本文段落较多，内容较复杂，不利于考生快速确定文章中的主要要点。这就要求考生研读每一个段落并抓住段落主旨，然后根据段落主旨确定摘要写作的要点。各段段落大意简要如下：

第一段：病人心理作用影响药物疗效，有必要研究药物心理学

第二段：药物产生两种效应：生理作用和心理效应

第三段：药物心理效应的定义

第四段：药物和心理状态的关系：形象比喻

第五段：药物信誉

第六段：服药心理对药效的影响

第七段：药物心理学对人体的作用

第八段：心理暗示有效缓解自觉症状

第九段：医护人员的语言、举止和行为对病人的用药心理影响很大

第十段：药物心理学的重要组成部分是暗示疗法和安慰剂

　　根据这些段落主旨考生可以提炼或总结概括摘要的要点，不难看出这篇文章的要点如下：药物产生的两个效应、药物心理学定义及重要性、药物心理效应对人体的作用、药物心理学的重要组成部分。具体相关细节参见文章划线部分。

2. 摘要的中文大纲

　　第一部分（第1～3段）：药物作用于人体的病变部位，而病人的心理作用会或多或少地影响药物的作用。现代医药学认为：药物能产生两种效应：生理作用即通过药理作用治病，和心理效应，它可促使药物取得更好的疗效。药物心理效应是指医生的威信，病人对药物的信任感，接受药物治疗的体验、评价和治疗时外界的暗示及药物的广告效应等共同作用而产生的综合效应。

　　第二部分（第4～6段）：在治病过程中，药物的心理效应起到十分微妙的作用。服药心理关系最密切的是药物的信誉。药物的良好信誉，能树立人对药物治病救人的坚定信念。不良心态会影响内分泌、心脑血管系统等功能，从而减弱人体的抗病能力。相反积极的服药心理可激活内分泌和潜在的免疫功能，使药物发挥最佳疗效。

　　第三部分（第7～10段）：药物心理学的重要组成部分是暗示疗法和安慰剂。安慰剂通过心理暗示作用而影响病人的心理状态，进而影响机体的生理功能，从而起到积极的治疗作用。医护人员的语言、举止和行为对病人的用药心理影响很大。对于那些有神经质、意志薄弱、心理缺陷和易受暗示的人，或是有自觉症状的慢性病人，安慰剂可通过心理暗示作用于疼痛部位，从而减轻疼痛，缓解症状。

3. 供参考的表达式

药物心理学	pharmacopsychology
病变部位	the site of pathological changes
药理作用	pharmacological effect
威信	prestige
信任感	sense of trust
心理暗示	psychological implication
综合	comprehensive
药物信誉	credibility of medicine
内分泌	endocrine
心脑血管系统	cardiovascular and cerebrovascular system
抗病能力	resistance to diseases
免疫功能	immune function
疗效	efficacy
安慰剂	placebo
生理功能	physiological function
神经质	neurotic person
意志薄弱	weak will
心理缺陷	mental defect
自觉症状	self-sense symptom

4. 参考范文

Medicine imposes effects on the body's disease and patients' psychology can more or less affect the result of medicine. Medicine can produce two effects: physiological effect and psychological effect. The former one means diseases can be cured by pharmacological effects, while the latter one can promote the medicine more effective. Psychological effect of medicine refers to the comprehensive effects including physicians' prestige, patients' trust on medicine and their experiences of treatments and their evaluation.

In the process of treatment, psychological effect of medicine performs the delicate roles. The credibility of medicine is closely related to patients' psychology. Unhealthy mental attitude would affect endocrine and cardiovascular and cerebrovascular functions, which will lower body's resistance to diseases. On the contrary, positive attitude can activate potential immune functions and increase the efficacy.

The two important components of pharmacopsychology are implication and placebo. Placebo will influence patients' mental state and body's physiological functions through psychological implication, and then enhance the effectiveness of drugs. In this case, medical staff's words and behavior will greatly influence patients' medication attitude. For those people with weak will or psychological defects or those with self-sense symptoms, placebo can impose effect on the pains through mental hints, which will relieve pains and symptoms.

（202 words）

七、写作专项练习与解析

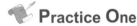 **Practice One**

一说心脏病这个话题就有点沉重，据世界心脏联盟预计，<u>2025 年前，在全世界范围内，25 岁以上的成年人中，每 3 人就有 1 人将罹患心血管疾病。心血管疾病的死亡率远远高于包括癌症、艾滋病在内的其他疾病，堪称威胁人类健康的"第一杀手"。在中国，每年大约有 260 万人死于心脑血管疾病。</u>在专家看来，目前预防心脏病意识提高的主要集中在老年人，在过去 15 年里，中国 35 岁至 44 岁年龄组患冠心病的人数增长了 150%，心脏病发病正在年轻化，发病风险最高的是 40 岁至 50 岁的人群。<u>9 月 28 日是世界心脏病日，而高血压、糖尿病、肥胖都已成为引发心脏病高发的潜伏杀手。今年世界心脏日活动主题也因此命名为"了解您的危险因素"，目的是敦促人们了解威胁自己心脏健康的危险因素。</u>

许多医学专家指出，要想拥有健康的心脏，必须了解并远离形成心血管疾病的危险因素。<u>目前得到公认的冠心病危险因素包括两方面。一是依据现有的医疗水平不能认为控制的，如年龄和遗传因素。二是目前医疗手段可以控制的危险因素如吸烟、肥胖、高血压、血脂异常、高血糖等。胡吃乱喝、不运动是导致慢性非传染性疾病患病率上升的主要原因。</u>这其中，城市居民禽肉类及油脂消费过多，谷类食物消费偏低。除此以外，现代人的不健康生活方式也是成为威胁人们健康的杀手之一，如吸烟酗酒、经常熬夜、不合理营养、长期不运动、紧张压抑等。"总有人会说工作太忙、应酬太多、竞争太激烈，导致自己不能有健康的生活方式，但我说，健康是一颗空心玻璃球，一旦掉下去就会粉碎；工作只是一个皮球，掉下去后还能再弹起来。"中华医学会会长、中国工程院院士钟南山在接受记者采访时说。钟南山强调，快节奏、高强度的工作，抽烟、酗酒、经常熬夜吃夜宵、饮食不合理、长期不运动等不健康的生活方式，使越来越多的都市人处于亚健康的灰色地带，"都市人患病70% 是不合理的生活方式所致"。

那么，我们应该如何预防心血管疾病呢？我们首先要从健康的生活方式做起。①合理安排饮食，避免肥胖和超重。每天进食的总热量不能过高，一般要求的60岁以上老年人，男性2000～2500千卡，女性1700～2100千卡；70岁以上老年人，男性1800～2000千卡，女性1600～1800千卡；80岁以上老年人，男性1600千卡，女性为1400千卡。应选择低脂肪、低胆固醇、富含维生素的食物，限制含糖食物的摄入。应以蔬菜类、粗粮、水果为主，可常食富含钙、钾、碘、铬、钴的食物，因它具有降血压、保护心脏，减少冠心病发病率的良好作用，如牛奶、虾皮、黄豆、核桃、蒜苗、鲜雪里红等。所食油类应尽量用花生油、棉籽油、豆油、菜籽油、玉米油等植物性油类。②保持血压正常，若出现高血压，应积极采取措施，包括药物及非药物措施，使血压降至正常范围。③参加一定量的体育锻炼，促进机体新陈代谢，消耗过多的脂肪，防止肥胖，又可增强心血管系统的调节功能，防止冠心病的发生与发作，如慢跑、散步、练气功、游泳等。④戒烟。香烟中含有大量有害物质随烟雾被吸入肺内，进而进入血液中，通过作用于心脏、血管、神经系统，从而促进动脉硬化及冠心病的发生。⑤生活起居要有规律，保证充足睡眠，保持心情愉快，避免情绪激动。

保护心脏不分早晚、不分年龄大小，改善生活方式和饮食习惯越早越有益。为拥有健康的心脏，应从现在做起。

（1295字）

↗ 写作解析

1. 分析中文原文

本文的中心思想是远离危险因素，拥有健康的心脏。而且文章结构清晰，易于考生提炼完成英文摘要的提纲。每段的大意如下：

第一段：心血管疾病已成为人类健康头号杀手，今年世界心脏病日活动主题目的是敦促人们了解威胁心脏健康的因素

第二段：威胁心脏健康的因素

第三段：如何预防心血管疾病

第四段：总结

2. 摘要的中文大纲

第一部分（第1段）：据估计，2025年前，在全世界范围内，25岁以上的成年人中，每3人就有1人将罹患心血管疾病。心血管疾病的死亡率远远高于包括癌症、艾滋病在内的其他疾病，堪称威胁人类健康的"第一杀手"。在中国，每年大约有260万人死于心脑血管

疾病。9月28日是世界心脏病日，而高血压、糖尿病、肥胖都已成为引发心脏病高发的潜伏杀手。

第二部分（第2段）：目前得到公认的冠心病危险因素包括两方面。一是依据现有的医疗水平不能认为控制的，如年龄和遗传因素。二是目前医疗手段可以控制的危险因素如吸烟、肥胖、高血压、血脂异常、高血糖等。胡吃乱喝、不运动是导致慢性非传染性疾病患病率上升的主要原因。除此以外，现代人的不健康生活方式也是成为威胁人们健康的杀手之一，如吸烟酗酒、经常熬夜、不合理营养、长期不运动、紧张压抑等，这些会使越来越多的人处于亚健康的灰色地带。

第三部分（第3～4段）：为了预防心血管疾病，我们首先要从健康的生活方式做起。①合理安排饮食，避免肥胖和超重。②保持血压正常。③参加一定量的体育锻炼，促进机体新陈代谢，如慢跑、散步、练气功、游泳等。④戒烟。⑤生活起居要有规律，保证充足睡眠，保持心情愉快，避免情绪激动。

3. 供参考的表达式

心血管疾病	cardiovascular disease
死亡率	mortality
肥胖	obesity
潜伏杀手	invisible killer
遗传因素	hereditary factors
血脂异常	dyslipidemia
高血糖	high blood glucose
不合理营养	unbalanced diet
长期不运动	inactive; sedentary
压抑	depression
新陈代谢	metabolism
充足睡眠	adequate sleep
愉快心情	cheerful mood

4. 参考范文

It is estimated that one in three adults aged above 25 will have developed heart diseases by the end of 2025. Thus cardiovascular mortality is much higher than the mortality of other diseases including cancers and AIDS. Up to now, heart diseases have become the top killer, claiming 2.6 million deaths annually in China.

In terms of risks of heart diseases, it is acknowledged that there are two aspects: one aspect contains some uncontrolled factors, such as age and hereditary factors; the other aspect involves some controlled risks, for instance smoking, obesity and high blood pressure. In addition, unhealthy lifestyle is another potential risk: unbalanced diet, lack of physical exercise, pressure and depression, which result in sub-health.

In order to prevent heart disease, we had better start with healthy lifestyle. Firstly, have a well balanced diet and avoid obesity and overweight. In order to control the total amount of calories we intake, low-fat, low-cholesterol and high-fiber food are recommended, such as vegetables, fruit and cereals. Secondly, regular and moderate physical exercise, such as jogging, swimming, can promote metabolism, prevent overweight and lower the incidence of heart attack. Thirdly, stop smoking. Last but not least, healthy living habits are equally significant. Adequate sleep and cheerful mood are beneficial too.

（212 words）

 Practice Two

很多人不重视早餐，常常是随便凑合一下或者干脆不吃。其实早餐对保障人体健康、维持体能、提高学习和工作效率有着至关重要的作用。不仅如此，专家还认为，应该根据人的不同年龄和体质状况，科学合理地搭配早膳，以满足人体健康的需要。

幼儿的早餐　幼儿正值生长发育的旺盛时期，应当注重补充丰富的蛋白质和钙（calcium），尽量少吃含糖较高的食物，以免引起龋齿（decayed tooth）和肥胖。如果在条件许可的情况下，幼儿的早餐通常以适量的牛奶、鸡蛋和面包为佳。当然，也可以用果汁或粥来代替牛奶，或者用饼干、馒头代替面包。

青少年的早餐　青少年时期身体发育较快，是肌肉和骨骼生长的重要时期，需要足够的钙、维生素C、维生素A等营养成分，尤其是要保证充足的热量供应。青少年比较合理的早餐是一杯牛奶、适量的新鲜水果或蔬菜、100克干点（面包、馒头、大饼或饼干等含碳水化合物（carbohydrate）较高的食品）。所含的热量要充分满足青少年脑力活动与体力活动的需要。

中年人的早餐　人到中年，肩挑工作、家务两副重担，身心的负荷相当重，加上中年时期组织器官的功能和生理功能日渐减退，其体力和精力都不如青少年。为了减缓中年人衰退的过程，推迟"老年期"的到来，除了要保持乐观的思想情绪和进行必要的体育锻炼之外，合理地搭配膳食也非常重要。中年人的饮食，既要含有丰富的蛋白质、维生素、钙、磷（phosphorus）等，还应保证低热量、低脂肪并适当地控制碳水化合物的摄入量。中年人较理想的早餐是：鸡蛋、豆浆或粥、干点（馒头、大饼、饼干和面包均可）和适量的蔬菜。

老年人的早餐　老年人的新陈代谢（metabolism）已经明显衰退，但必需的营养成分不能减少，尤其是要保证钙的供应，以防止老年人的骨质疏松（osteoporosis）。老年人的早餐除了供应牛奶和豆浆以外，还可多吃粥、面条、肉松和花生酱等既容易消化、又含有丰富营养的食物。除此之外，老年人的早餐应注意少吃油炸类食品。因为这类食物脂肪含量高，胃肠一般难以承受，容易出现消化不良，并易诱发胆、胰疾患，或使这类疾病复发、加重。多次使用的油里往往含有较多的致癌物质，如果常吃油炸的食品，可增加患癌症的危险。老年人还要少吃甜食，因为多余的糖在体内转化为脂肪，容易引起无机盐缺乏。动物内脏类如肝、肾、脑等胆固醇（cholesterol）含量甚高，老年人如经常食用，会使血中胆固醇增高，从而容易引发冠心病、肝病、动脉硬化、高血压等心脑血管疾病，或使原有的疾病加重。

（953 字）

↗ 写作解析

1. 分析中文原文

本文因为有副标题，故文章结构清晰，要点明确。各段大意如下：

第一段：早餐很重要

第二段：幼儿的早餐

第三段：青少年的早餐

第四段：中年人的早餐

第五段：老年人的早餐

2. 摘要的中文大纲

第一部分（第1段）：很多人不重视早餐，甚至不吃早餐。其实早餐对保障人体健康、维持体能、提高学习和工作效率有着至关重要的作用。不仅如此，专家还认为，应该根据人的不同年龄和体质状况，科学合理地搭配早膳，以满足人体健康的需要。

第二部分（第2段）：幼儿的早餐　幼儿处于生长快速阶段，应当注重补充丰富的蛋白质和钙（calcium），尽量少吃含糖较高的食物，以免引起龋齿（decayed tooth）和肥胖。幼儿的早餐通常以适量的牛奶、鸡蛋和面包为佳。当然，也可以用果汁或粥来代替牛奶，或者用饼干、馒头代替面包。

第三部分（第3段）：青少年的早餐　青少年时期身体发育较快，是肌肉和骨骼生长的重要时期，需要足够的钙、维生素C、维生素A等营养成分，尤其是要保证充足的热量供应。青少年比较合理的早餐是一杯牛奶、适量的新鲜水果或蔬菜、100克干点（面包、馒头、大饼或饼干等含碳水化合物（carbohydrate）较高的食品）。

第四部分（第4段）：中年人的早餐　为了减缓中年人衰退的过程，中年人的饮食，既要含有丰富的蛋白质、维生素、钙、磷（phosphorus）等．还应保证低热量、低脂肪并适当地控制碳水化合物的摄入量。中年人较理想的早餐是：鸡蛋、豆浆或粥、干点（馒头、大饼、饼干和面包均可）和适量的蔬菜。

第五部分（第5段）：老年人的早餐　老年人的新陈代谢（metabolism）已经明显衰退，但必需的营养成分不能减少，尤其是要保证钙的供应，以防止老年人的骨质疏松（osteoporosis）。老年人的早餐除了供应牛奶和豆浆以外，还可多吃粥、面条、肉松和花生酱等既容易消化、又含有丰富营养的食物。除此之外，老年人的早餐应注意少吃油炸类食品。因为这类食物脂肪含量高，肠胃一般难以承受，容易出现消化不良。老年人还要少吃甜食，动物内脏类如肝、肾、脑等。

3. 供参考的表达式

不吃早餐	skip breakfast
补充	supplement
蛋白质	protein
钙	calcium
青少年	adolescent

碳水化合物	carbohydrate
粥	porridge
消化	digest

4. 参考范文

Many people tend not to attach the importance to breakfast, and even skip breakfast. Actually breakfast plays vital roles in people's health and their efficiency in work and study. Proper breakfast should be based on their physical conditions and age.

Infants are in the stage of rapid growth, so they should consume plenty of protein and calcium and intake less high-sugar food to avoid decayed teeth and obesity. Milk, eggs and bread are optimal food for breakfast.

Adolescence is a critical period for the growth of muscles and bones. Adequate calcium, Vitamin C and Vitamin A are necessarily required. Milk, fresh fruit and vegetable along with food with carbohydrate can meet the requirement of mental and physical activities.

Due to the age, many middle-aged people suffer from decline in organ function and they have less energy than before. In this case, food for breakfast should be high in protein, vitamin, calcium and phosphorus and they should control the intake of carbohydrate properly. It is suggested that they have eggs, soybean milk, porridge together with bread and vegetable for breakfast.

Old people's metabolism has declined greatly but the adequate nutrients should not be reduced, especially the supply of calcium, in order to prevent osteoporosis. In addition to milk, soybean milk or food easily digested are recommended, such as porridge, noodles.

（219 words）

Practice Three

抑郁症是精神疾病中危害人群最大的一种精神疾病。目前有 1.21 亿人患有抑郁症，该病患病人群仍在不断增加。患抑郁症的人通常会感到异常忧伤、觉得人生毫无价值、对原本感兴趣的活动失去兴趣、精力丧失、疲劳无力、消极悲观、烦躁、甚至会产生自杀的念头。身体症状一般表现在：食欲减退、体重减轻和睡眠障碍。食欲减退、体重减轻：多数病人都有食欲不振，胃口差的症状，美味佳肴不再具有诱惑力，病人不思茶饭或食之无味，常伴有体重减轻。睡眠障碍：典型的睡眠障碍是早醒，比平时早 2～3 小时，醒后不复入睡，陷入悲哀气氛中。

那么什么样的人容易患上抑郁症呢？追求十全十美的人。这类人因为要求自己所做的每一件事都完美无缺，所以把全部精力都放在事物上，从另一个角度而言，即有很强的占有欲、控制欲，在临床上常称这些人具有强迫倾向。过分追求完美的人在某些事情未完成时，就会产生相当强烈的焦虑感，觉得浑身不对劲，所以，不论在任何情况下，他都必须今日事今日毕，一旦碰到什么事没法马上做完时就会紧张万分。倘若跟别人一起做事时，别人不根据他的标准来做的话，他也会觉得如坐针毡。这类人往往更易患焦虑障碍。具有自卑倾向的人。这类人常常会有强烈的不安全感，有些人深信自己的容貌、身体特征、口才、表情、学业成绩、体能状况处处不如人，由于坚信不疑以致这种观念根深蒂固，每当与别人在一起时，这种想法就蜂拥而出，使其无法放松来与别人交谈和交往，总觉得自己处处不如人。有些人在感觉到别人投过来的视线时，脸上的肌肉就会马上僵硬起来，嘴巴张不开，甚至连喉咙也会发生阻塞感。过分自卑往往易发展为社交焦虑障碍。过度关心自己的人。这类人会变成焦虑倾向。这些人通常以自我为中心，非常关注自己健康的状况。当他发现自己有任何的身体症状时，他会非常紧张而马上采取各种医疗行为。一些轻微的不适，如头痛、颈酸、腹痛等也会引起他们对严重疾病的强烈恐惧，并有可能发展成为严重的焦虑障碍。

针对如何治疗抑郁症，专家提出以下建议：

给自己安排的计划要现实合理。即使你在慢慢恢复，但也不要总把自己的时间安排得满满的。

试着摆脱由抑郁症引起的如失败感等此类的消极想法，这些想法会随着抑郁症的减轻而逐渐消除。

参加一些你喜欢的、能让自己感到愉快的活动。

当你情绪低落的时候，避免去做人生中的重大决定。如果一定要做出决定，最好向可信赖的朋友或家人寻求帮助。

不要喝酒精饮料或服用非医生开具的药物，因为这可能会与抗抑郁类药物发生严重反应，而且可能会使病情加重。

多锻炼身体，每周锻炼四至六次，每次至少 30 分钟。

（1001 字）

↗ 写作解析

1. 分析中文原文

本文结构很清楚，属于分析问题—解决问题型的文章，故摘要结构可依据这种结构完成。

第一段：抑郁症的症状

第二段：易患抑郁症的人群

第三至九段：如何治疗抑郁症

2. 摘要的中文大纲

第一部分（第 1 段）：抑郁症是精神疾病中危害人群最大的一种精神疾病。目前有 1.21 亿人患有抑郁症，该病患病人群仍在不断增加。患抑郁症的人通常会感到异常忧伤、觉得人生毫无价值、对原本感兴趣的活动失去兴趣、精力丧失、疲劳无力、消极悲观、烦躁、甚至会产生自杀的念头。身体症状一般表现在：食欲减退、体重减轻和睡眠障碍。

第二部分（第 2 段）：一共有三类人容易患上抑郁症。第一类是追求十全十美的人。这类人因为要求自己所做的每一件事都完美无缺，所以把全部精力都放在事物上，从另一个角度而言，即有很强的占有欲、控制欲，在临床上常称这些人具有强迫倾向。一旦碰到什么事没法马上做完时就会紧张万分。第二类就是具有自卑倾向的人。这类人常常会有强烈的不安全感，有些人深信自己的容貌、身体特征、口才、表情、学业成绩、体能状况处处不如人，使其无法放松来与别人交谈和交往。第三类人是过度关心自己的人。这些人通常以自我为中心，非常关注自己健康的状况。当他发现自己有任何的身体症状时，他会非常紧张而马上采取各种医疗行为。

第三部分（第 3～9 段）：针对如何治疗抑郁症，专家提出以下建议：给自己安排的计划要现实合理；试着摆脱由抑郁症引起的如失败感等此类的消极想法；参加一些你喜欢的、能让自己感到愉快的活动；当你情绪低落的时候，避免去做人生中的重大决定。最好向可信赖的朋友或家人寻求帮助；不要喝酒精饮料或服用非医生开具的药物；多锻炼身体。

3. 供参考的表达式

抑郁	depression
威胁	endanger; threaten
劳累	tiredness; fatigue
悲观	pessimism
烦躁	irritation
食欲不振	poor appetite
消瘦	weight loss
失眠	insomnia
十全十美	perfection
自卑	be inferior to
没安全感	insecurity
以自我为中心	self-centered

4. 参考范文

Depression is the biggest mental disease which endangers people. At present, there are 121 million people suffering from depression and the number is increasing. Depression can make people feel extremely sad, worthless and lose enjoyment in what they used to be interested before. Besides loss of energy, fatigue, pessimism and irritation poor appetite, weight loss, and insomnia are typical symptoms.

It is said three kinds of people are liable to depression. People pursuing perfection strictly require everything be perfect. If something is unfinished, they tend to feel very anxious. People who feel inferior to others, have strong insecurity and they are convinced that they are inferior to others in all aspects. People who concern about themselves excessively are very self-centered and they concern about their health. Even a slight headache may arouse their fear.

There are some helpful tips for the treatment of depression. Firstly, set a reasonable schedule for yourself. Don't arrange a tight schedule for yourself. Secondly, try to remove the negative thoughts. Thirdly, try not to make decisions when you are gloomy. If you have to, you may turn to your friends or parents for help. Fourthly, don't drink alcohol or take unprescribed drugs, which may make your mental health worse. Last but not least, take physical exercise as possible as you can.

（217 words）

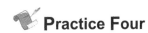 **Practice Four**

失 眠 症

　　睡眠是每个人的健康需要，也是本应享有的基本权利，但快节奏的生活却"吞噬"着人们越来越多的睡眠时间。在 3 月 21 日"世界睡眠日"之际，世界卫生组织公布的最新数字显示，全球近 1/4 的人受失眠困扰，每年近 8.6 亿人患失眠抑郁障碍。流行病学调查显示，33% 的美国人失眠，欧洲 4%～22% 的人受此影响。美国全国睡眠基金会 3 月最新调查显示，美国人每天平均工作 9 小时 28 分，仅睡 6 小时 40 分。全美约 7000 万人失眠。其中，女性更为严重，2/3 的女性睡不好，近 30% 的女性常吃安眠药。来自法国的数据显示，53% 的人"想在白天躺会儿"，30% 的人出现过睡眠紊乱，而 2006 年，这一比例仅为19%。澳大利亚睡眠协会的调查则显示，约 6% 的澳大利亚人存在失眠、打鼾等睡眠问题，40% 的人经过一夜睡眠后仍浑身乏力。在日本，每隔 5 年就有一次面向 8 万户家庭 18 万人的睡眠情况调查。结果显示，从 1986 年起，日本人睡眠一直在减少。其中，45～49岁之间的人睡眠时间最少。中国台湾失眠人口高达 28%，位居亚洲第一位，每年安眠药花费新台币 11 亿元。在大陆也有统计显示，有 20%～30% 患有失眠症，超过 50% 的人有睡眠问题。现代研究证实，有近 90 种疾病与长期失眠相关。有专家表示，虽然当今失眠现象较普遍，但如何正确认识和有效防治失眠，尚未引起人们的高度重视。

　　上海市中医失眠症医疗协作中心副主任施明提出，中国人目前 50%～55% 的失眠与精神情志因素有关。据有关资料显示，35～55 岁是当今失眠症发病率最高的年龄段，而且失眠有向青年人群蔓延的趋势。失眠人群的职业以经营、管理、财务、文教等脑力劳动人员为主。有专家指出，导致失眠的原因主要有以下几种：1. 疾病：有明确疾病存在的患者，睡眠往往不好。2. 心理因素：如紧张、焦虑、抑郁、兴奋、恐惧、烦闷、忧伤等情绪都会引起失眠。3. 生活习惯：饮用含咖啡因的饮料、抽烟和睡前饮酒，这些都会影响睡眠。晚餐过晚或过饱等不良生活习惯也会造成失眠。4. 生理因素：如老年人与更年期女性的失眠，多数与生理现象有关。5. 环境因素：城市的声光污染、气味、床铺舒适度、室温高低等都会干扰睡眠。6. 生物节律的干扰与紊乱，最常见的是倒时差与倒班。7. 药物：某些慢性病患者，长期服用一些毒副作用较强的药物也会影响正常睡眠。

　　失眠不仅给患者本人造成很大痛苦，还将给整个社会带来诸如医疗资源消耗增加、事故发生率上升和生产力下降等负面问题。有统计显示，45% 的车祸和失眠有关，55% 的工地事故是人们睡眠不够导致的，约 30% 的高血压和 20% 的心脏病是由不良睡眠引发的。失眠者中患抑郁症的人是睡眠正常人的 3 倍，超过 90% 的焦虑症和抑郁症患者同时伴有失眠。不过如果发生一天或几天睡眠不好的情况，并不算是得了失眠症，一般通过自身调整，睡眠自然就会恢复正常。

　　针对不同病因，治疗失眠的方法也有所不同。主要方法有：药物治疗、心理治疗、自我调节治疗、器械治疗等。自我调节治疗主要是保持情绪稳定，改变睡前饱食、喝酒、看刺激书刊等影响睡眠的习惯。器械治疗则是指使用有助于健康的床垫、枕头等辅助治疗。除此以外，中医针灸或点按穴位也是治疗失眠比较安全有效的方法。

（1186 字）

↗ 写作解析

1. 分析中文原文

此文主要讨论了导致失眠的原因、失眠的危害以及主要治疗方法。各段中心意思如下：

第一段：失眠问题很普遍

第二段：失眠的高危人群和原因

第三段：失眠危害

第四段：治疗方法

2. 摘要的中文大纲

第一部分（第1段）：失眠问题：当今失眠现象在全世界十分普遍，但如何正确认识和有效防治失眠，尚未引起人们的高度重视。

第二部分（第2段）：失眠的高危人群和原因：35～55岁是当今失眠症发病率最高的年龄段，失眠人群以脑力劳动人员为主。导致失眠的原因主要有以下几种：1. 疾病：有明确疾病存在的患者。2. 心理因素：如紧张、焦虑、抑郁、兴奋、恐惧、烦闷、忧伤等情绪。3. 生活习惯：饮用含咖啡因的饮料、抽烟和睡前饮酒，晚餐过晚或过饱等不良生活习惯。4. 生理因素：如老年人与更年期女性。5. 环境因素：城市的声光污染、气味、床铺舒适度、室温高低等。6. 生物节律的干扰与紊乱，最常见的是倒时差与倒班。7. 药物：长期服用一些毒副作用较强的药物。

第三部分（第3段）：失眠的危害：失眠不仅给患者本人造成很大痛苦，还将给整个社会带来诸如医疗资源消耗增加、事故发生率上升和生产力下降等负面问题。

第四部分（第4段）：失眠的治疗方法：针对不同病因，治疗失眠的方法也有所不同。主要方法有：药物治疗、心理治疗、自我调节治疗、器械治疗、中医针灸或点按穴位治疗等。

3. 供参考的表达式

失眠	insomnia; sleeplessness; sleep disorder
发病率	incidence
心理因素	psychological factors
生理因素	physiological factors
更年期妇女	female climacteric syndrome patients
生物节律	biological rhythm
倒时差	have jet lag
倒班	shifts
心理治疗	psychotherapy
中医针灸	acupuncture
按穴位	point-pressing

4. 参考范文

Insomnia

Insomnia is becoming a common problem throughout the world now. However, people have neither paid enough attention to the problem nor taken effective measures to cope with it.

The highest incidence of insomnia is found in individuals aged from 35 to 55 and mainly in brainworkers. There are six factors contributing to insomnia. Firstly, people with diseases tend to have such a problem. Secondly, psychological factors such as tension, anxiety, depression and sorrow probably lead to sleep disorder. Thirdly, unhealthy living habits, for instance, drinking alcohol before sleep, late dinner, may affect sleep. Fourthly, insomnia of elderly and female climacteric syndrome patients results from certain physiological factors. Fifthly, insomnia has something to do with environmental factors, for example, pollution, temperature in rooms and comfort degree of bed. Sixthly, people in different shifts or with jet lag can't sleep well. Lastly, medicine with toxic side effects taken by chronic patients is another contribution to insomnia.

Undoubtedly insomnia has many negative effects on patients as well as society. It not only brings great pain to the patients, but also causes many social problems, such as increased medical cost, high accident rates, and reduced production, etc.

Based on various causes, treatments for insomnia can be quite different. Apart from medicine and psychotherapy, self-adjusting and changing in living habits may be beneficial to patients. In addition, acupuncture and point-pressing are strongly recommended.

（227 words）

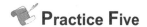 **Practice Five**

喝　　水

　　水是生命之源，人体一切的生命活动都离不开水。对于人体而言，水在身体内<u>不但是"运送"各种营养物质的载体，而且还直接参与人体的新陈代谢，因此，保证充足的摄水量对人体生理功能的正常运转至关重要。</u>但是，很多人对喝水的理解仅仅限于解渴。其实喝水也是一门学问，正确地喝水对维护人的健康非常重要。

喝水多少因人而异

　　深圳市第二人民医院肾内科主任何永成博士告诉记者，<u>一般而言，人每天喝水的量至少要与体内的水分消耗量相平衡。人体一天所排出的尿量约有 1500 毫升，再加上从粪便、呼吸过程中或是从皮肤所蒸发的水，总共消耗水分大约是 2500 毫升左右，而人体每天能从食物中和体内新陈代谢中补充的水分只有 1000 毫升左右，因此正常人每天至少需要喝 1500 毫升水，大约 8 杯左右。</u>

　　通常每个人需要喝多少水会根据活动量、环境，甚至天气而有所改变。正常人喝太多水对健康不会有太大影响，只是可能造成排尿量增多，引起生活上的不便。但是对于某些特殊人群，喝水量的多少必须特别注意，<u>比如浮肿病人、心脏功能衰竭病人、肾功能衰竭病人都不宜喝水过多，因为喝水太多会加重心脏和肾脏负担，容易导致病情加剧。而对于中暑、膀胱炎、便秘和皮肤干燥等疾病患者，多喝水则可对缓解病情起到一定效果。此外，人在感冒发烧时也应多喝水，因为体温上升会使水分流失，多喝水能促使身体散热，帮助病人恢复健康。而怀孕期的妇女和运动量比较大的人水分消耗得多，也应多喝水。</u>

温开水是最好的饮料

专家说，从健康的角度来看，白开水是最好的饮料，它不含卡路里，不用消化就能为人体直接吸收利用，一般建议喝30摄氏度以下的温开水最好，这样不会过于刺激肠胃道的蠕动，不易造成血管收缩。含糖饮料会减慢肠胃道吸收水分的速度，长期大量地喝含糖饮料，对人体的新陈代谢会产生一定不良影响。何博士告诉记者，像橙汁、可乐等含糖饮料口感虽好，但不宜多喝，每天摄入量应控制在一杯左右，最多不要超过200毫升，而对于糖尿病人和比较肥胖的人来说，则最好不要喝这类饮料。

纯净水和矿泉水等桶装水由于饮用方便深受现代人青睐，但是何博士提醒，喝这些水时一定要保证其卫生条件，一桶水最好在一个月内喝完，而且人们不应把纯净水作为主要饮用水。因为水是人体的六大营养素之一，水中含有多种对人体有益的矿物质和微量元素，而纯净水中的这些物质含量大大降低，如果平时人们饮食中的营养结构又不平衡，就很容易导致营养失调。有的人担心自来水硬度太大会不利于身体健康，但何博士介绍说，水的硬度对人体健康基本没有影响，而且现在国内的自来水都符合生活饮用水的标准，饮用煮沸了的自来水是安全的。茶和咖啡具有提神效果，但何博士提醒人们，喝茶宜喝淡茶，并且切忌酗咖啡，咖啡因会影响钙的吸收。

喝水不要大口吞咽

很多人往往在口渴时才想起喝水，而且往往是大口吞咽，这种做法也是不对的。喝水太快太急会无形中把很多空气一起吞咽下去，容易引起打嗝或是腹胀，因此最好先将水含在口中，再缓缓喝下，尤其是肠胃虚弱的人，喝水更应该一口一口慢慢喝。

至于喝水时间，专家则告诉记者，喝水切忌渴了再喝，应在两顿饭期间适量饮水，最好隔1小时喝一杯。人们还可以根据自己尿液的颜色来判断是否需要喝水，一般来说，人的尿液为淡黄色，如果颜色太浅，则可能是水喝得过多，如果颜色偏深，则表示需要多补充一些水了。睡前少喝、睡后多喝也是正确饮水的原则，因为睡前喝太多的水，会造成眼皮浮肿，半夜也会老跑厕所，使睡眠质量不高。而经过一个晚上的睡眠，人体流失的水分约有450毫升，早上起来需要及时补充，因此早上起床后空腹喝杯水有益血液循环，也能促进大脑清醒，使这一天的思维清晰敏捷。

（1463字）

↗ 写作解析

1. 分析中文原文

本文从喝水量、喝什么水、如何喝水、饮水时间四个方面简述喝水的重要性。因为有副标题，故文章结构很清楚，便于确定摘要结构。各段大意如下：

第一段：水的重要性

第二、三段：一般而言，人每天喝水的量至少要与体内的水分消耗量相平衡。因此正常人每天至少需要喝1500毫升水，大约8杯左右

第四段：通常每个人需要喝多少水会根据活动量、环境，甚至天气而有所改变

第五、六段：白开水是最好的饮料，少喝含糖饮料

第七段：桶装水要注意卫生，喝茶要喝淡茶，切忌酗咖啡

第八、九段：避免大口吞咽

第十段：喝水的时间

2. 摘要中文大纲

第一部分（第 1 段）：人体一切的生命活动都离不开水。因此，保证充足的摄水量对人体生理功能的正常运转至关重要。但是，很多人对喝水的理解仅仅限于解渴。其实正确地喝水对维护人的健康非常重要。

第二部分（第 2～4 段）：人每天喝水的量至少要与体内的水分消耗量相平衡。人体一天总共消耗水分大约是 2500 毫升左右，而人体每天能从食物中和体内新陈代谢中补充的水分只有 1000 毫升左右，因此正常人每天至少需要喝 1500 毫升水，大约 8 杯左右。对于中暑、膀胱炎、便秘和皮肤干燥等疾病患者、感冒发烧患者、孕妇和运动量较大的人应多喝水。但是，对于浮肿病人、心脏功能衰竭病人、肾功能衰竭病人都不宜喝水过多，会加重心脏和肾脏负担。

第三部分（第 5～7 段）：温开水是最好的饮料。长期大量地喝含糖饮料，对人体的新陈代谢会产生一定不良影响。纯净水和矿泉水等桶装水不应作为主要应用水，容易导致营养失调。喝茶宜喝淡茶，切忌酗咖啡，咖啡因会影响钙的吸收。

第四部分（第 8～9 段）：口渴时才想起喝水以及大口吞咽，容易引起打嗝或是腹胀，因此最好先将水含在口中，再缓缓喝下。

第五部分（第 10 段）：喝水应在两顿饭期间适量饮水，最好隔 1 小时喝一杯。人们还可以根据自己尿液的颜色来判断是否需要喝水，睡前少喝、睡后多喝也是正确饮水的原则。

3. 供参考的表达式

营养物质	nutrient
新陈代谢	metabolism
生理功能	physiological function
解渴	relieve thirst
浮肿	dropsy
心脏功能衰竭	heart failure
肾功能衰竭	kidney failure
中暑	heat stroke
膀胱炎	cystitis
便秘	constipation
孕妇	pregnant women
纯净水	purified water
矿泉水	mineral water
桶装水	barreled water
提神	refresh oneself

吸收	absorb
打嗝	hiccup
腹胀	abdominal distention
尿液	urine
大口吞咽	gulp; swallow
长期的	long-term; chronic

4. 参考范文

No living activities of our body can go without water. Therefore, adequate water supply plays a crucial role in maintaining proper physiological functions.

The amount of water we drink each day need to be equivalent to the water we consume. Our body consumes approximately 2,500ml water a day, while it can supplement only about 1,000ml water from food and metabolism. So, a normal person should drink at least 1,500ml water, about 8 glasses. People who suffer from heat stroke, cystitis and constipation, and pregnant women are recommended to drink more, while patients with dropsy, heart failure and kidney failure should not drink too much water.

The best drinking water is warm boiled water. Long-term drinking of beverage with sugar affects the body's metabolism. Purified water and mineral water should not be the main drinks, which might cause malnutrition. Light tea is highly recommended, but drinking too much coffee will affect the absorption of calcium.

Try to avoid gulping, because it tends to cause hiccup and abdominal distention. The correct way is to keep water in the mouth and then wash it down slowly.

You should drink moderate water between two meals and drink a glass every one hour. Besides, you can determine whether you need to drink according to your urine color. Furthermore, less water before sleep and more water after sleep is the correct way.

（226 words）

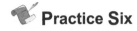 **Practice Six**

艾滋病和 HIV 的传播

我们自以为熟知如何应付的一种威胁正在迅猛地扩散。在今年 12 月 1 日的世界艾滋病日之际，世界卫生组织发现，全球的艾滋病病毒感染者人数达到了历史最高值：40300000，比 10 年前翻了一倍。4000 多万，这意味着全球每 160 个人当中就有一个艾滋病病毒感染者。

艾滋病（AIDS）不是一个单纯的病，而是一种综合征，叫作获得性免疫缺陷综合征。1981 年在美国首次报道艾滋病病例，后来这个综合征演变成了全球范围的流行病。艾滋病是由人类免疫缺陷病毒（HIV）所引起。这种病毒进入人体后通过杀死或损害人体免疫系统的细胞，逐步损伤机体抵抗感染和某些肿瘤的能力。由于免疫功能的下降，艾滋病人很容易并发一种致命的感染性疾病，叫作条件致病性感染。所谓的条件治病性感染就是，一些病毒或是细菌通常不会导致健康的人感染，但是可以导致艾滋病人患病。

　　艾滋病的确是一种传染病。但艾滋病本身不会传染，只是 HIV 病毒具有传染性。HIV传染的最常见的方式是通过与艾滋病患者或者已经感染 HIV 病毒的性伴侣进行无保护措施的性交。在性接触过程中这种病毒可通过阴道、外阴、阴茎、直肠、口腔等进入体内，导致感染。人们也可以通过接触被 HIV 感染的血液导致感染。在献血还没有经过 HIV 感染筛查的年代，HIV 通过输入感染的血液或血液制品进行传播。如今，献血和输血已经有了严格的管理措施，所以输血或血液制品传播 HIV 的危险性已经非常小了。然而，HIV 在吸毒者之间传播还是常见的，他们通常是通过共用注射针头或是被 HIV 感染过的注射器相互之间传染病毒。偶尔也有医务人员被 HIV 污染的针头或其他的医疗器械传染。还有一种传染方式是在感染 HIV 病毒母亲和子女之间进行。感染 HIV 的孕妇可以在怀孕或是分娩期间将病毒传给她们的孩子。尽管如此，艾滋病或 HIV 感染的妇女在得到一定的医学措施护理时，也是可能生下健康的孩子的。如果医务人员为这类孕妇进行适当的治疗和行剖宫产术来分娩婴儿，那么孩子感染 HIV 的概率将降到百分之一。

　　虽然艾滋病是一种可怕的疾病，但是人们在日常生活中也不必过于害怕，因为 HIV 不会通过一般性接触传染。一般说来，与艾滋病人共用餐具、毛巾、寝具、电话或是坐便等是不会传染这种疾病的。昆虫叮咬一般也不会传播 HIV。

↗ 写作解析

1. 分析中文原文

　　本文一共四段，在阅读中文原文后，我们可以确定每一段的段落大意，并在原文划出相应的关键细节内容。关键细节内容请见原文划线部分。各段的段落大意简要如下：

第一段：艾滋病的威胁迅猛扩散
第二段：什么是艾滋病
第三段：HIV 病毒传播的途径
第四段：在日常生活中不必过于害怕

2. 摘要中文大纲

　　第一段：世界卫生组织发现全球艾滋病病毒感染者人数达到历史最高：40300000，这意味着全球每 160 人当中就有一个艾滋病病毒感染者。并且几乎在全球所有国家里，艾滋病病毒感染者数量都在上升。

　　第二段：艾滋病叫作获得性免疫缺陷综合征。1981 年美国首次报道艾滋病病例，后来该病演变成全球范围流行病。艾滋病是由 HIV 病毒引起，这种病毒进入人体后通过杀死或损害人体免疫系统的细胞，逐步损伤机体抵抗感染和某些肿瘤的能力。实际上艾滋病本身不会传染，但 HIV 病毒具有传染性。

　　第三段：HIV 病毒传染最常见的方式是通过与艾滋病患者或者已经感染 HIV 病毒的性伴侣进行无保护措施的性交。此外，人们也可以通过接触被 HIV 感染的血液导致感染。HIV 病毒在吸毒者之间通常是通过共用注射针头或是被 HIV 感染过的注射器相互之间传染病毒。偶尔也有医务人员被 HIV 污染的针头或其他的医疗器械传染。最后，HIV 病毒可以在母婴之间传播。

第四段：虽然艾滋病是一种可怕的疾病，但人们在日常生活中不必过于害怕，HIV 病毒不会通过一般性接触感染，如共用餐具、毛巾、寝具、电话；昆虫叮咬也不会传播 HIV。

3． 供参考的表达式

全球范围流行病	worldwide epidemic disease
抗感染	infectious resistance
感染的血液	infected blood
孕妇可以将病毒传染给孩子	mothers can infect their babies with virus

4． 参考范文

WHO has found patients with HIV have reached the peak: 40,300,000, which means there is one with HIV among 160 people around the world.

AIDS (acquired immunodeficiency syndrome) was first reported in the United States in 1981 and has become a major worldwide epidemic disease. AIDS is caused by HIV virus, which destroys the body's ability to fight infections and certain tumors by killing or damaging cells of the body's immune system. In fact, AIDS is not transmitted, but the virus is.

HIV is spread commonly by having unprotected sex with an infected partner. It is also spread through contact with infected blood. HIV is frequently spread among injection drug users by the sharing of needles or syringes contaminated with infected blood. It is rare, however, for a patient to give HIV to a health care worker by accidental sticks with infected needles or other medical instruments. Women can transmit HIV to their babies during pregnancy or birth.

Although AIDS is a terrible disease, but people don't need to feel scared excessively. HIV is spread neither through casual contact such as the sharing of food utensils, towels and bedding, swimming pools, telephones, etc, nor insects biting.

（196 words）